TECHNIQUE OF INTERNAL FIXATION OF FRACTURES

BY

M. E. MÜLLER

M. ALLGÖWER   H. WILLENEGGER

WITH CONTRIBUTIONS BY

W. BANDI · H. R. BLOCH · A. MUMENTHALER
R. SCHNEIDER · S. STEINEMANN · F. STRAUMANN
B. G. WEBER

REVISED FOR THE ENGLISH EDITION BY

G. SEGMÜLLER

WITH 244 FIGURES

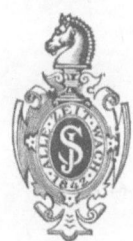

SPRINGER-VERLAG
BERLIN · HEIDELBERG · NEW YORK
1965

First published under: Technik der operativen Frakturenbehandlung

By M. E. MÜLLER, M. ALLGÖWER, H. WILLENEGGER

Springer-Verlag, Berlin · Göttingen · Heidelberg 1963

© by Springer-Verlag, Berlin · Heidelberg 1965
Softcover reprint of the hardcover 1st edition 1965

Library of Congress Catalog Card Number 65—14819

ISBN-13: 978-3-642-88358-3   e-ISBN-13: 978-3-642-88356-9
DOI: 10.1007/ 978-3-642-88356-9

The use of general descriptive names, trade names, trade marks, etc. in this publication, even if the former are not especially identified, is not to be taken as a sign that such names, as understood by the Trade Marks and Merchandise Marks Act, may accordingly be used freely by anyone

Titel-Nr. 0438

Foreword

It is to the great and lasting credit of LORENZ BÖHLER and his school that they have in the last decade developed and demonstrated so thoroughly the techniques for the conservative management of fractures.

Nevertheless there have always been many, including some from BÖHLER's school, who have found considerable place for surgical management, and with the significant progress in general surgery seen in postwar years, a new stimulus has been given to this part of traumatic surgery, especially since bone injuries have become more complex and frequent.

The concept of internal fixation is not new. The serious criticisms that have been levelled at it retain today their basic significance. Progress in the fields of asepsis, corrosion-free metal implants, operative experience and postoperative care has diminished the dangers but has not relieved the surgeon of responsibility.

The *Association for the Study of the Problems of Internal Fixation* (AO) has devoted itself over a number of years to the basic principles and best methods of open treatment of fractures by means of extended clinical and scientific studies in order to determine in each individual case the most promising line of treatment. At the same time a well designed and tested instrument set has been developed with precise instructions for the appropriate techniques. As a result, the new observations about primary bone healing which have emerged from the practice of rigid internal fixation are as interesting as the uses to which they can be put in allowing early mobilization.

This book is intended to serve as a guide to the choice of procedure and to the proper execution of operative fracture treatment. Only if one is familiar from the outset with the details of indications, techniques and aftercare can failures be prevented. Under these circumstances internal fixation is a responsible and rewarding medico-surgical endeavour.

Freiburg i. Br., December 1964   H. KRAUSS

Preface

Early in 1958, fifteen Swiss general and orthopaedic surgeons joined together to re-examine the common procedures then in use for the operative treatment of fractures. This group formed the *Association for the Study of the Problems of Internal Fixation (AO)**. Basic research workers, metallurgists and the *Laboratory for Experimental Surgery* at Davos, Switzerland, have cooperated in evaluating the results.

This book contains the guiding principles about open fracture treatment which have been crystallized during an experience covering 5 years in which 4000 fractures have been treated surgically and documented. Its purpose is to describe established procedures from our own clinical experience and also to emphasize the dangers and failures that have occurred.

This book is not basically intended to distinguish between the indications for surgical and conservative treatment. Indeed, in the case of fractures of the shaft of the humerus, we tend to be overwhelmingly conservative. Nevertheless, the surgical treatment of the fractured humerus will be discussed in detail as well.

It should also be mentioned that the operative procedures described here relate to mature bone. Occasionally a non-rigid fixation, for example with parallel KIRSCHNER wires, may be indicated in the case of periarticular fractures in children, to prevent later growth trouble or in the case of articular fractures to restore good joint alignment. In general, however, the indications for opening a closed fracture on a growing skeleton are rare indeed.

Our clinical experiences repeatedly emphasize the significance of the stability and blood supply of the fractures we operated on. When these two objectives were attained, firm and rapid union of the fractures resulted in all cases. The quantity of metal used does not appear to be of primary significance.

The healing of the bone, however, represents only part of the problem. The practice of emphasizing the bone lesion to the exclusion of the soft tissue damage should be firmly abandoned. Modern fracture treatment has as its goal the restoration of full function to the injured extremity. In our view, internal fixation can only be satisfactory when the fracture is mechanically neutralized so that the patient can actively and without pain move muscles and joints of the broken extremity at the earliest possible moment after surgery.

---

* This in German is „Arbeitsgemeinschaft für Osteosynthesefragen" and will be referred to as AO.

Open treatment of fractures is a valuable but difficult method which involves much responsibility. We cannot advise too strongly against internal fixation if it is carried out by an inadequately trained surgeon, and in the absence of full equipment and sterile operating room conditions. Using our methods, enthusiasts who lack self-criticism are much more dangerous than skeptics or outright opponents. We hope therefore that readers will understand our efforts in this direction and that they will pass on any constructive criticisms to us.

December 1964   M. E. MÜLLER
                                                       M. ALLGÖWER
                                                       H. WILLENEGGER

Acknowledgements for the German Edition

We have to express our gratitude to those without whose help publication of this book would not have been possible. First we are indebted to Miss E. WIESSNER for her editorial skill, to Mr. SCHUMACHER, scientific illustrator, Mr. HOLLIGER, photographer, Mr. E. FREI, technical assistant of the Laboratory for experimental Surgery, Davos. We also recall with gratitude the help and efforts of our publisher Springer Berlin-Göttingen-Heidelberg and the firm Cliché Lang in Basle. It was certainly not an easy task in so short a time to bring out a multiple author book with so many illustrations.

Acknowledgements for the English Edition

We are particularly indebted to Mr. and Mrs. DONALD L. HERSHEY, Philadelphia (USA) and to Dr. HARALD VASEY, St. Gallen (Switzerland) who made the first draft for the translation, and to Dr. RICHARD L. BATTEN, F.R.C.S., Birmingham (England) who added his own large experience in traumatic surgery and his editorial skill to make this English edition possible. All views expressed however remain the only responsibility of the editors of the German and English edition.

Table of Contents

General Technique

Special Fractures

Supplement

Contributors

M. ALLGÖWER, M.D.   Associate Professor of Surgery, University of Basle Medical School, Surgeon-in-Chief, Dept. of Surgery, Kantonsspital, Chur/Switzerland

W. BANDI, M.D.   Surgeon-in-Chief, Dept. of Surgery, Bezirksspital, Interlaken/ Switzerland

H. R. BLOCH, M.D.   Surgeon-in-Chief, Dept. of Surgery, Kantonsspital, Glarus/ Switzerland

M. E. MÜLLER, M.D.   Professor of Orthopaedic Surgery and Chairman of the Dept. of Orthopaedic Surgery, University of Berne Medical School, Chief of the Dept. of Orthopaedics and Traumatology, Kantonsspital, St. Gallen/Switzerland

A. MUMENTHALER, M.D.   Dept. of Orthopaedics and Traumatology, Kantonsspital, St. Gallen/Switzerland

R. SCHNEIDER, M.D.   Surgeon-in-Chief, Dept. of Surgery, Bezirksspital, Grosshöchstetten/Switzerland

S. STEINEMANN, Ph.D.   Laboratory for Metallurgy of Prof. Dr. Ing. h. c. R. Straumann, Waldenburg/Switzerland

F. STRAUMANN, Ing.   Laboratory for Metallurgy of Prof. Dr. Ing. h.c. R. Straumann, Waldenburg/Switzerland

B. G. WEBER, M.D.   Dept. of Orthopaedics and Traumatology, Kantonsspital, St. Gallen/Switzerland

H. WILLENEGGER, M.D.   Associate Professor of Surgery, University of Basle Medical School, Surgeon-in-Chief, Dept. of Surgery, Kantonsspital, Liestal/Switzerland

Responsible for the English Edition:

G. SEGMÜLLER, M.D.   Dept. of Surgery, Kantonsspital, Chur/Switzerland

General Technique

A. Introduction

I. Historical Review

The date of the first use of internal fixation is unknown. As early as 1862, in a book by GURLT, a number of cases were reported in which the freshening and reduction of fractured bone ends as well as the nailing, screwing and wiring of bones were attempted. At that time open reduction of fractures was indicated only in those cases where prolonged conservative treatment had failed. Thus, open fracture treatment was only a supplementary measure — actually a sensible attitude since asepsis had not been developed, and BARDENHEUER, the father of extension therapy, was in practice. Exceptions were only made in fractures that occurred in subcutaneous bones such as the patella and the olecranon process. The wiring of a fractured patella is thus one of the oldest forms of internal fixation (LISTER, 1877).

Toward the end of the last century, with the development of asepsis, operative fracture treatment emerged more and more from its position as a supplementary measure. One reason was that far better results were achieved with early and even primary internal fixation. Among the pioneers of this technique were the German surgeon FRITZ KOENIG, ELIE and ALBIN LAMBOTTE of Belgium, LANE of England and SCUDDER of the USA.

FRITZ KOENIG and the two LAMBOTTE brothers may be called the actual originators of internal fixation. FRITZ KOENIG recognized the importance of internal fixation while working as an assistant of ORTH, the then famous anatomist, and he published his first concept in a paper in 1902.

Of particular help in advancing this new concept were the postgraduate facilities available at the so-called Doctor's Club in Altona, where, in 1895, KOENIG began his first independent surgical practice as chief-physician of the Municipal Hospital of Altona-on-the-Elbe. In his memoirs he wrote of these decisive years as follows:

"The postgraduate facilities enhanced my studies and I emerged as an absolute adherent of the principle of open treatment in all cases at an early stage. Before the large Physicians' Association of Hamburg which discussed this question for four successive evenings, I convincingly substantiated this conviction and retained it during my entire surgical career with the best of results. KÜMMEL was particularly impressed."

The controversy over internal fixation was topical even then. KOENIG wrote:

"To recommend internal fixation at the Congress of the German Society for Surgery in 1901 was like skating on thin ice. Ten years earlier, a daring surgeon PFEILSCHNEIDER, did so by presenting patients who had been treated surgically. His views were completely rejected. ERNST VON BERGMANN especially, who was later my teacher, disapproved strongly of PFEILSCHNEIDER's actions, partly because of his poor substantiation and partly because of the incidence of suppuration. The effects of this rejection were still felt in 1902 and 1904. Only REHN's school in Frankfurt adopted my approach without reserve."

KOENIG's efforts were directed toward defining the indications for the conservative versus the operative method of management, and toward the use of rigid internal fixation in order to permit functional postoperative mobilization by reducing the need for plaster

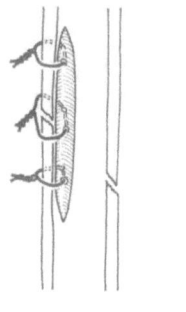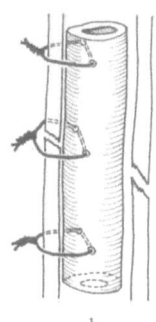

a   b

Fig. 1a and b. Stabilization of bone sutures with ivory pegs
a or bone inserts b after FRITZ KOENIG

cast fixation. At the same time, KOENIG was aware of the inadequacy of materials
available for internal fixation. Methods carried over from the 19th century were bone
suture and bone screwing as suggested by ELIE LAMBOTTE. KOENIG, from the point of view
of bone nutrition, advocated hemi-cerclage-wiring on principle. He also tried to produce
improved stability by using ivorypegs (Fig. 1a) and bone inserts (Fig. 1b). On the
Belgian side, the writings of ALBIN LAMBOTTE gave internal fixation an especially prolonged stimulus. His first monograph was prepared in 1907 under the title: "The Open
Reduction of Recent and Old Fractures". LAMBOTTE's own conception of internal fixation
could be traced back to his brother ELIE, who was hardly known in medical literature
but who (at the *Schaerbeek Military Hospital*) systematically treated oblique fractures of
the lower leg by open reduction and fixation with wire sutures or screws. One of the
first descriptions of this procedure is found in the *Presse Médicale Belge* of 1890. ALBIN
LAMBOTTE wrote:

"The basically simple nature of this surgery has impressed me vividly and the excellence of the results
obtained has convinced me that this is in fact the rational therapy for a fracture with displacement of the
bone ends."

Despite these good results, ELIE LAMBOTTE met with almost unanimous rejection.
Discouraged by this criticism, he withdrew completely, largely because he could not
entirely substantiate his method. His brother ALBIN, however, pursued internal fixation
further during his studies at the *Stuivenberg Hospital*. Even more strongly than KOENIG,
LAMBOTTE emphasized the possibility of early movement when using internal fixation; and, while placing less importance on the traditional wire suture, he advocated
internal fixation with a plate and with external clamps which subsequently were named
after him (Fig. 2 and 3). In addition he improved the technique for screw fixation and
attempted, by creating curved and Y-shaped plates, to enlarge the field for rigid internal
fixation for periarticular fractures (Figs. 5b, c, 7). In 1913, LAMBOTTE's second revised
and enlarged monograph appeared, entitled: "The Operative Treatment of Fractures".
In that volume the functional principles of internal fixation were very impressively
treated. For LAMBOTTE early movement without weight bearing was by far the most
important positive factor in weighing the pros and cons of internal fixation. He was
thus particularly concerned with the rigid fixation of periarticular fractures (Figs. 4—9).
For small intraarticular fragments he developed the thin nail ("embrochage"). LAMBOTTE
may then also be given the credit for the conception of internal fixation of the scaphoid
(Fig. 10).

In 1931 the Springer Publishing House presented the first and only monograph in
German by FRITZ KOENIG entitled "Operative Surgery of Fractures". Elsewhere in
German literature internal fixation attained a position which MATTI in the first edition
(1918) of his book described as follows:

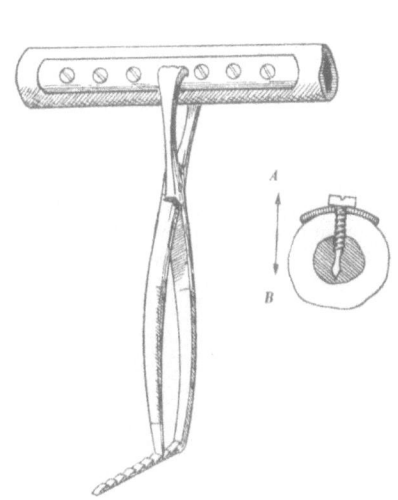

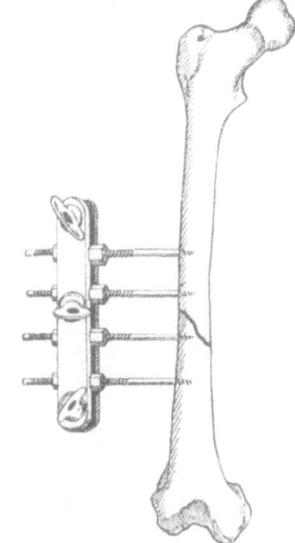

Fig. 2. Forceps and plates, after LAMBOTTE

Fig. 3. External fixation clamps, "fixateur externe", after LAMBOTTE

"Despite groundless and arbitrary rejection covering several years, open reduction of fractures has won its own well-defined place."

This opinion was also supported in MATTI's second edition and by HELFERICH (1921) and K. H. BAUER (1927).

The progress of internal fixation was decisively advanced at the German Congress of Surgeons in 1940 where KÜNTSCHER presented the V-shaped medullary nail.

The further development of the medullary nail is well-known. During that very first year KÜNTSCHER developed the rigid, slotted medullary nail with the cloverleaf cross-section for use in the femur. In 1950 HERZOG modified this nail to produce a forward curve and thereby introduced the era of rigid medullary nailing for fractures of the tibia. In 1956 he developed a slotted nail to allow rotational control with the help of accessory wires. The concept of reaming the bone resulted from MAATZ's demand in 1942 for a perfect fit between metal and bone and this was developed in 1951 by KÜNTSCHER who used thicker nails to increase stability both for pseudarthroses and for fresh fractures. A recent modification of medullary fixation is HACKETHAL's use of bundles of wires.

The Belgian orthopaedic surgeon DANIS contributed materially to internal fixation in his monograph entitled "Theory and Practice of Internal Fixation" (1947). He was primarily concerned with the theoretical principles involved:

a) To combine stability and compression he designed a special compression plate which, particularly in forearm fractures, paved the way for early mobilization, something which had hardly been known previously.

b) He advocated tapping the threads for screwing into hard bone.

c) He advanced mechanical principles for the accurate placing of screws in butterfly fractures.

DANIS's lasting contribution, however, lies not so much in the perfection of devices for internal fixation as in the biological concepts he originated. He pointed out that with axial compression and rigid fixation of fractures of the shaft of the radius and ulna, healing occurred without radiological signs of callus formation. He called this type of

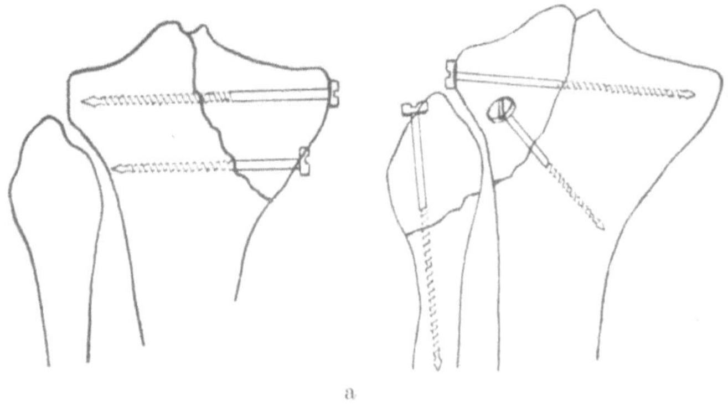

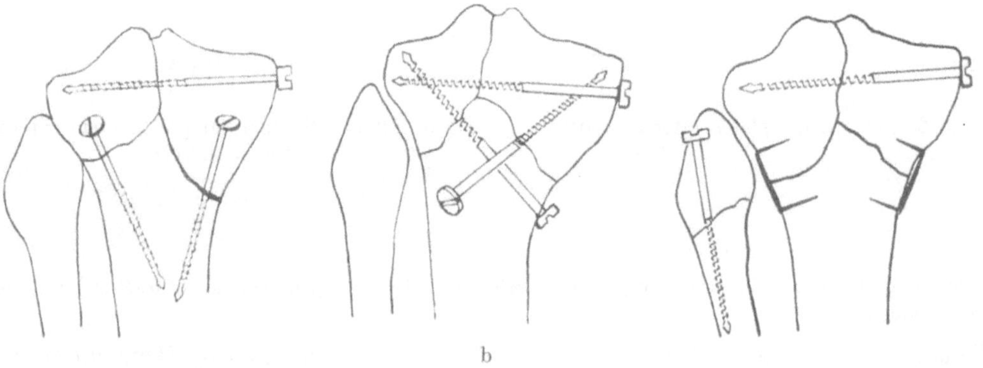

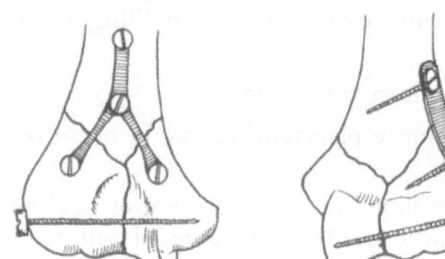

Fig. 4a and b. Internal fixation of fractures of the upper end of the tibia, after LAMBOTTE

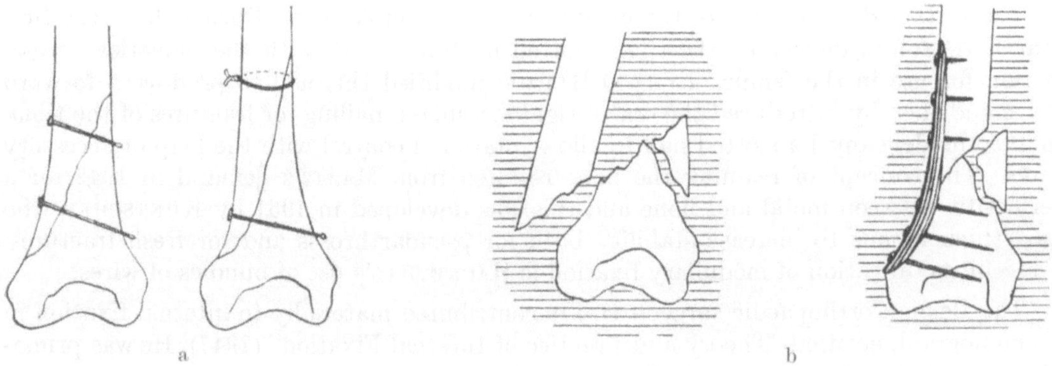

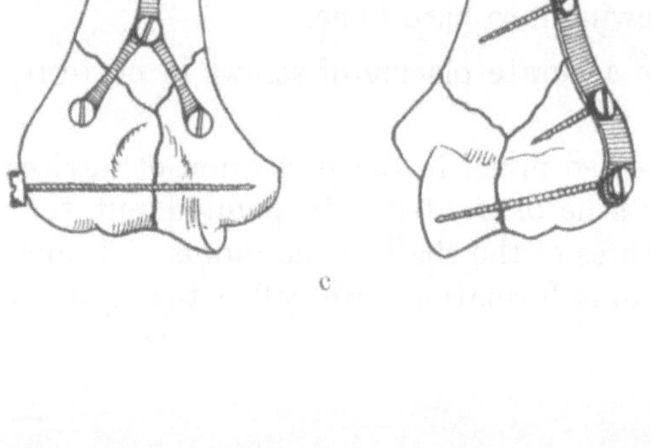

Fig. 5a—c. Internal fixation of the lower end of the humerus, after LAMBOTTE

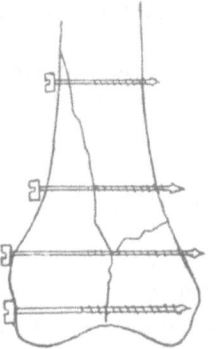

Fig. 6. Internal fixation of the lower end of the femur, after LAMBOTTE

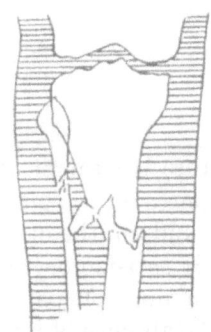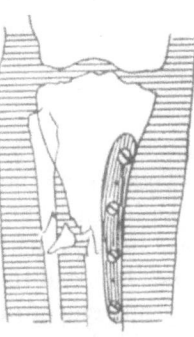

Fig. 7. Internal fixation of a fracture of the upper tibial shaft with a plate, after LAMBOTTE

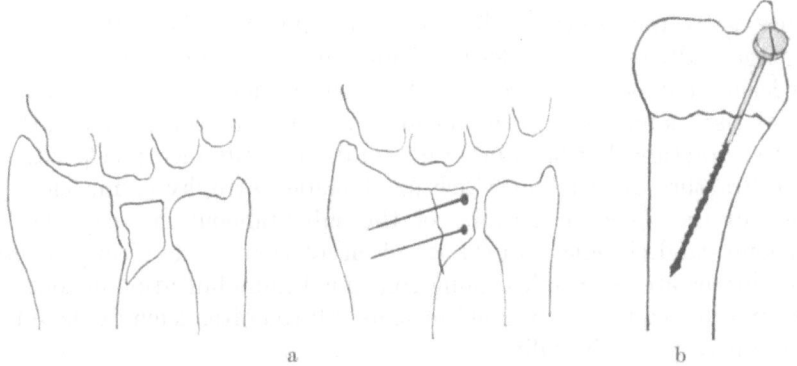

a   b

Fig. 8a and b. Internal fixation of fractures of the lower end of the radius, after LAMBOTTE

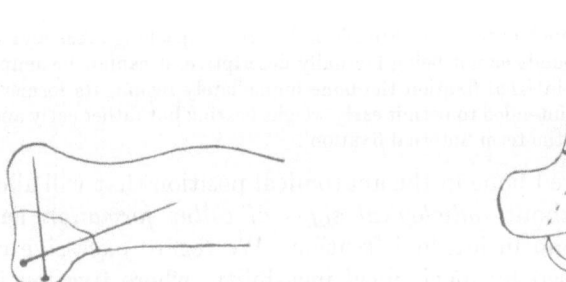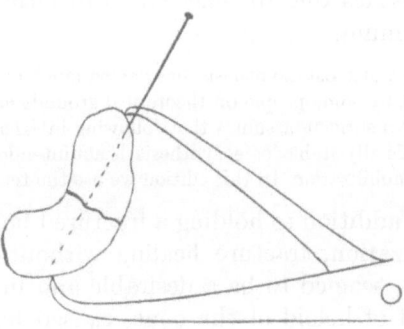

Fig. 9. Internal fixation of fractures of the radial head, after LAMBOTTE

Fig. 10. Method of fixing a scaphoid fracture proposed by LAMBOTTE

bone healing "soudure autogène" (primary bone healing) and assumed that the cortex, under the effect of longitudinal compression, was capable of primary bone union. He believed that with rigid fixation the healing process must follow a different course from that which occurs in conservative treatment where the biological basis for union is visible callus formation. The recognition of these fundamental differences gave internal fixation a scientific background which is still the focus of basic research.

II. Objectives and Hazards of Internal Fixation

No two fractures can be treated alike (HELLNER).
The aims and basic principles, however, remain the same.

Today's methods of fracture treatment aim at complete restoration of all functions of the injured limb. This requires on the one hand rapid ossification of the fracture after it has been properly reduced, and, on the other hand the integrity of the surrounding soft parts. Internal fixation is only satisfactory when it can neutralize the fracture and allow early movement of the surrounding soft parts and joints. When an anatomical reduction is obtained in a fracture, in the absence of internal fixation, external methods of splintage must be used. Open reduction by itself without appropriate internal fixation should not be attempted in any case where conservative treatment may be expected to produce union of the fracture in a satisfactory alignment. Here the risk of opening a closed fracture without proceeding to internal fixation would be injustifiable.

In fracture cases, the injury to the soft parts must be taken into consideration and treated as energetically as the bone lesions found on x-ray. Injuries such as torn cartilages and ruptured ligaments are the direct result of an accident, whereas indirect damage to joints and soft tissues may also occur during and after treatment. The latter conditions may be due to a fracture that has united in an anatomically incorrect position or to what DANIS called "fracture disease," in which are included atrophy of muscle and cartilage, decalcification of the skeleton, atrophy of the subcutaneous fat, capsular contraction, stiffening of joints and chronic disturbance of circulation in the form of edema. In most cases, the conditions are the result of long continued immobilization of joints adjacent to the fracture, and inadequate early relief of pain. All too often such damage is irreversible and may cause permanent disability.

Functionally stable internal fixation unites the fragments so rigidly that external fixation may be omitted from the beginning, and *both muscles and joints of the injured limb can be mobilized without discomfort immediately after surgery*. Thus the damage to soft tissues due to inactivity can either be completely avoided or at least reduced to a minimum.

The word 'osteosynthesis' has gained much currency in French and German speaking areas and while it is rejected by some people on theoretical grounds as not being factually descriptive, it cannot be simply wished away. No surgeon assumes that following internal fixation the bone immediately regains its former strength, a functionally stable 'osteosynthesis' is not intended to permit early weight bearing but rather early and painless active mobilization. In this edition we use the term 'internal fixation'.

In addition to holding a fractured bone in the anatomical position that will allow early mobilization, fracture healing without *radiological signs of callus formation* has, since DANIS, seemed to be a desirable aim in internal fixation. We regard excessive callus as a kind of keloid of the bone, caused by mechanical instability, where fixation is either inadequate in the first place or becomes so in time as a result of the disrupted blood supply of the bone ends. The so-called "per primam" ossification of a fracture is considered the mark of perfect rigidity and testifies to the quality of the method used and the mastery of its technique. In more than two thirds of our cases, fracture union without visible periosteal or endosteal callus can be observed. Visible callus formation indicates instability and is regarded by us as a warning sign which if ignored may lead to delayed union, to secondary displacement of the fragments or even to nonunion.

Internal fixation should considerably shorten the length of hospitalization and the period of disability. It must be a reliable method of treatment not only for relatively simple oblique or spiral fractures but also for large comminuted fractures and in multiple injuries, since early mobilization of all joints is especially important in such cases. Internal fixation, however, is an extremely difficult method of treatment which is dangerous if performed by an orthopaedic surgeon without adequate training and experience, correct judgement, technical dexterity and three-dimensional thinking. It follows that internal fixation, in spite of all its advantages and successes when used properly, can never be recommended indiscriminately as a universal method of fracture treatment.

Not every surgeon will attain equally good results with internal fixation. It is our concern, therefore, that everyone should critically examine the fractures he has treated surgically so that he may recognize not only the limitations of the method used, but also his own personal limitations. If he does not improve the functional results of the cases he treats with internal fixation, he should then content himself with fracture management by plaster cast or traction.

The surgeon should not only supervise the postoperative treatment but also carry out an uninterrupted follow-up of all fractures treated by internal fixation. Long term follow-up demands a great deal of effort and money and needs a special organization. Our method of assessment will therefore be discussed in detail.

In open fracture treatment bone infection represents a very grave complication. The factors involved include not only the sterility of the operating theatre where this form of treatment is practised, but also the importance given by the surgeon to the careful management of the tissues during the operation (p. 21). Even the virtuoso cannot hope for perfect results unless he has the right instruments which will permit him to carry out any operation that may be needed in bone surgery. All metal implants must be compatible with body fluids, mechanically strong and free from the risk of corrosion (see page 28). A full stock of such appliances must always be available at the hospital.

Thus, we felt it was our first duty to evolve a set of instruments that would satisfy the most demanding needs. These tools, however, are only the mechanical prerequisites and are only useful in hands that know how to use them skilfully and artistically. The surgeon should not only know how and when the special instruments should be used, but, of course, he must also be able to handle them properly; and it is this technique that we shall describe. Each surgeon must develop for himself the necessary skills.

III. Theoretical and Practical Principles of Rigid Internal Fixation

To obtain rigid internal fixation that will last for the duration of the healing process, three criteria must be fulfilled:

a) Anatomical reduction must be accurate in restoring the original shape of the bone.

b) A mechanically stable unit must be achieved. This can be done either by *interfragmentary compression* with lag screws, compression plates, traction absorbing wiring or external compression clamps, or by *an internal support* in the form of a thick medullary nail inserted into a marrow cavity that has previously been reamed out.

c) The blood supply of the bone fragments must be preserved or conditions provided that will enable revascularization to occur easily.

a) Anatomical Reduction

To obtain maximal rigidity an anatomically exact reduction of the fracture is essential. In articular fractures, an accurate reconstruction of the articular surface is necessary if unequal loads are not to fall on certain parts of the joint, producing later osteoarthritis.

In the leg, an axis deviation may produce unequal loading on the joints distal to the fracture. In the lower leg, for example, an internal rotation of 10^0 or a varus deformity of more than 5^0 may cause, in our experience, pain in the subtalar joint similar to that experienced in untreated talipes equinovarus. On the other hand the foot seems to be able to compensate for valgus positions of as much as 10^0.

b) Rigid Fixation of the Fragments

To hold a reduction rigidly, the fracture must be converted into a stable unit. Only if this rigidity is maintained during the whole healing process, can patients remain free from pain even while exercising muscles and joints. The slightest movement at the fracture site will result, according to HICKS, in joint stiffness produced by pain. Pain and any resulting psychogenic problem can only be eliminated when no movement at all is possible at the fracture site. The rigidity of internal fixation therefore determines the success of open fracture treatment: the mechanical stability obtained has to permit early active postoperative mobilization. It follows that the different methods of internal fixation advocated must be able to withstand the stresses involved in these early movements. The desired aim is not immediate weight bearing, but early mobilization of muscles and joints after operation without bearing weight.

Firm surgical fixation of the fracture does not mean that the bone has regained its previous strength. Living bone is a compound structure like reinforced concrete (KNEESE 1958). Only when the collagen fibres with their coating of calcium apatite have been placed under tension, and successive lamellae have been laid down along the lines of stress, does the bone regain its previous strength. Under optimal conditions this process takes about 12 months.

We can achieve sufficient rigidity by the application of two principles: by *compressing the fragments* together or by *medullary fixation*, the latter being used especially for certain fractures of the shaft of the tibia or the femur. It is only in a few fractures in cancellous bone that stabilization of the fragments by wire pins, as in fractures in the neighborhood of joints in children, or by blade-plates as in femoral neck fractures, can be regarded as adequate.

Internal splintage using medullary nails, RUSH-pins or multiple wires has become so well known in German speaking areas, especially through the work of KÜNTSCHER, MAATZ, and HACKETHAL, and through the work of LOTTES in the English speaking countries, that it will be dealt with fully in the chapter on medullary nailing. The *principle of compression* on the other hand is little known in the English and not known at all in the German speaking areas.

DANIS held the view that axial compression promoted osteogenesis and thereby the healing of any type of fracture. CHARNLEY supplied proof that in the case of cancellous surfaces, as in arthrodesis of the knee, compression could cause extremely rapid ossification. In the case of fractures of the shaft, however, he found that increased pressure produced by his external clamps remained ineffective. He did not mention that absolute stability and thus constant compression could not be achieved with his instruments.

WATSON-JONES on the one hand admits that bone stability is increased by compression but on the other hand shares LENGGENHAGER'S opinion that compression is destructive to bone. As examples he refers to a vertebra eroded by an aortic aneurysm, to bone eroded by the pressure of a neuroma, and to the unfavourable effect of early weight bearing on fracture healing. The difference between constant and intermittent pressure is not mentioned at all. KÜNTSCHER also believes that mechanical forces can only disturb bone formation.

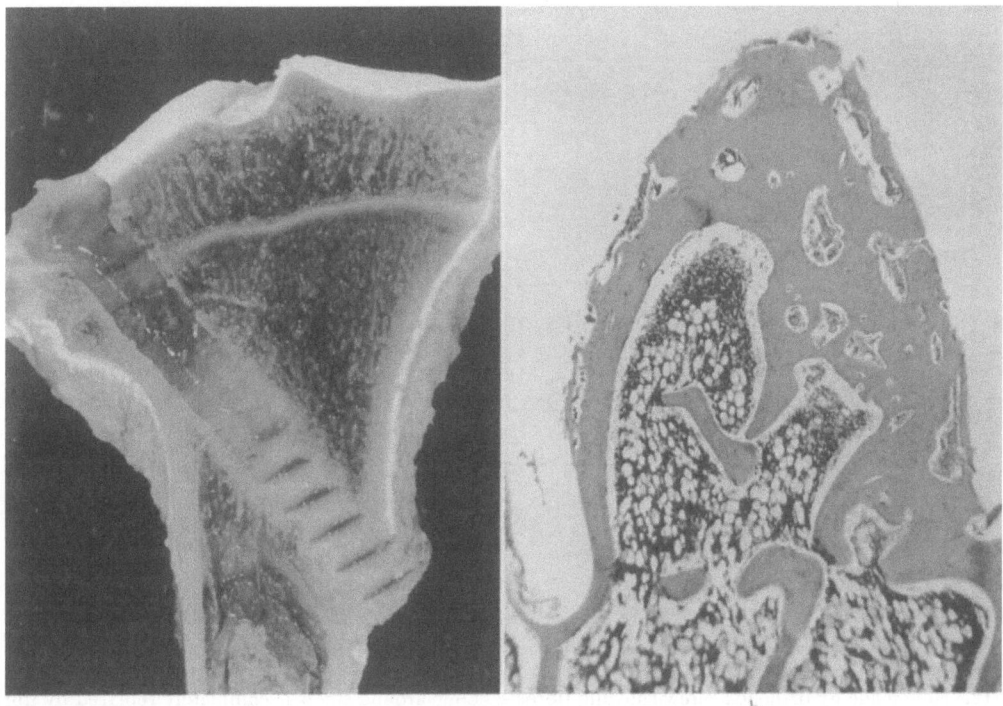

Fig. 11a and b. Adaptation of the bony tissue to the pressure of a screw: a An AOI cancellous screw placed in the upper end of a dog's tibia is subjected to continuous pressure due to the growing epiphysis. In the region of the unthreaded part of the screw hemopoietic bone marrow shines through the thin bony wall. In the region of the threaded part of the screw, areas of bone sclerosis have occurred as functional adaptation to the constant pressure (sawn section, enlarged twice). b Section through the bone that has been in contact with the screw thread. The compressing force of the screw was acting from right to left. Cancellous bone has become condensed on the side where the pressure of the screw thread was falling (the right side). The screw had been embedded in the bone for 5 months (paraffin section 10 μ thick, enlarged × 28), (from Wagner, H.: New screws for internal fixation and their compatibility with the tissues, Verh. Dtsch. Orthop. Ges., Zurich, 1962)

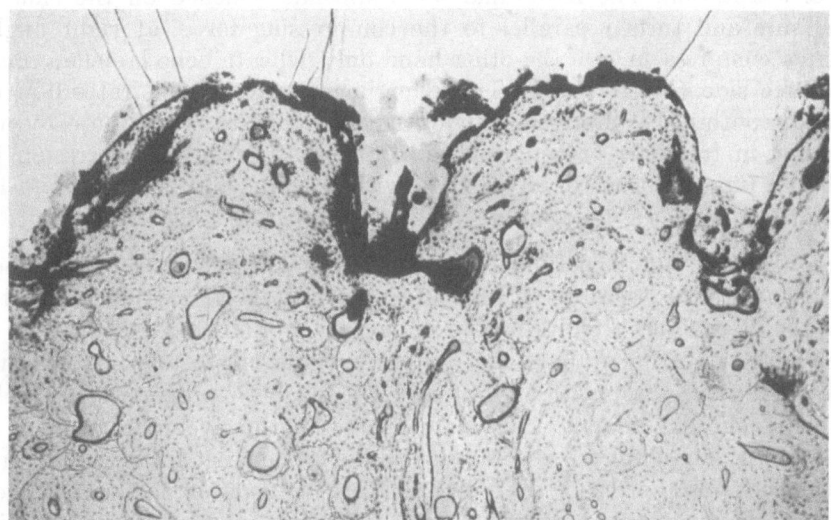

Fig. 11c. Adaptation of bone to the pressure of a screw: the bony bed in the tibial cortex which was the seat of an AOI cortex screw. The tibia has been sectioned exactly transversely, so that the Haversian systems surrounding the bed of the screw are shown in cross-section. In those parts of the bone that were in contact with the screw threads the lamellae have changed direction in accordance with the forces acting on them due to pressure from the threads of the screw. On the surface of the bone there is some discoloration due to the histological preparation, but there are no osteolytic changes. The screw was in the bone for 9 months. The section is of non-decalcified bone, 35 μ thick, magnified × 27 (preparation by H. Wagner)

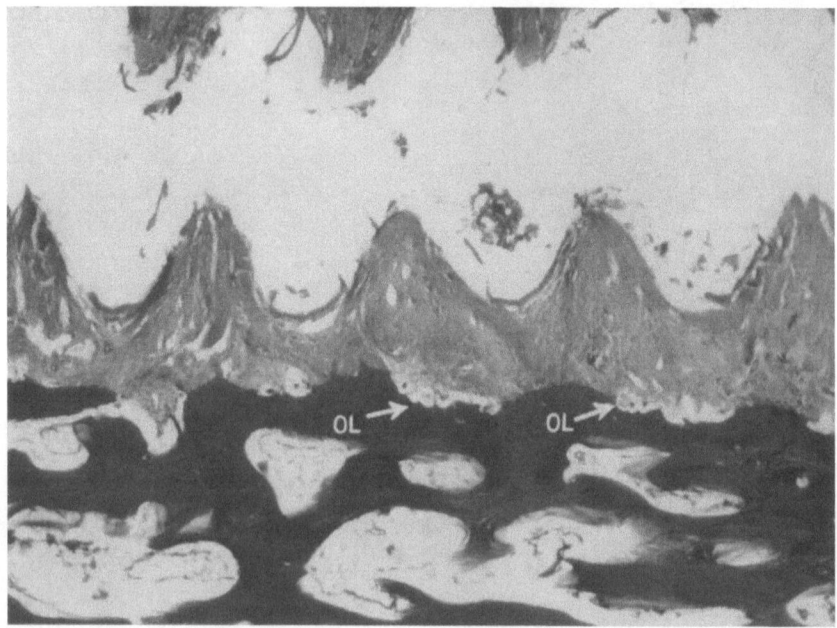

Fig. 12. Hole made by orthodox screw showing fibrosis. Bone around screw is completely replaced by fibrous tissue. Osteolytic activity (OL) between connective tissue and bony layers continues with many giant cells eroding lacunae into the bone. The screw was present for 4 months. (Paraffin section 10 μ mag. $\times 27$. Preparation by H. WAGNER)

WAGNER, however, showed that the bone reacts to constant pressure not by lysis but by osteogenesis. He inserted a cancellous screw through the epiphyseal line of the head of the tibia in a young dog. The screw retarded bone growth and constant pressure was exerted. The bone reacted with a condensation of tissue, and histology revealed a functional adaptation. The individual bone lamellae widened on the side of the increased pressure and turned parallel to the compressing force, at right angles to the surfaces under compression. On the other hand only delicate bone lamellae could be seen on the opposite side (Fig. 11a—c). This experiment only demonstrates how cancellous bone reacts to continued compression. KROMPECHER tried to prove the osteogenic effect of compression in fractures or osteotomies of the shaft. With compression he always obtained better fixation of the fracture than with traction, but the results of his experiments cannot be taken as a valid proof.

At the Laboratory for Experimental Surgery at Davos, WILLENEGGER and SCHENK in collaboration with the STRAUMANN Institute have been trying for over a year to measure the pressure at the fracture site during the whole period of healing. In this they have been using sheep as the experimental animal. Following transverse osteotomy of a metatarsal, the surfaces were compressed with an iron plate the magnetic properties of which were determined before the experiment. This plate itself is naturally under traction and daily measurements with a Ruhmkorff coil can determine the magnetism remaining in the plate and thus the continuing pressure that is applied to the fracture surfaces. Together with PETROKOV similar experiments are being carried out on dogs, the results of which will be published in a special monograph.

BASSETT showed that in vitro pluripotent mesenchymal cells could, under compression, differentiate into osteoblasts, whereas under distraction they differentiate into connective tissue cells. Thus it seems to be proved in vitro that pluripotent cells can be induced to differentiate either to osteoblasts or connective tissue cells, according to the mechanical

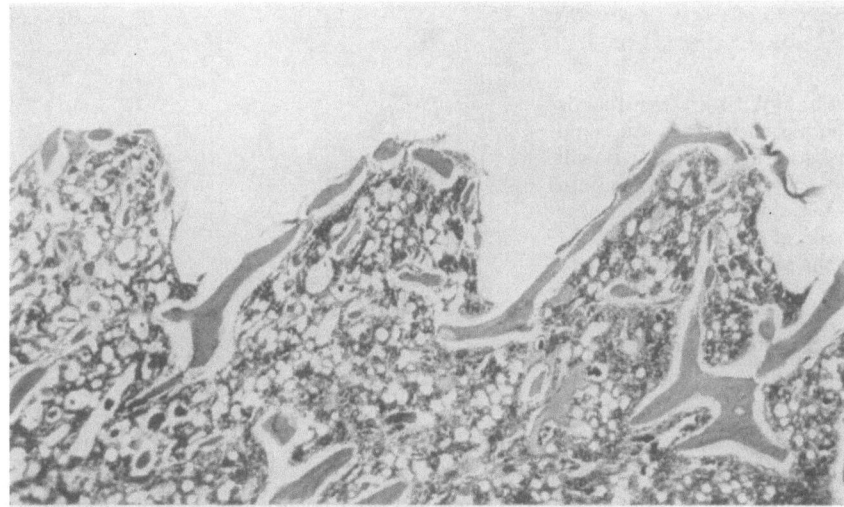

Fig. 13a. Hole made by an AOI cortex screw. Osseous tissue lies in close contact with the metal. Hemopoietic marrow is only separated from the screw by a fine bone lamella and in part it is in direct contact with the metal. There is no bone destruction and no fibrous tissue formation in the marrow. The screw had been in the bone for 2 months. (Paraffin section 30 μ mag. $\times 27$. Preparation by H. Wagner)

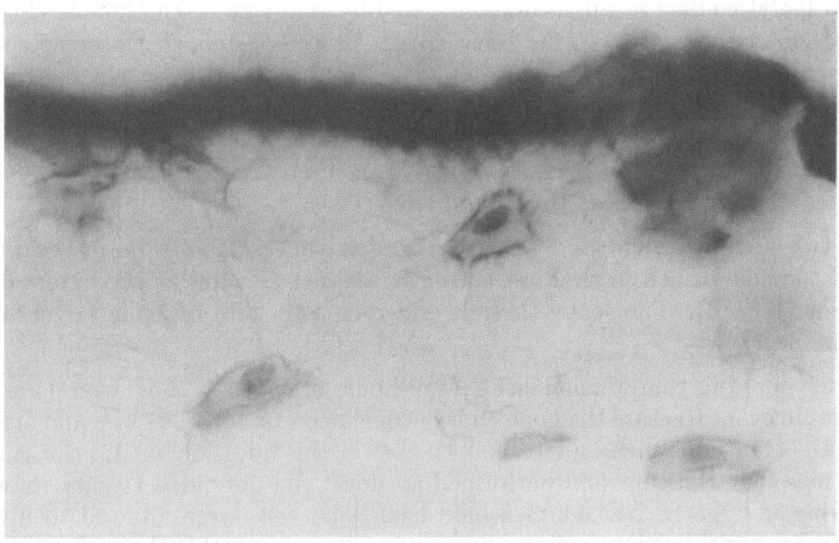

Fig. 13b. Hole made by an AOI cortex screw in the tibia. The surface of contact between bone and metal which is actually very thin appears as a broad band in the photograph due to a deposit of dye in the preparation. Live osteocytes are visible in the bone even in close proximity to the metal and the cell membranes actually reach the surface of the screw without any osteolytic changes being present. The screw had been in the bone for 9 months. (Non-decalcified section, 30 μ, magnified $\times 1300$. Preparation by H. Wagner)

stress applied to them. These examples are not intended to provide the final proof for the osteogenic effects of pressure, but to show that pressure is constructive rather than destructive in its effect on bone. More important appears to be the fact that compression increases the rigidity of fracture stabilization. This is true both with the use of lag screws and plates.

However, screws are taboo, especially in German speaking areas. Lange wrote as late as 1962:

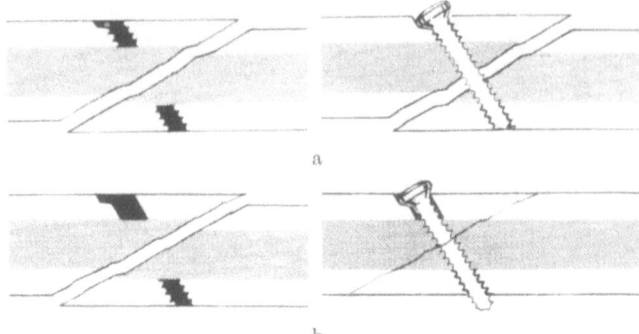

Fig. 14a and b. a With a screw that is biting into both cortices there can be no compression between fragments. It will break before the fragments come into contact. b When the hole in the near cortex is made as wide as the outside diameter of the screw, the thread has to be tapped into the far cortex only. When the screw is tightened the fractured surfaces are placed under compression

"It is utopian to believe that a simple screw will give permanent support to a bone. Zones of resorption soon form around the screw even if it was at first firmly anchored in the bone, with the result that the screw becomes loose and then behaves just like a simple nail. Fracture fixation is then lost and the loose screw can later be removed simply with a pair of tweezers."

It is clear from the example given in Fig. 12 that some self-tapping screws in common use, which are probably made from not entirely corrosion-proof metal, will convert osseous tissue into fibrous tissue. It is, however, indisputable that an atraumatic AOI[1] screw shows no osteolytic effect at all, as demonstrated by WAGNER's experiments (Fig. 13a and b). Thousands of internal fixations have shown us that osteoporotic areas surrounding screws develop only when the screw cannot resist external forces or when slight infection has occurred. If one considers that with self-tapping screws temperatures in excess of 90° C can develop, it is evident that burnt bone cells must first be replaced by connective tissue. In our method the screw hole is drilled slowly and then threaded with a very sharp tap. This reduces the damaging heat to a minimum.

When two bone fragments are screwed together they can only be placed under compression if the hole drilled in the first cortex is at least as wide as the external diameter of the screw (Fig. 14). The screw threads will then only bite into the far cortex pulling it up to the near cortex.

How long does this compression last? A few hours or days say those who share BÖHLER's opinion that in every fracture the bone ends become necrotic for 2—5 mm. and are resorbed. Is lysis of the bone ends then inevitable? To answer this question we did the same experiments on pigs that BASSETT had performed on dogs. We intended to show how a defect in the radius as large as 20×5 mm. would heal if no cells were allowed to invade from the endosteum, periosteum or surrounding areas. To achieve this the endosteal cells were scraped out through the gap with a sharp curette and a vertical cut made in the bone on each side of the defect. Through these vertical slots a Millipore filter was inserted (Millipore is a material that is permeable to body fluids but not to cells). The defect was thereby completely sealed off (Fig. 15a).

30 days after the experiment the defect showed newly formed bone directly adjacent to the old bone, and a few Haversian canals led straight into the newly formed osseous tissue without any evidence of resorption. It thus seems to be proved that to bridge a bone defect or a fracture gap neither periosteal nor endosteal cells are necessary. We offer no opinion as to whether this is direct ossification originating in the Haversian canals or whether blood elements invading the defect were transformed into osteoblasts or osteocytes. This experiment does demonstrate, however, what we mean by primary bone healing.

---

[1] AOI refers to the type of instrument or implant developed by AO (see Page 34).

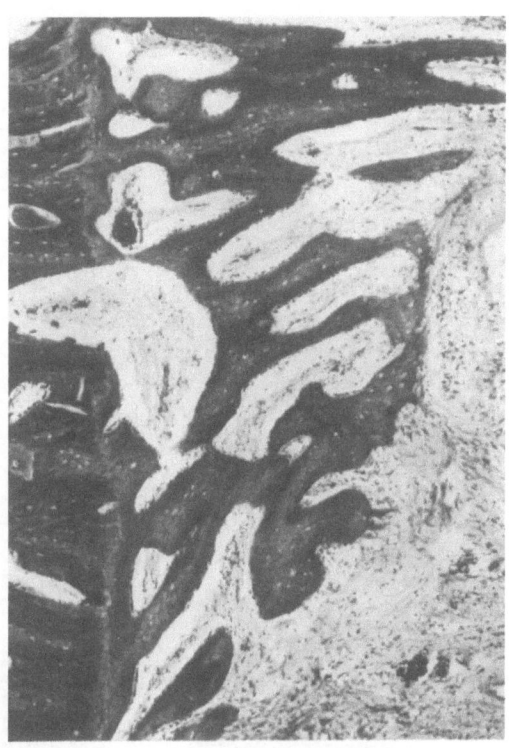

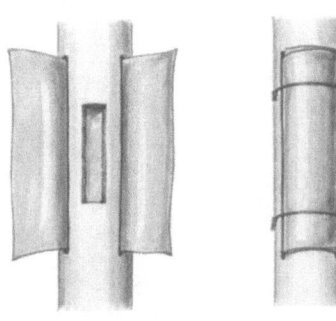

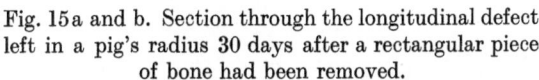

Fig. 15a and b. Section through the longitudinal defect left in a pig's radius 30 days after a rectangular piece of bone had been removed.
a Experimental Technique: to prevent access of endosteal or periosteal cells a Millipore membrane is introduced. b Magnification ×40. No zone of necrosis is visible. There is direct communication between original and newly-formed lamellae

b

The conclusions that Schenk draws from studying the ossification of this defect in a pig's radius are as follows:

1. The defect sealed off by the Millipore filter first contains blood that is soon replaced by granulation tissue. Assuming that the invasion of cells from the periosteum and medullary canal is truly prevented, this granulation tissue probably proliferates from the open Haversian canals. It is my impression that this was the case in the experiment.

2. Immediately after surgery, parts of the bone edges are certain to have been damaged and the contents of the Haversian canals destroyed over a short distance. These elements have excellent powers of regeneration. Necrotic portions of bone are of course subject to osteoclastic resorption. This produces marked localized enlargement of the Haversian canals. In Fig. 15b, for example, three osteoclasts are seen in situ. In general however the edges of the defect are in surprisingly good condition.

3. Bone regeneration certainly originates from granulation tissue. In the granulation tissue collagen fibers develop so that one must agree with Krompecher's concept of "desmal ossification". As osteoblasts can only function in close proximity to blood vessels, bone regeneration takes place mainly in the vicinity of capillaries proliferating outwards from the Haversian canals. In this way the direction of their growth determines the spatial arrangement of the newly formed bone substance. Regeneration thus takes place from the periphery of the defect, producing bone that resembles the cortex both in spatial arrangement and structure.

Even if some periosteal or endosteal cells entered the opening, we would speak of primary bone healing in all cases where no callus formation is seen in x-ray tomographs (Fig. 16d, e).

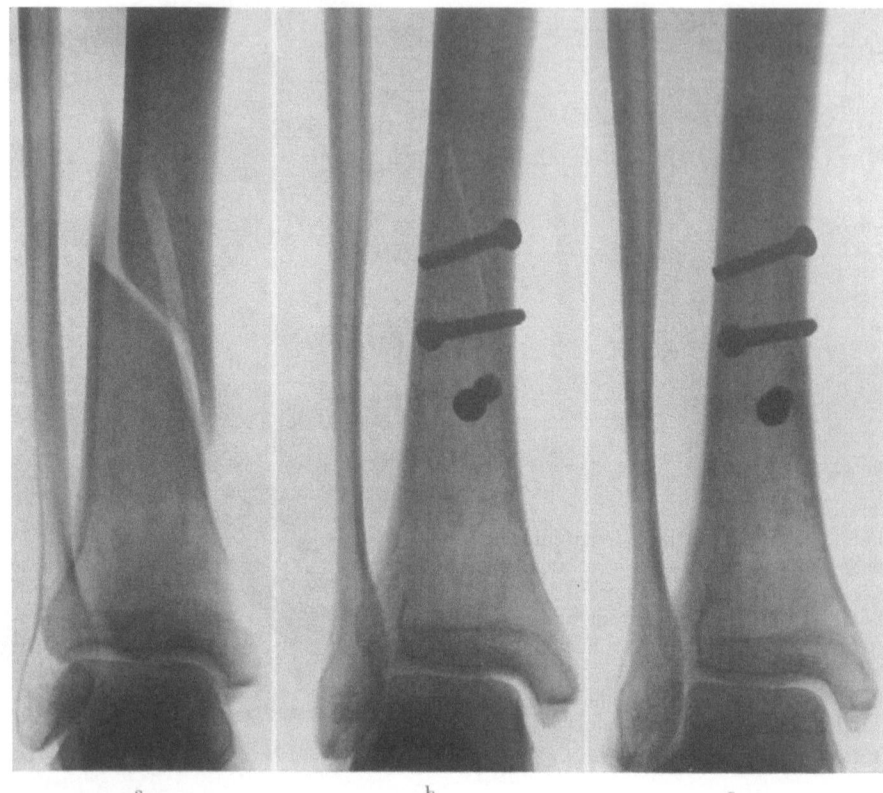

Fig. 16a—c. Spiral fracture of the tibia, treated with primary screwing. a Immediately after the accident. b 5 weeks later. c 25 weeks after internal fixation. There is "primary" union of the fracture, i.e. no radiologically visible callus formation

It must be admitted that histological processes cannot be observed radiologically and that a minimal layer of callus is required to bridge the microscopically small gap in any bone which remains in spite of compression. Whether this callus originates from blood elements or from the Haversian canals, or whether it proliferates from the periosteum or endosteum does not really matter. The important fact is that certain osteolytic processes, invisible radiologically, take place as well, producing simultaneous resorption and regeneration referred to as "creeping substitution".

Primary healing of bone has become a clinical and radiological concept. It is called "fracture union without visible callus formation". We even believe that any excess callus should be considered deleterious, be regarded as a kind of keloid of the bone (Danis) and that it indicates movement at the fracture site. We therefore regard any radiologically visible callus formation during fracture healing after internal fixation as a warning which should initiate appropriate action. Union without radiologically visible callus, on the other hand, appears to us to be the most desirable form of healing. The healing of a fracture without callus can be regarded as radiological evidence of continuous rigid fixation. Well over half of all fractures treated according to AO principles heal with minimal or radiologically invisible periosteal and endosteal reaction (Fig. 16).

Screws can only give rigid fixation to a shaft fracture if the length of the fracture line is at least twice that of the shaft diameter. The development of a plate was therefore urgent. We were aware that the earlier Lane's plate, which was used in England and

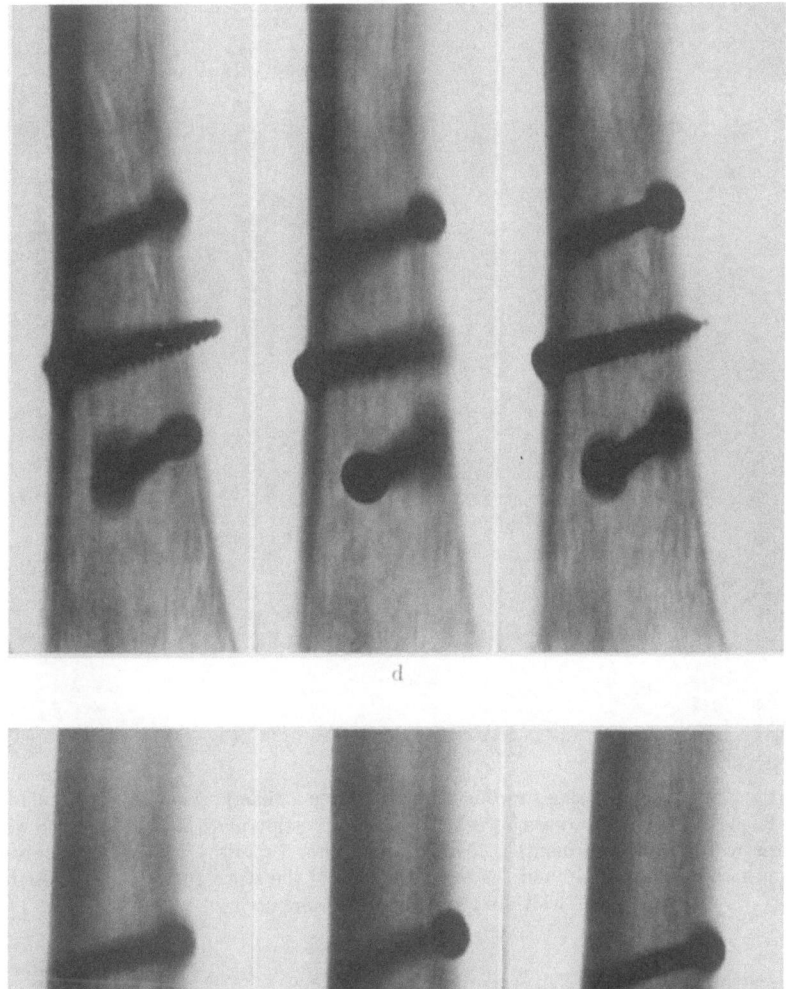

d

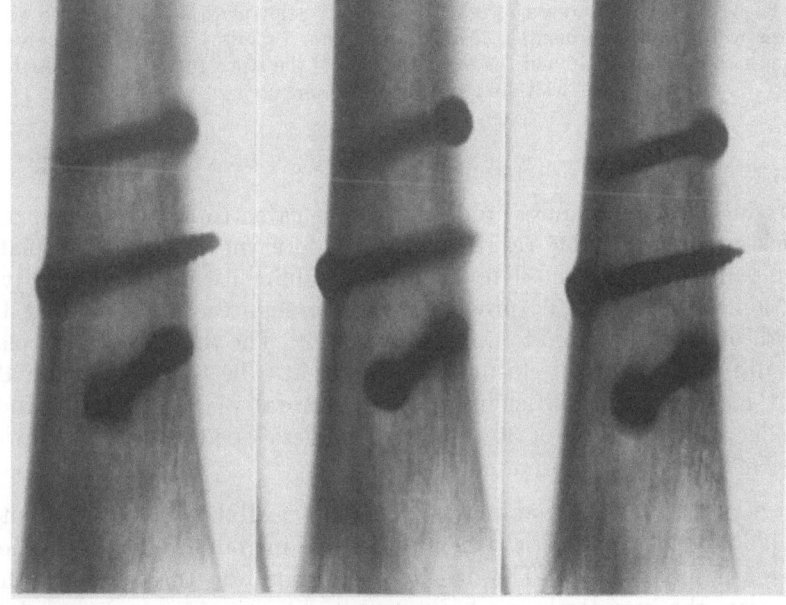

e

Fig. 16d and e. Tomographs showing: d Appearance at 5 weeks, e 25 weeks after fixation with screws. The fracture line at first barely visible has disappeared entirely at 25 weeks. There is no perceptible periosteal or endosteal callus formation

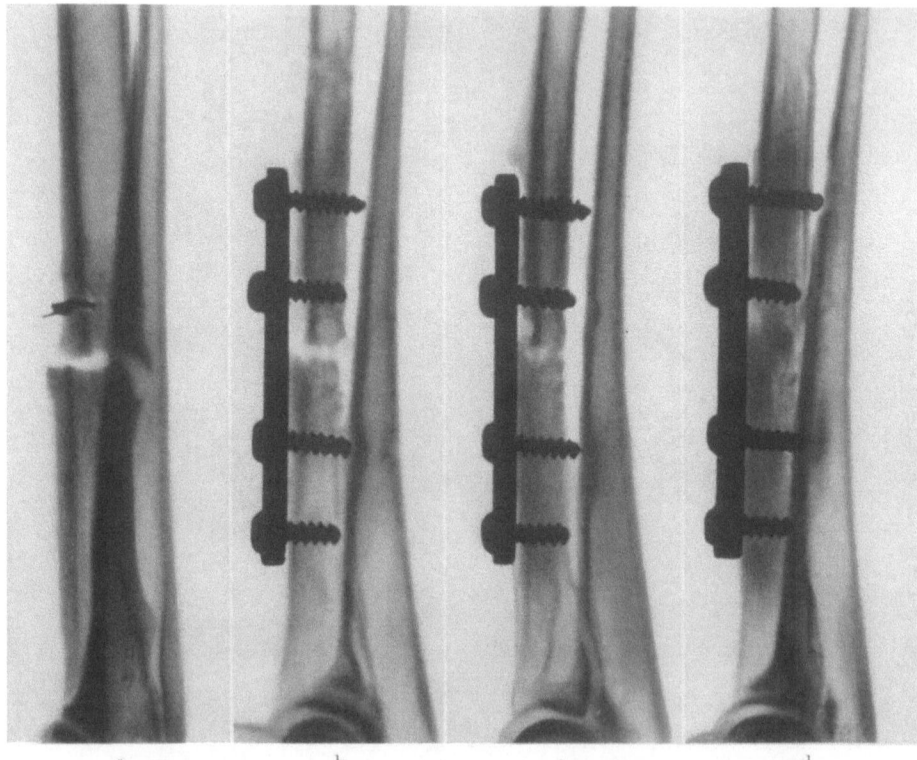

Fig. 17a—d. a Pseudarthrosis in a dog's radius 3 months after a silastic sheet has been introduced between the osteotomized bone ends. b Appearance 3 weeks after a compression plate has been applied without resecting the pseudarthrosis. c The same at 4 months. d Bony union after 7 months without appearance of any excess callus. There was no bone atrophy around the screws in spite of the stress the bone was submitted to and the width of the screws that were used

Germany, produced many failures and even some catastrophies. DANIS, on the other hand, demonstrated gratifying results with his forearm compression plate. Lately, JERGESEN of San Francisco and HICKS of Birmingham have more strongly advocated internal fixation with plates. To prevent even the slightest movement at the fracture site HICKS and collaborators tried to use thicker plates. The thickness of the plate however gives rise to difficulties in skin closure. It should also be noted that the Birmingham school cannot recommend a sufficiently strong femoral plate. In order to place bone fragments under a compression of 30 to 60 kg., we developed the AOI compression plate with a device of temporary compressing.

This plate was first tested in animal experiments. After transverse osteotomy of the radius of an adult dog, a "silastic" membrane was introduced between the fragments so as to cause a pseudarthrosis. The dog hopped around on three legs for three months during which time the pseudarthrosis became quite loose. A compression plate was then applied and two days later the dog ran about quite normally. Nevertheless the pseudarthrosis ossified in the course of five months and the screws showed not the slightest loosening. Rigidity was thus maintained for the entire duration of the healing of the pseudarthrosis (Fig. 17).

Experiments carried out by BOYD and ANDERSON at the Campbell Clinic have yielded the same satisfactory results, so that they now regularly use compression plates in the treatment of fractures of the forearm and of nonunions of the long bones.

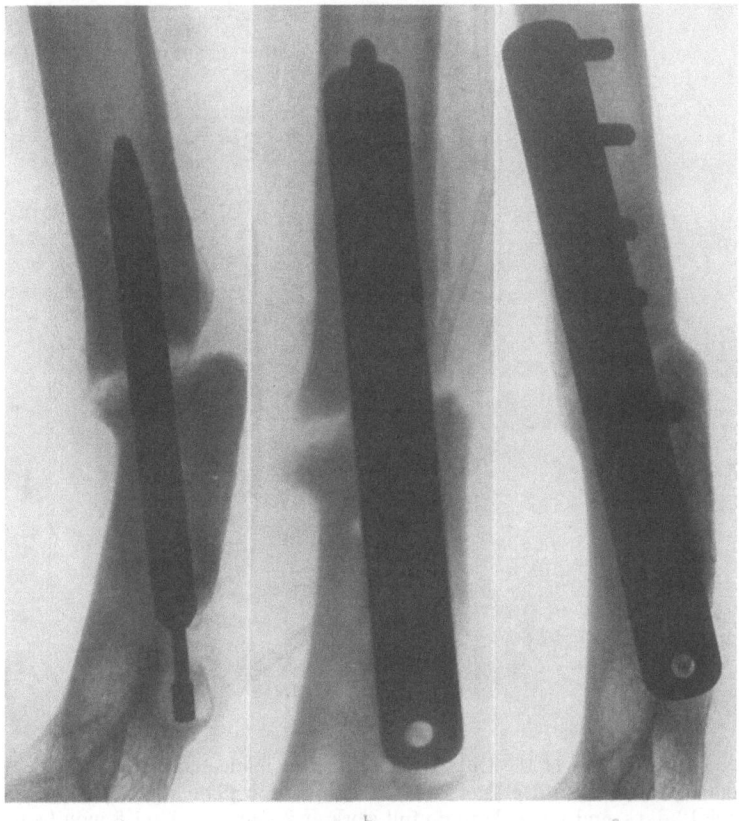

Fig. 18a—c. a Pseudarthrosis of the humerus treated with too short a compression plate after DANIS. b Appearance immediately after an AOI compression plate has been applied. No freshening of the fracture ends has been performed and no external fixation. c At 4 months the pseudarthrosis has united

The technique of applying compression plates is shown in Fig. 60. The systematic and accurate use of this plate, particularly on the forearm, has regularly produced perfect bone healing. Immediately after the operation the patients can move and use the fractured extremity without discomfort and may return to work shortly after internal fixation.

c) Vascularization of the Bone Fragments

When two necrotic bone fragments are held together by internal fixation, a loosening of the fixation will occur and the healing process is either retarded or stopped. The result is a so-called avascular pseudarthrosis with devitalized bone fragments, an especially dreaded complication of internal fixation. Usually this devitalization is caused by faulty operative technique. If, however, only a single bone fragment is cut off from its blood supply, rapid ossification may be expected, especially if the fragments have been impacted or placed under compression (FRIEDENBERG and FRENCH 1952).

It is known that rapid union may be expected with a perfectly fixed femoral neck fracture whether the femoral head is necrotic or has an intact blood supply. PETROKOV's experiments in dogs showed that homografts placed under compression are incorporated without radiologically visible change. The process of destruction and regeneration takes place simultaneously. Equally many clinical observations show that small avascular

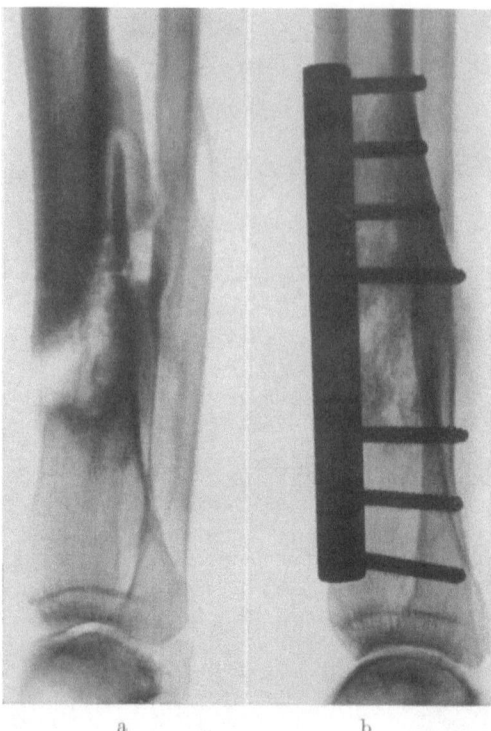

Fig. 19a and b. a Pseudarthrosis of the tibia 18 months after inadequate fixation with 4 Vitallium screws followed by 6 months treatment in a plaster cast. b Compression plate without a plaster cast, the patient was hospitalized for 12 days, and was able to do full work at 2 months. After 8 months union was complete

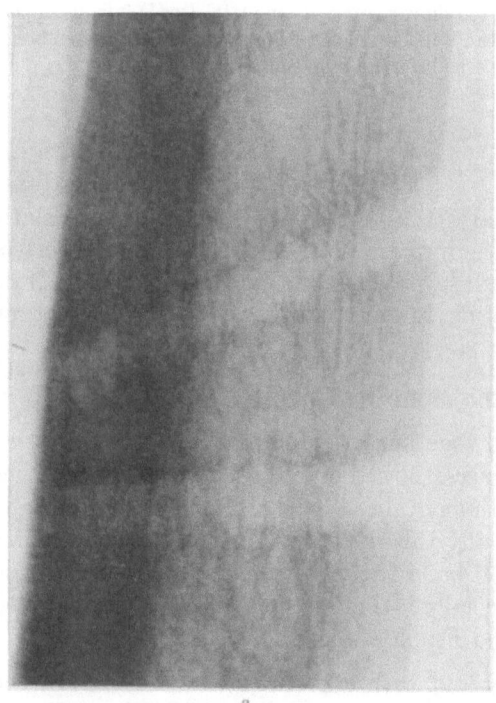

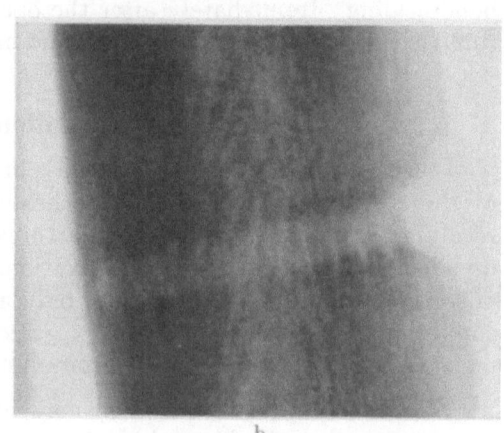

Fig. 20a and b. After removal of the screws from the bone the enlarged screw hole in the first cortex soon fills with bone. Osteoblasts seem to have originated from the Haversian canals. a Overall view. b Enlargement of the screw hole in the first cortex

bone fragments carefully repositioned and placed under compression will become incorporated and thus promote healing.

Circulation can be impaired by removal of the periosteum or by heat, as for example in prolonged reaming of the medulla. A nailed fracture subsequently treated with a plate can often lead to the final disruption of periosteal and endosteal circulation. In principle, therefore, a medullary nail removed from a pseudarthrosis should be replaced by a thicker medullary nail.

Functionally stable internal fixation requires not only mechanical skill but also corresponding biological understanding. It is essential that the surgeon concern himself with the blood supply during the whole operation. On no occasion should a large loose fragment be disconnected from its adhering soft tissues. If, in spite of all precautions, it is concluded that two adjacent bone fragments have become devitalized, a large cancellous autograft may be necessary to promote revascularization.

B. Operative Technique and Postoperative Management

I. Basic Principles of Operative Technique

Without the strictest asepsis, open reduction of a fracture should not be undertaken. In closed fractures even one single case of osteitis occurring in one hundred internally fixed fractures is a tragedy for which the method used must be held responsible. It is often overlooked that even with the conventional treatment of fractures using extension, osteitis of the femur or the os calcis may occasionally occur, and that there have even been cases where amputation was necessary.

a) Asepsis is a problem of organization, which can be solved only if aseptic standards can be rigidly enforced from the preoperative period until the wound is healed. The prevention of wound infection alone is not enough, for a wound, under the best conditions, can never be kept absolutely sterile. There is practically always some bacterial invasion. Hematomata and necrotic tissues form excellent nutrient media for invading pathogens. Consequently an atraumatic technique combined with meticulous asepsis is vital for operative fracture treatment. Osteitis and necrosis of wound edges are clearly infectious, but any postoperative tissue induration should be regarded also as potentially infectious. Even after an extensive exposure of a fracture the resulting scar should be free of irritation and movable on its bed 10 days postoperatively. As soon as one or more infections, however slight, occur, a careful investigation should be carried out involving everyone concerned in order to discover the source of infection.

b) Operating Theatre. If possible a special operating room where no other surgery — especially abdominal surgery — is carried out, should be reserved for internal fixation operations. To keep the theatre as germ-free as possible, filtered slightly humidified fresh air should be introduced under positive pressure. "Air sterilization" devices such as ionization equipment have shown some good results though they do not actually sterilize but merely reduce the number of bacteria. Beds from the wards must always be regarded as septic and must under no circumstance be brought into the theatre. Patients should be placed on a litter or the actual operating table in the preparation room whence they are wheeled into theatre, and following surgery they should be returned to the preparation room on the operating table. Sheets and linen from the wards have no place in the theatre, nor do cabinets with dressings and instruments or case histories and x-ray envelopes. Dust particles are excellent germ carriers and must be meticulously eliminated. Floors should be washed daily with an antiseptic solution, and walls and cylinders in the theatre and adjacent rooms should be thoroughly washed once a week.

c) Staff. No one should be admitted to the theatre in street clothes or shoes, nor without a mask or cap. As more than a third of all people are pathogen carriers, care must be taken that surgical masks fit closely around the mouth and nose. To avoid the contact of an unsterile part of a coat with the instrument table, the backs of operating gowns should also be sterile.

Presterilized packs of theatre linen have produced better results than keeping these materials in drums that have to be repeatedly opened. There should be as little conversation as possible in the theatre itself, not only to maintain asepsis but to allow the surgeon to concentrate fully on the operation.

d) Disinfection of Hands. Hands are disinfected according to general surgical rules and if Phisohex is used, cultures of the solution must be made at regular intervals. Saprophytes may develop in containers that are not regularly sterilized. It is to the surgeon's advantage to wear cotton gloves over his rubber ones. Not only does this reduce the danger of perforation of the rubber gloves but the moistened cotton gives the surgeon a feeling of increased safety when handling instruments. With a little experience he will be able to use them even for the most delicate procedures.

e) Care of the Soft Tissues. Careful anatomically correct surgery of the soft tissues is just as important as the mechanical treatment of the bone. Scalpels, scissors and osteotomes should be razor-sharp and kept in this state. Only the most delicate forceps and sutures should be used. The assistant too, by the careful use of hooks and retractors, must take care to avoid damaging soft tissue and thereby increasing the danger of infection. Fragments of fascia, periosteum or other necrotic looking tissue must be excised. At intervals of half an hour we rinse the wound with sterile Ringer solution, which reduces the bacterial count, prevents desiccation of the tissues and washes out loose necrotic particles. A local antibiotic, suitable for topical application, may be added to the Ringer solution, e.g. Neomycin and Bacitracin in a concentration of $^1/_4$ to $^1/_2{}^0/_{00}$. We have given up the non-touch technique; a securely covered finger can provide information about conditions which evade the eye. Fracture reduction itself can also be facilitated by the pressure of a finger on the right place. In general, however, fingers have no business in the wound. The surgeon should also cultivate the habit of touching as little as possible the metal parts that are introduced into the bone.

If diathermy is used, blood vessels should only be coagulated singly since coagulated tissue is necrotic tissue, and necrotic tissue provides a good nutrient medium for bacteria.

f) Local Preparation. For emergency operation, the skin must be washed with soap and a brush, shaved with a sterilized razor and painted with an antiseptic solution. Although preparation is chiefly the duty of a nurse or orderly, we require the final painting to be done by a doctor.

In elective surgery a skin test for sensitivity to the adhesive used (e. g. Mastisol) must be made 24 to 36 hours before the operation, since we found that between 1 and 2% of all patients show some allergy to Mastisol. On the day before operation the skin is washed, brushed and covered overnight with a clean cloth.

g) Draping. To cover the skin, a polyethylene or other plastic film is fixed in place with an adhesive. This hermetically seals the pores of the skin. Since polyethylene breaks down at a temperature of 100°C, it cannot be autoclaved, but it can be boiled. For this purpose the films are covered with cotton gauze and rolled into a thick tube, quite conveniently around a medullary nail. The whole is then boiled for 15 minutes (Fig. 21).

The adhesive we have used over many years is the solution advocated by LEVEUF. This solution, which needs to be filtered twice by the pharmacist, must be very fluid and is stored only in small bottles containing enough for one day's use.

The formula is: Rp. mastix 200.0, colophonium 400.0, oleum ricini 10.0, dichloramine T 1.0, ether 580.0.

h) Skin Incisions. Standard incisions are used according to the type of operation. They should avoid dividing nerves as much as possible. Long straight incisions provide better exposure. Incisions are usually made longitudinally for shaft fractures and transversely for articular fractures, following normal skin creases.

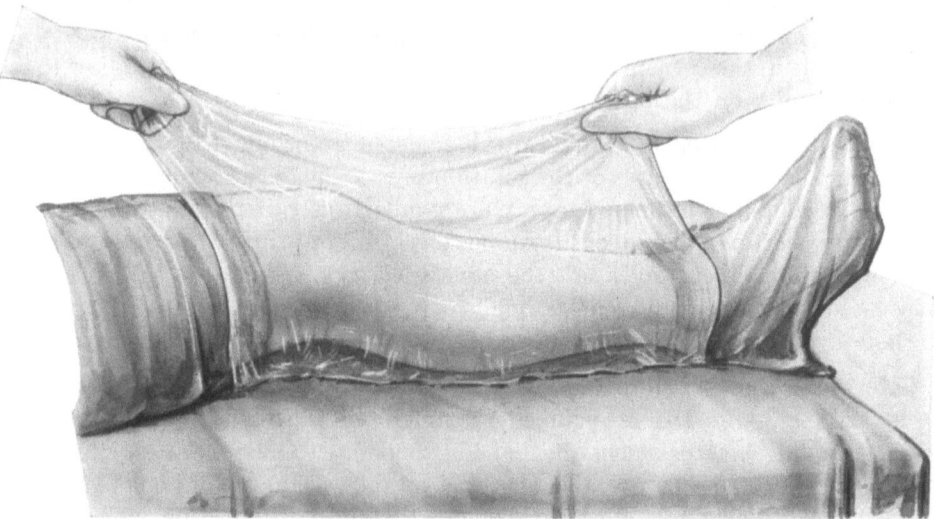

Fig. 21. Draping of the lower leg with a sheet of polyethylene

i) Open Reduction. It is usually done with the help of longitudinal traction by an assistant. Only with fractures of the shaft of the femur has it become customary to stretch the leg in an extension device. In all other cases the fragments can usually be reduced without great effort especially with the help of relaxants given by the anesthetist.

k) Temporary Fixation. This can be achieved in cancellous bone with the help of KIRSCHNER wires and in cortical bone with a cerclage wire or suitable bone holding forceps. Whichever method that requires the least exposure and is most gentle to soft tissues should be preferred.

l) Choice of Procedure. In every case a method should be chosen that will offer the greatest rigidity with the least length of exposure and destruction of soft tissues. For this reason the surgeon should master all the techniques of internal fixation and have available the full range of necessary instruments. Quite often the best procedure can only be determined after the fracture has been visualized and its complexity assessed. If one procedure is found to be unsuitable during the course of the operation, the surgeon should not hesitate to adopt another method that is better suited to the particular case.

m) Drainage. JOST-REDON's automatic suction drainage has proved useful when adopted systematically for operative wounds (Fig. 23). It prevents hematoma formation and reduces the danger of infection. We usually use a thin polyethylene or silicon rubber drainage tube directly over the bone and a second one subcutaneously. Each is brought out through a stab incision between 10 and 15 cm. from the wound. The drains are left in place until no more blood is extracted and this usually is between 24 and 48 hours. A late hematoma is aspirated under sterile conditions.

II. Principles of Postoperative Care

a) Dressing and Position. In very few cases is a plaster cast applied after operation. An exception is made for malleolar fractures which can usefully be immobilized for about a week in a double gutter splint with the foot in maximum dorsiflexion (Fig. 22). In all other cases the leg is loosely bandaged and then elevated as far as possible on a foam rubber splint. In fractures of the femoral shaft the knee is flexed at a right angle to prevent postoperative contraction of the extensors. Since using the foam rubber splint we have had no case of peroneal paralysis such as can occur with BRAUN's splint (see Figs. 23, 24).

After 24 to 48 hours the suction drains are removed. One or two days later the dressings are removed also, so that the earliest possible open wound care can be instituted.

b) Postoperative Mobilization. This is one of the basic requirements of AO. It can

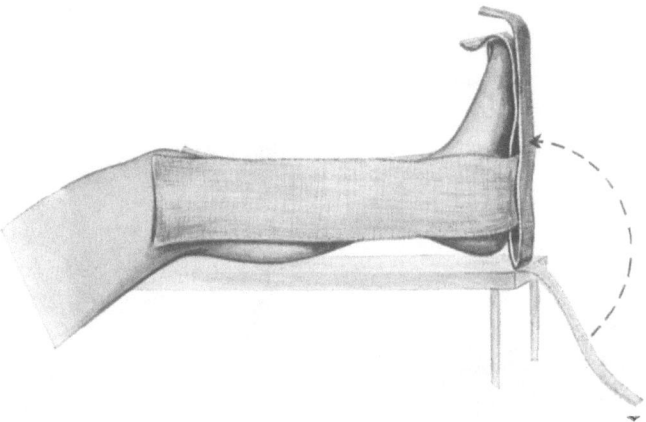

Fig. 22. Double gutter splint constructed from 2 plaster slabs. The foot remains free

be argued whether the patient should be systematically given exercise on the first day or whether wound healing should first be allowed to proceed for four to six days. Excellent results have been achieved with both methods. In cases of medullary nailing or in fractures near joints we usually wait for about a week, while in all shaft fractures that have been internally fixed with screws or plates the joints of the injured extremity can be moved within 24 hours.

c) Walking Calipers. As soon as the joints can be moved freely and actively a below-knee caliper is fitted to allow walking without weight bearing in fractures of the lower leg. After discharge patients are instructed to keep the injured limb elevated and to move the joints frequently. The walking caliper made of Plastoid 015 was developed in cooperation with the RÖCK Company. The four standard sizes can be fitted quite easily by heating the plastoid. The body weight is carried by the upper end of the tibia and the patella. Patients are usually able to walk between 10 and 14 days after the operation as the caliper prevents any weight being transmitted through the fracture (see page 103 and Fig. 113).

After an open fracture it is important to make sure that no infection is developing before active movements are started. In these cases we wait for about a week.

III. Follow-up

Regular postoperative examinations of our patients are of great value not only for the patients themselves but also for the surgeon and his assistants. By a careful follow-up we can correctly evaluate the virtues of the method used, and many mistakes have been recognized in the course of these examinations. The follow-up examination also gives a chance of detecting an imminent nonunion in good time so that it can be promptly treated. This review, however, requires a lot of patience and good organization and involves considerable expense.

The 20 surgeons of the *Association for the Study of the Problems of Osteosynthesis (AO)* have created a documentation centre in Davos. A *yellow code sheet* which is completed after the first discharge from the hospital is sent there together with x-rays taken before and after the operation. Based on this first code sheet, two cards are punched and reduced prints of the x-rays are pasted on the back of the cards. One of these cards is returned to the surgeon and the second remains in Davos (Fig. 25). After four months a *blue code sheet* with the four months follow-up and new a.p. and lateral x-rays, together

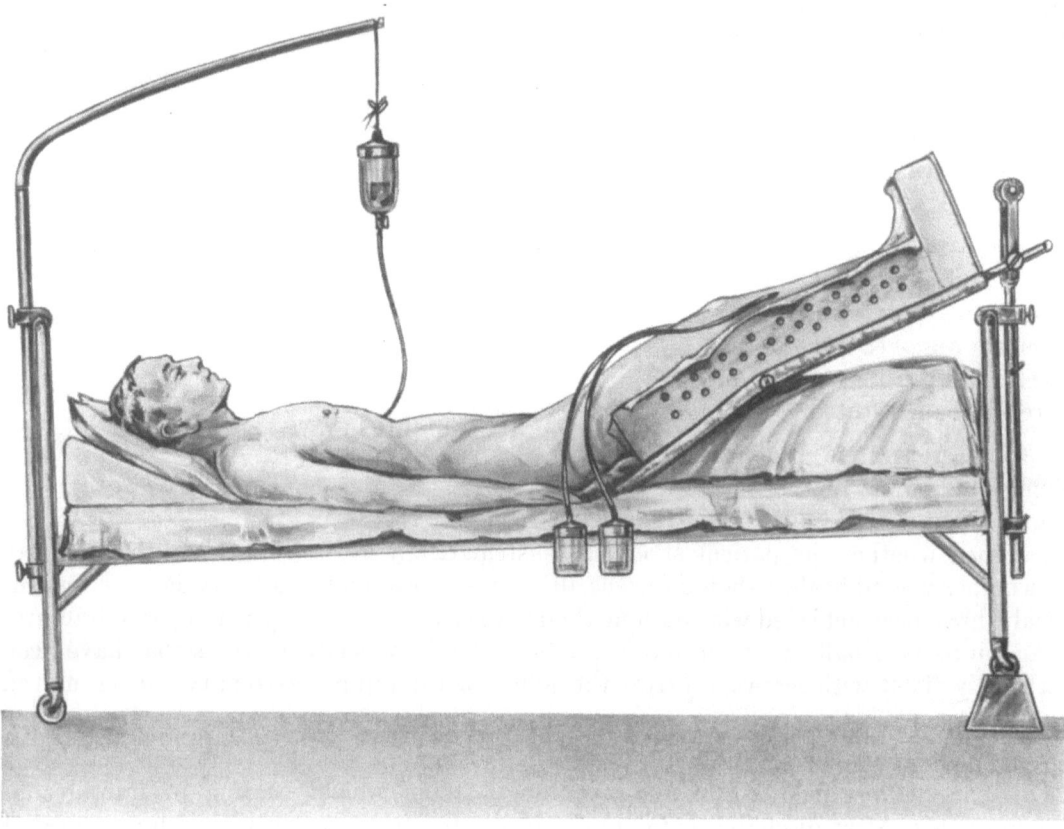

Fig. 23. Elevation of the leg in a foam rubber splint and suction drainage

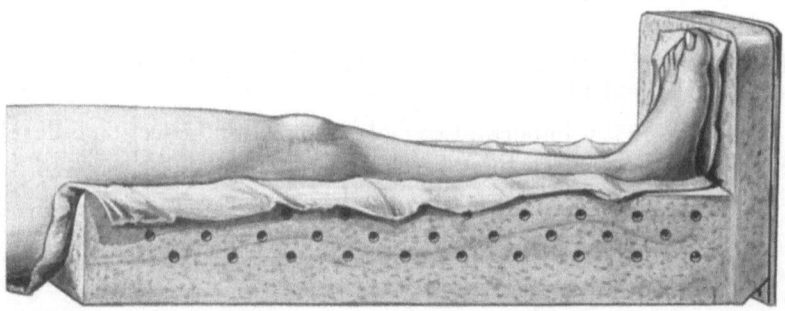

Fig. 24. Foam rubber splint with a wooden board reinforcing the sole. A clean cloth is first placed on the
splint to prevent it being soiled with sweat and blood

with the punched card, are returned by the surgeon to Davos. Copies of these x-rays are
fixed to the punched card and one of the two cards with the original x-rays is returned to
the surgeon. After the one-year follow-up a *red code sheet* is completed on the assumption
that the case can now be closed. If this is not the case the surgeon makes a note that
an additional examination will be required after another six months.

The review of the case at four months has proved desirable, as it is at this time that
the fracture has usually fully united, so that the patient in most cases has resumed his
normal activities. The final examination is usually undertaken after the removal of the

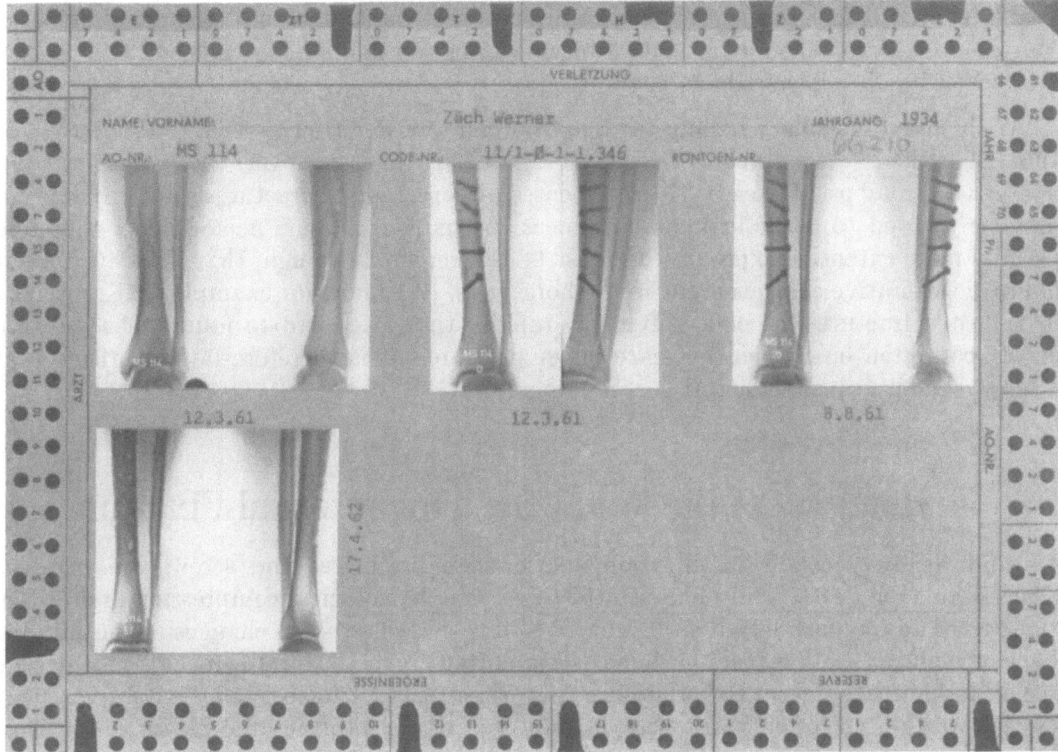

Fig. 25. The AO punched card: Fracture of the tibia before and after internal fixation and at the 4 months and 12 months review

plates, screws or wires, when full work has been resumed, i.e. at the conclusion of the case. Should subsequent complications occur, follow-up examinations must of course be carried out.

IV. Timing of the Operation

Both with open and closed fractures, especially in cases where the skin is contused, we recommend surgery within eight to ten hours, even when this is outside normal operating room hours in the evening or at night. Experience shows that the danger of infection increases materially after this time, particularly when the skin is contused or a sharp piece of bone is pressing the skin up. This is especially true with a transverse fracture of the medial malleolus where the skin is stretched over the sharp bony edge and damaged from the inside. Generally, therefore, a transverse fracture of the medial malleolus is either operated upon within the ten hour period or it is treated primarily by closed reduction and operated on in three to five days. If the operation cannot be performed within the eight hour limit one should wait for four to eight days by which time local hyperemia may have produced more favourable conditions. Generally speaking, the earlier surgery is performed, the better is the healing rate and the appearance of the resulting wound. Reduction of the fracture is also more difficult after 24 hours, as inflammatory reaction has then already set in.

When for medical or other reasons the operation must be postponed, a fracture should be reduced with the help of a wire or Steinman pin extension if the bone lies subcutaneously, especially in the tibia, if there is great danger of overlapping fragments, e.g. in the femur or if a pointed bone spike could produce internal soft tissue damage. In any case of skin contusion operation should not be performed after ten hours have elapsed. This is also true when fracture blisters have begun to form.

With closed medullary nailing the operation may be deferred — as KÜNTSCHER (1950, 1951) suggested — for three to five days. After this time, however, the danger of postoperative thrombosis increases. In some cases of comminuted fractures, local hyperemia may be allowed to occur first, as it reduces the danger of bone necrosis and therefore permits more extensive exposure. It must be remembered, though, that after even a few hours, degenerative changes occur in the bone ends. We know for example that especially in malleolar fractures the bone softens so rapidly that after two to four weeks the thin cortex can often be crushed by mere finger pressure. It is therefore not surprising that a screw cannot grip in these soft surroundings.

V. Removal of the Metal Used for Internal Fixation

Under normal conditions in young patients, nails, plates and screws are removed after 12 to 14 months, partly because they exert unphysiological compression and distention forces on the bone which according to WOLFF's laws result in changes of the internal bone structure. As long as the bone is supported by plates and screws it can neither regain its normal internal structure nor its former elasticity (see page 8). Furthermore as time passes, corrosion may occur in any case where two metallic pieces are in close contact.

Metal is usually left in elderly patients but even then it will be removed if symptoms occur.

Before the metal is removed it should be ascertained, which is not always easy, that the fracture has completely united. Especially with internal fixation of comminuted fractures using two plates, the circulation may have been so disrupted that one fragment may still be in the process of revascularization. In such a case the circulation in the bone must be studied by chiselling off a very thin surface layer before removal of the second plate. If there is no good evidence of healthy circulation especially in fractures of the femoral shaft, one plate should be left in place and at the same time extensive superficial cancellous autografts applied.

When two methods of internal fixation are combined, e.g. cerclage wiring and medullary nail, it is advisable to remove the wire suture at a very early stage — i.e. after six to ten weeks. Where the circulation is deficient, a cancellous bone graft may be indicated at the same time.

Periarticular fractures in cancellous bone are usually consolidated after two months so that screws, wires and nails can easily be removed after the third month. Experience shows that in children wires and screws in cancellous bone can be removed without any risk after 3 weeks. In the exceptional case where the internal fixation is carried out in an adolescent the metal may also be removed after four to six months.

C. Instruments and their Use

I. Metallurgical Considerations

NICOLE (1940, 1947) was one of the first to carry out comprehensive scientific research in metals used for internal fixation. He concluded that complete success could only be guaranteed when two conditions were fulfilled: keeping a balance between mechanical and physiological requirements on one hand, and on the other, avoiding any damage caused by the metal during the whole period of bone healing. Favourable biomechanical conditions depend largely on the surgical technique applied to an individual case. Prevention of damage by the metal depends upon the specific material used. It is remarkable that these two factors were appreciated in NICOLE's time, since metallurgical and chemical technology had not produced the same quality of corrosion resistant metals as are available today. NICOLE realized that a foreign body implanted according to biomechanical criteria could produce perfect fracture healing in spite of corrosion and toxic effects of the metal, or, as he expressed it "the body is capable of overcoming the ill-effects of metal to a certain extent". NICOLE wrote that "the development of high quality in metal implants is an important field for research but the central problem of internal fixation is to guarantee a balance between physiological and mechanical requirements until the fracture has consolidated".

In the development of the AOI instrument set it was our primary aim to produce standardized materials for internal fixation that fulfilled as closely as possible the biomechanical requirements. The general and specific problem of corrosion and toxic effects will be discussed here in brief to make the surgeon familiar with the behaviour and effects of metal implants.

The term "metal damage", as used here, includes a number of basically biological and metallurgical processes besides structural failure in the implant's supporting role. Two distinct types of processes occur in the metal itself:

a) Processes concerned with the material itself as it is immersed in a corrosive medium (intrinsic factor).

b) Processes that are concerned with factors external to the metal (extrinsic factors), such as biochemical processes (fluctuating pH, varying oxygen concentration) and unfavourable mechanical stress with reference to NICOLE's work, these factors are listed in Table 1. This table is confined to the more inert modern metals, so the most severe types of chemical damage to the metal and toxic effects on the host are eliminated at the outset. Other phenomena such as the formation of localized currents caused by variations in oxygen tension, corrosion due to contact and fretting or to pitting may occur instead. In stainless steel, pitting is a special characteristic, the existence of which the surgeon must take into account. Clinically significant effects can be seen from this table: On the one hand are the toxic effects on the tissues of the host, and on the other the damage to the implant which may range from loss of strength to complete collapse.

Table 1. *The different types of corrosion on the implant and their sequelae*

Internal (intrinsic) causes of corrosion:

    Active metal

    Instability of the passive layer

    Localized currents: various metals, metal struc-
       ture altered through processing, metal trans-
       fer due to differences in alloys

    Faulty material (rolled in foreign matter, etc.)

External (extrinsic) causes of corrosion:

  I. *Conditions in the tissue:*
     Changes in pH
     Variations in oxygen concentration

 II. *Unfavourable mechanical stress*

Mechanical and biological sequelae:

   I. *Type of corrosion:*
     Crevice corrosion
     Contact corrosion
     Fretting corrosion
     Pitting (characteristic of stainless steel)
     Stress corrosion   }
     Fatigue corrosion } — (complete collapse)

  II. *Local effects of corrosion in the tissue*
     (Metallosis):
     Damage to soft tissues due to size of implant.
     Impregnation of the tissue with metal par-
     ticles
     Decreased tissue viability

 III. *Loosening*, weakening, or complete collaps
     of implant

1. Corrosion Resistance of Metals

The process by which a metal in the electrolyte solution of the body fluid tends to corrode is electrochemical in nature. This develops as the result of anodic and cathodic areas arising on the metal surface, and the flowing of electrical currents between these areas. At an anodic point some of the metal dissolves (corrosion). On a cathodic surface components of the electrolyte are deposited or loose their electrical charge. There are several explanations to account for the cathodic course of reaction. With metals in a highly acid environment, there is a release of hydrogen ions at the cathode into electrically neutral gas and this is known as the hydrogen corrosion type. In our case, however, where the environment is usually slightly alkaline the so-called redox process at the cathode plays the decisive role: the combination of oxygen with water to form hydroxyl ions is the best known reaction of this kind and gives rise to the term "oxygen corrosion type".

The nature of corrosion can be explained along the lines of the theory involving localized currents in the presence of cathodic (inert) and anodic (active) areas on the surface of the metal. We must imagine that the size of such a localized electrochemical cell can range from one of atomic dimension to one visible to the naked eye. In Figs. 26 and 27, diagrams show the most likely situations in which localized electrochemical cells can develop resulting from either internal (intrinsic) or external (extrinsic) types of corrosion. In addition it provides clues to the special phenomenon of pitting.

Metals show varying degrees of resistance to such processes and can be classified accordingly. Theoretical classifications are made according to galvanic currents. The engineer and surgeon, however, must classify metals according to their corrosive potential. This classification demonstrates the astonishing fact, furthermore, that nearly all metals are capable of being in two states as regards their susceptibility to corrosion, namely active and passive. The term metal passivity can be used to describe the condition in which the tendency to react to the corrosive environment has been inhibited, resulting in a chemically passive state of the metal.

To retain a passive state a thin protective layer is necessary and this is invisible to ordinary observation, being only about $1/_{200,000}$ mm. (approximately 30 atoms) thick. This forms an intact covering of the whole surface of the metal as FARADAY correctly surmised at the beginning of the 19th century. Chemically this layer probably consists of a real union of oxygen with the metal, and oxygen is necessary for it to occur. Under suitable conditions, as in nitric acid, the protecting layer forms in a small fraction of a second.

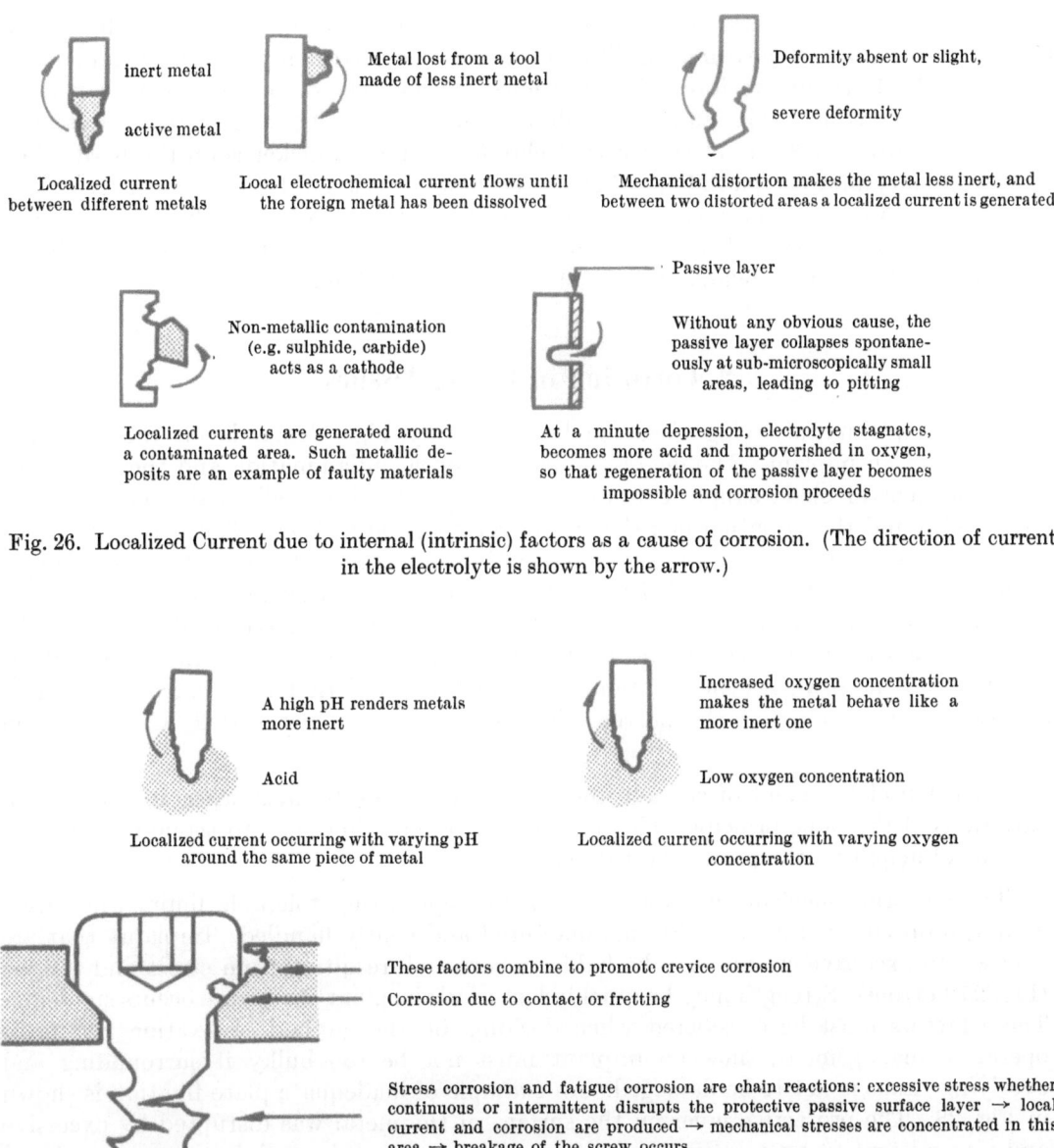

Localized current
between different metals

inert metal

active metal

Metal lost from a tool
made of less inert metal

Local electrochemical current flows until
the foreign metal has been dissolved

Deformity absent or slight,

severe deformity

Mechanical distortion makes the metal less inert, and
between two distorted areas a localized current is generated

Non-metallic contamination
(e.g. sulphide, carbide)
acts as a cathode

Localized currents are generated around
a contaminated area. Such metallic de-
posits are an example of faulty materials

Passive layer

Without any obvious cause, the
passive layer collapses spontaneously at sub-microscopically small
areas, leading to pitting

At a minute depression, electrolyte stagnates,
becomes more acid and impoverished in oxygen,
so that regeneration of the passive layer becomes
impossible and corrosion proceeds

Fig. 26. Localized Current due to internal (intrinsic) factors as a cause of corrosion. (The direction of current
in the electrolyte is shown by the arrow.)

A high pH renders metals
more inert

Acid

Localized current occurring with varying pH
around the same piece of metal

Increased oxygen concentration
makes the metal behave like a
more inert one

Low oxygen concentration

Localized current occurring with varying oxygen
concentration

These factors combine to promote crevice corrosion

Corrosion due to contact or fretting

Stress corrosion and fatigue corrosion are chain reactions: excessive stress whether
continuous or intermittent disrupts the protective passive surface layer → local
current and corrosion are produced → mechanical stresses are concentrated in this
area → breakage of the screw occurs

Active force

Fig. 27. Localized Current due to external (extrinsic) factors as a cause of corrosion

Surgical implants are manufactured from such metals as are capable of being made inert and all materials used for internal fixation in surgery are provided with this protective layer. As soon as the metal enters the living environment it is exposed to corrosive influences. At first these corrosive fluids attack the protective layer on the surface as though attempting to remove it as being a state contrary to nature. The metal seems to defend itself against this by the production of a very small continuous corrosion current which rebuilds the protective layer (a process called passivation). This may also occur when the surface layer is mechanically damaged, as may happen during the introduction of the implant. It is possible that even soft tissues may injure the protective layer.

The more such a process of passivation occurs, the more inert becomes the metal. CLARKE and HICKMAN measured in different metals the corrosion potential, meaning the anodic back electromotive force (ABE) in horse serum. There appeared to be a parallel between corrosive potential and compatibility with tissues. The older stainless steel of V2A type (AISI type 302 or 304) with 18% chromium and 8% nickel is on the border line of corrodibility and compatibility, whereas the newer steels of the type V4A (AISI 316 according to American specifications or British B.S.I. type EN58J) with a higher nickel content and the addition of molybdenum are so inert in practice that they meet almost all compatibility requirements. This is also true for Vitallium.

2. Corrosion in Living Tissues

The complexity of living tissue makes especially high demands on the corrosion resistance of an implant. The degree of postoperative inflammation and the quality of local and general blood supply can vary the oxygen level as well as the movement of electrolytes and the variation of pH values over a period of time. This means that the implant is exposed to a series of influences which may cause the formation of localized electrochemical cells (Fig. 27). With the less corrodible modern metals these local currents become less significant over large distances but can still have local effects in the small crevices between a screw and a plate where little movement of the electrolyte is possible and the oxygen concentration is so much reduced that local corrosion (crevice corrosion) can occur, and the surrounding tissues become permeated with corrosion products.

Corrosion at the point of contact and fretting corrosion between areas in contact are variations of the same principle. This type of corrosion is harmless to tissue with metals capable of acquiring the protective passive film.

The corrosion mechanisms described can be kept within tolerable limits when used with appropriate metals carefully manufactured and gently handled. Implants that are exposed to excessive strains may be liable to corrosion resulting from stress and fatigue (Fig. 27 bottom). Strength may be quickly lost until the point of rupture occurs suddenly. These factors must be considered when deciding on the method of fixation and post-operative management, since an implant must not be too bulky if surrounding and overlying tissue is not to be damaged. An example of inadequate plate fixation is shown in Fig. 28. The protective layer on the surface of the metal was disrupted by excessive and intermittent forces resulting in fatigue. Electrically active points were exposed and gradually deep fissures formed (Fig. 29). A sectional view of the implant (Fig. 30) shows the nature of the fissure.

3. Local Effects of Corrosion on the Tissues

The two most important local effects are the impregnation within or between cells of solid disintegration products of metal and the impairment of cell vitality. For the latter, soluble disintegration products are mainly responsible. NICOLE first, and other authors (FERGUSON et al.) showed spectroscopically that disintegration products invade adjacent tissues. To study this quantitatively, FERGUSON and his co-workers buried small metal cylinders of Vitallium and stainless steel in the muscle of rabbits and later removed them, together with pieces of tissue of equal size. The quantity of elements found in the tissue was then measured for stainless steel and Vitallium (see Table 2).

In the *Association for the Study of the Problems of Osteosynthesis*, HULLIGER was able to show in connective tissue cultures that soluble salts of toxic metals (cobalt and nickel) caused little if any disturbances of growth in very low concentrations. The dilutions tested

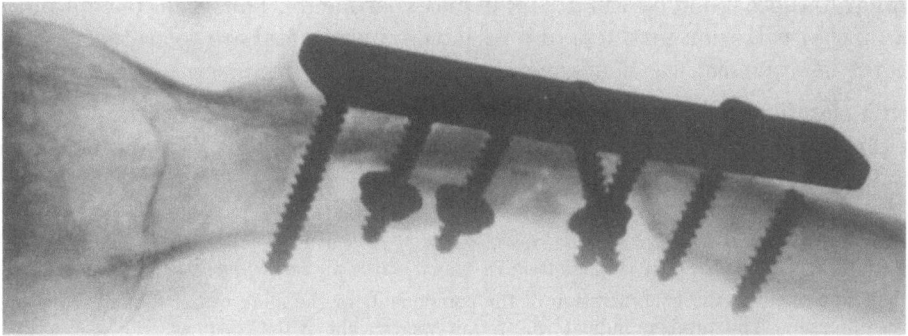

Fig. 28. Inadequate fixation. Too little purchase has been obtained on the distal fragment so that excessive strain is thrown on the end screw. Fatigue corrosion occurs, followed by breakage

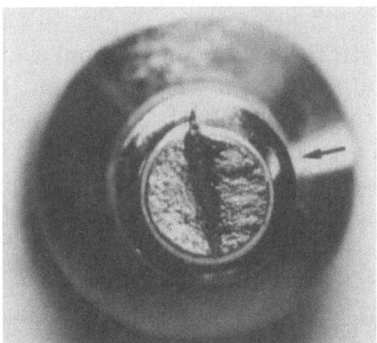

Fig. 29 a. Section through the break at the top thread of the screw. Disruption of continuity at the right (shown by the arrow) is due to fatigue corrosion, but that at the left is due to sudden strain of breakage

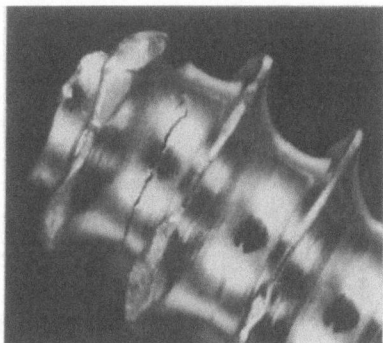

Fig. 29 b. Fissure caused by stress in the broken off part of the screw

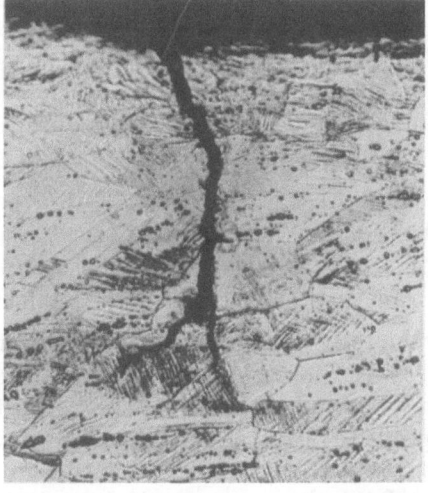

Fig. 30. Section of the screw made through the fissure shown in Fig. 29b. As this crack obviously developed during a very short period of time it has taken a trans-crystalline course rather than running along the granular edges as would be characteristic in a corrosion fissure which develops slowly

were similar to those found by FERGUSON in his experiments. Thus, the concept put forward by NICOLE that corrosion products of a relatively inert metal are tolerated without much damage to the organism was confirmed.

With a significant amount of corrosion, corrosion products of a certain degree can be seen in the tissues under the microscope or electron microscope. In animal experiments

Table 2. *Quantitative analysis of local tissue concentration of the various components of Vitallium and stainless steel, after implantation in muscle tissue for several months:*

In less than four months the concentration of the components of the alloy in the tissue becomes stabilized. The numbers indicate mega-units per weight of the tissue ashes

	Nickel	Chromium	Iron	Molybdenum	Cobalt	Total mega-units of the alloy
Vitallium	—	60	—	6	65	131
AISI 316	30	65	40	3	—	138

(sheep, rat, rabbit) corrosion could not be demonstrated in the metal from which AOI instruments are made, nor when single (screw) implants were removed from humans. Only where powerful extrinsic factors were operating, could effects on the local tissues be shown (Fig. 31). By contrast, pure nickel, which is an important component of stainless steel, is extraordinarily susceptible to corrosion even without extrinsic factors. It produced severe local effects in sheep (Fig. 32). Nickel plating of material used in internal fixation, therefore, should be finally abandoned.

4. Metals Used in Practice

The development of the materials used in internal fixation today has taken a long time. Alloys such as Vitallium which contain cobalt have a uniformly high resistance to corrosion, whereas some stainless austenitic steel alloys have only reached the required degrees of resistance and uniformity with the advance of modern technology.

It must be appreciated that the ideal metal for implants combining tissue compatibility and great mechanical strength does not exist. The search is for one that best combines the qualities of mechanical strength, tissue compatibility, workability and economy. The following factors must be considered: Maximal rigidity is most easily obtained with metals of great strength. The stainless steel of the AOI implants as used reaches a strength of 100 to 120 kilograms per square millimetre (roughly between 60 and 70 tons per square inch) and is stronger than cast Vitallium which reaches a maximum of 80 kilograms per square millimetre (48 tons per square inch).

The local effects of stainless steel of the A.I.S.I. 316 type appear to be tolerated by the body as well as those of Vitallium. The contact of the screw with the bone, as examined by WAGNER and FERGUSON's trace analysis in the tissue was no better with Vitallium, although Vitallium has a somewhat higher corrosion potential (ABE).

The many complex and precise processes involved in producing metal for internal fixation and designed to satisfy biomechanical criteria are only possible with stainless steel. Certain disadvantages of stainless steel, however, must not be ignored. Even the best stainless steel is susceptible to pitting in an electrolyte containing halogen and oxygen, so that after a few years it may produce some local tissue effects although the mechanical weakening is insignificant. Metal, therefore, should be removed after one to three years and it should not be used again. On the other hand, trouble may be caused by crevice, contact and fretting corrosion. By careful attention to the actual construction of the AOI

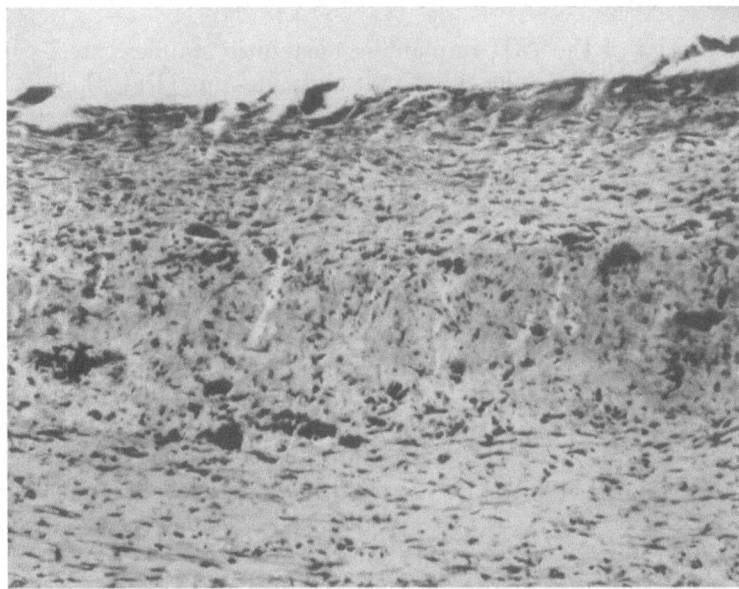

Fig. 31. Metallic products in the connective tissue surrounding crevice corrosion between screw and plate. The larger corrosion particles are found outside the cells and the smallest particles both intra- and extra-cellularly

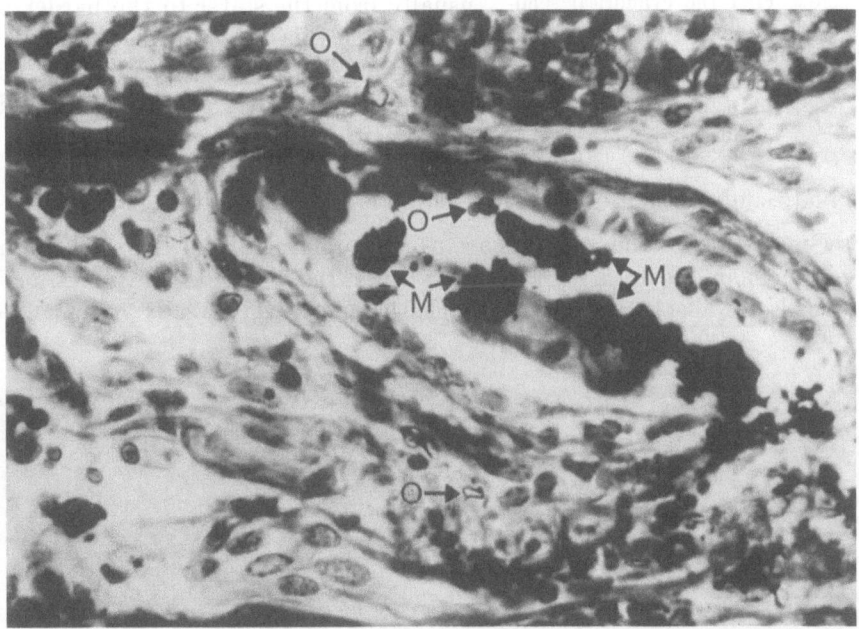

Fig. 32. Corrosion products produced by pure nickel. With this metal corrosion is very intense. Besides nickel oxide (O) there are also particles of pure nickel (M) seen here in a lymph vessel

instruments, these difficulties are largely overcome. In addition, by attention to details in technique the surgeon can make a positive contribution. For example, the precise centering of screws in the holes of the plate and tightly fitting them into the plate reduce the likelihood of corrosion occurring.

5. The Manufacture of the AOI Implants and Instruments

The basic material of the AOI implant is austenitic stainless steel type A.I.S.I. 316 with 17.5% chromium, 12% nickel, 2.5% molybdenum, less than 3% silicon and manganese combined, a maximum of 0.06% carbon, the remaining part being iron. The austenitic condition refers to a well defined crystalline structure of the metal atom. It is the non-magnetic state. This type of crystal structure only occurs at high temperatures in pure iron, but with the addition of nickel, austenite becomes a stable state at low temperatures. The completely austenitic metal provides a greater degree of resistance to corrosion.

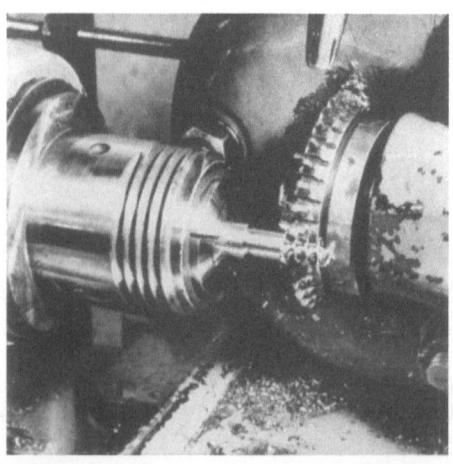

Fig. 33. Machining the deep threads of an AOI cancellous screw. First the cylindrical semi-finished screw is produced by turning from rods. In this picture, the machine-tool is cutting the thread into the semi-finished screw in one process, while it is being slowly turned and advanced

The instruments are made of the above chromium-nickel stainless steel, or, when greater strength and hardness are required, a stainless chromium steel is used. For tools like drills and screw drivers, where hard and long lasting edges are required, the decreased corrosion resistance is acceptable.

Some authors fear that transfer of small particles of metal from lower grade tools coming into contact with the implant might set up localized currents (Fig. 26). It is known, however, that the metal which becomes transferred by contact is usually from the softer to the harder metal and in our case this means from the implant to the tool, which is nearly twice as hard. Hard particles lost from the tool are uncommon and dissolve slowly with minor effects on the tissue. Examinations of the tissues adjacent to an intentionally scratched plate confirm that local tissue reaction is not enhanced by such surface damages.

The raw materials for the implants are usually obtained from the steel works as semi-finished products in the form of rods for screws, flat sections for plates, or tubes for medullary nails for instance. At this stage the steel has already been cold-drawn or

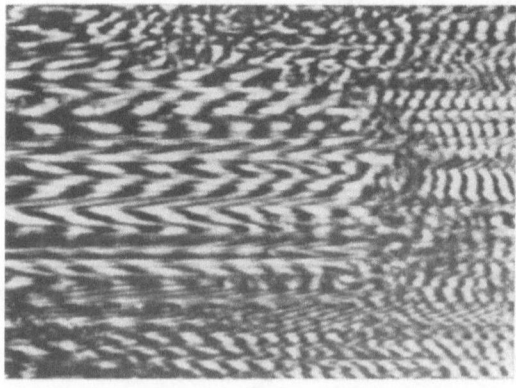
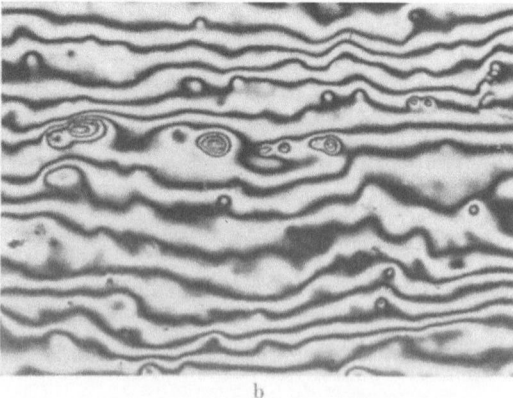

a   b

Fig. 34a and b. The surface of an AOI plate in a highly magnified optical interference photograph (interferences are caused by superimposing light waves from points at different height; the differences in the niveau between interferences is $^1/_{6000}$ mm.): a Milled surface, showing roughness by very irregular interferences; b Highly polished surface, following mechanical and electrolytic polishing, with regular and strong interference lines. Ring-shaped interferences point to tiny depressions caused by the removal of a few impurities rolled according to processes which will give it a uniform mechanical strength of 100 to 120 kilograms per square millimetre (or 60 to 70 tons per square inch).

All metals used for implants are examined under laboratory conditions for mechanical properties. Gross defects such as rolled-in foreign metal, oxides, etc., are excluded by careful inspection and testing. Tests for magnetism are also conducted. Chemical analysis, a corrosion test in boiling sulphuric acid/copper sulphate solution, together with inspection of cross sections by metallography give the necessary information on composition, heat treatment and purity, that is required to differentiate between varying degrees of corrosion resistance. From these tests we know typical defects which have to be avoided, especially in the form of too much rolled-in foreign matter (Fig. 26) and incorrect temperatures used in annealing before cold-working.

The final form is given by machining on automatic lathes, drills, or milling machines (Fig. 33). Machining, unlike pressing and rolling, does not appreciably alter the homogeneous structure of the metal so that one internal (intrinsic) corrosion factor is eliminated (Fig. 26). These mechanical processes are carried out on the AOI devices with the highest precision possible and we have found standardization valuable in that most items are interchangeable. Standardization of screw threads, for instance, has made it possible to change one screw for another in any hole cut by the appropriate tap.

Special care is given to finishing and electrolytic polishing. Turning, milling or boring produce irregularities on the surface of the metal. This deformed surface, which is thin but undesirable, is removed by polishing in order to expose the homogeneous basic metal. A smooth surface presents the smallest possible area exposed to the corrosive environment (Fig. 34). In this highly polished and corrosion resistant state the implant reaches the surgeon.

II. Instruments

1. General Considerations

There is, as yet, no universal procedure for the operative fixation of any two bone fragments. When a closed fracture is explored, the type of internal fixation indicated depends on the viability of the bone. Instruments on the market today are not uniform in design or material and it is never certain whether two dissimilar metals in contact may not generate electrical currents and destroy the bone and surrounding tissues. To avoid these defects, a screw has been developed for internal fixation that ensures maximal strength, is easily inserted and removed, has an even thread and is not self tapping (Figs. 38, 40, 42).

Over a period of several years, the need for a uniform set of instruments has become clear. Alloys suitable for implants will either be those containing cobalt, i.e. Vitallium, or stainless steel of the V4A type (A.I.S.I. 316).

Besides the chemical composition of the raw material, the metal processing itself plays an important part in securing tissue compatibility and resistance to corrosion (see page 34). Some screws on the market, for instance, have only been polished mechanically and not electrolytically and it is not surprising that, as shown by BRUSSATIS and WAGNER, the surface of this steel may corrode, producing inflammatory reaction in which the dead bone is replaced by fibrous tissue.

The A.I.S.I. 316 stainless steel and B.S.I. EN58 J steels are officially recognized in the U.S.A. and England as suitable for making metal implants for the human body. We now use only the A.I.S.I. 316 type of steel with a low carbon content of less than 0.08%. To obtain the smoothest possible surface all metal implants are polished mechanically,

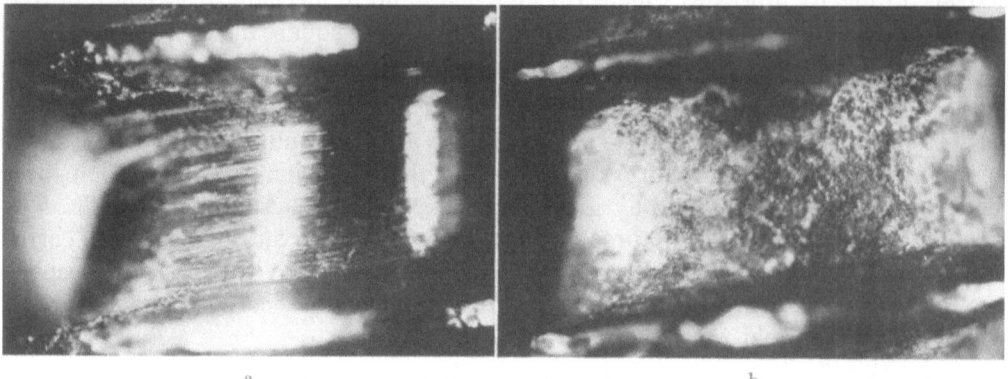

Fig. 35a and b. Threads of an ordinary wood screw (after Brussatis). a Before implantation. b 2 months after implantation in an animal experiment

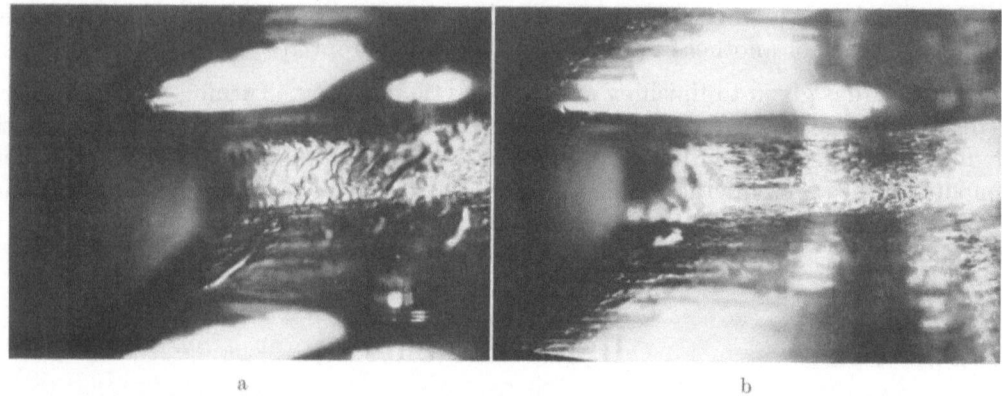

Fig. 36a and b. Appearance of an AOI screw which was only polished mechanically. a Before implantation. b 2 months after being implanted in an animal — there is clear corrosion on the surface

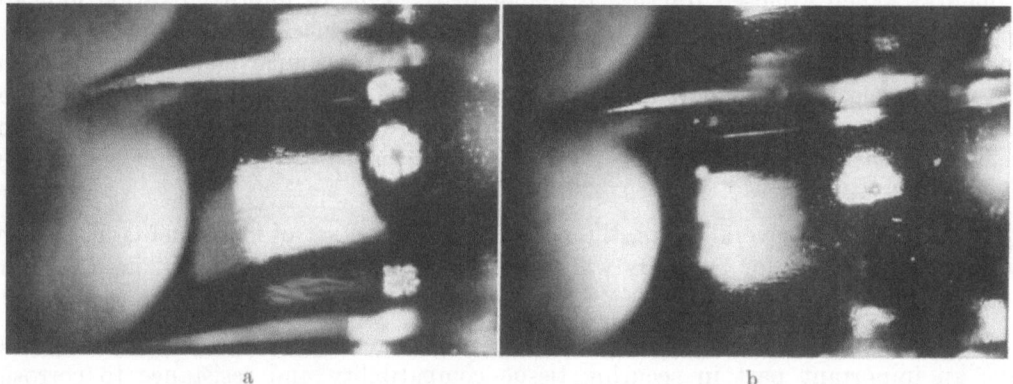

Fig. 37a and b. An AOI screw polished electrolytically (after Brussatis): a Before implantation. b 2 months after implantation, in an animal experiment — surface appearing smooth and unchanged

chemically and electrolytically. We hoped to use the same steel for the instruments, but it became clear that it was not strong enough to meet our requirements; consequently stainless steel that can be hardened and tempered is used for this purpose. The stainless steels used for the tools are not of exactly the same composition as that used for the implants. Hence if a drill or tap breaks, the lost particle must be found and removed from the wound.

In collaboration with ROBERT MATHYS we have, over the years, developed a standard instrument set for the surgical treatment of fractures. The *Straumann Institute for Metallurgical Research* tested the steels that were used and the *Laboratory for Experimental Surgery* in Davos, with the help of WAGNER and BRUSSATIS, examined their tissue compatibility.

The twenty members of the *Association for the Study of the Problems of Osteosynthesis* (AO) carried out systematic clinical trials and the *AO Documentation Centre* in Davos analysed all surgical cases treated with the newly developed instruments (see page 23). Our purpose was to produce an instrument set that would be suitable for any type of fracture and consistently good results can only be expected if the whole range of instruments is available.

In the following sections the various techniques and the corresponding instruments developed by AO, including wiring, screwing, plating and nailing are described.

2. Cerclage Wiring, Pinning with KIRSCHNER Wires and Traction Absorbing Wiring

These techniques only require a small amount of implanted material, but properly used, a firm fixation of bony fragments, especially in cancellous areas, can be obtained.

We do not put much reliance on cerclage wiring of shaft fractures, as has been advocated by FEHR in 1945, USADEL in 1950, KNÜPPER in 1952, SCHUMPELICK in 1953, BRUCK and MOSER in 1954, HOLDER in 1954, HÄUPTLI in 1956, HAUCK in 1956. Cerclage wiring can hold the bone fragments in position but cannot fix them rigidly, so that a long period in plaster is needed as well. The advantages of early movement are thereby lost and the time to union may be greatly prolonged (TRILLAT, 1955; EGGELING, 1959).

Cerclage wiring for fractures of the shaft combines the disadvantages of conservative treatment and of open reduction. It can therefore only be recommended as a supplementary measure, as in hemi-cerclage wiring of a lateral malleolus, or when cerclage is combined with a medullary nail. When it is used, there should be a minimal subperiosteal exposure of the fragments and the wire should be removed from the tibia before the eighth week. Several wires used in combination with a medullary nail often have catastrophic results as much of the periosteum becomes destroyed, thus jeopardizing the viability of the bone.

Cerclage wiring can be recommended, however, as a temporary fixation when screwing fractures of the shaft of the tibia (see page 85). It must be performed with great care for the soft tissues and with the least possible exposure.

Traction absorbing wiring has proved useful in achieving compression in fractures near joints, especially in the olecranon and the patella (see page 155). This technique has been described in detail by WEBER, 1962, with special reference to the olecranon.

Pinning with KIRSCHNER wires has not proved effective in shaft fractures, though BÖHLER's school as well as FRANK and KISSLER (1960) still recommend it for medullary wiring of transverse fractures in the tibia. DE WULF (1955) and LABES (1957) reported good results using KIRSCHNER wires for fractures of the clavicle and subluxations of the acromio-clavicular joint. In Monteggia fractures in children we have used KIRSCHNER wires successfully, as have DESENFANS (1950), PENROSE (1951) and WONDRAK (1958). In other cases, as was emphasised by BÖHLER, jr. (1955), WILLENEGGER (1961) and BLOCH (1963), KIRSCHNER wires are chiefly indicated for fractures in and around joints which in effect limit their use to cancellous bone.

TERLEP in 1958 and PENROSE in 1951 strongly recommend pinning for fractures of the head of the radius and FORGON (1954), HILL (1954), SIMON (1957) and WITT (1955), also recommend it for supracondylar fractures in children. For irreducible fractures of the lower end of the radius FORGON, BERENYI (1955) and SCHAEFER (1957) passed wires first through the ulna. The use of KIRSCHNER wires has also been discussed by VON SAAL (1953) for finger fractures, CORDREY (1960) for fractures of the capitate, MAXFIELD (1955) for the os Calcis, WHISTON (1953) for the pelvis, SPIGELMANN (1953), DUPUIS (1955) and BÖHLER jr. (1955) for fractures of the tibial plateau.

The advantages of pinning that have been suggested are the simplicity of the technique, the need for no special instruments, the small amount of metal used, the little damage to soft tissues and the minimal danger of infection. BÖHLER (1957) and LANGE (1953) have often advocated percutaneous pinning.

In children, internal fixation if used at all should be reserved almost exclusively for fractures around joints. In adults, cross wiring of small fragments may be useful, as in malleolar fractures. Traction absorbing wiring combined with KIRSCHNER wires used as pins, gives a very rigid internal fixation that resists traction forces. The pins here act as stabilizers. To obtain good results with this method, the KIRSCHNER wires used as pins need to be inserted parallel to the line of action of the traction forces in order to give the greatest purchase to the encircling wire. This is chiefly indicated in fractures of the olecranon, avulsion of the great trochanter, fractures of the patella and comminuted malleolar fractures.

In fractures of the tibial condyles, crossed wires can only be accepted if they can secure a really good articular surface. Here we usually prefer screws, sometimes combined with the use of plates and cancellous grafts, so that early mobilization can be carried out safely. KIRSCHNER wires can be used for temporary fixation during operations on trochanteric fractures, subcapital fractures of the femoral neck and fractures of the femoral condyles.

3. Screw Fixation

In 1907 LAMBOTTE coined the phrase: "For most fractures of the shaft of the tibia the screw is the basic element of rigid fixation." In 1949 DANIS gave a detailed description of tibial fixation using his special lag screw. WHITE (1953), DELAUNOY (1955), TRILLAT (1955), MERLE D'AUBIGNÉ (1959), ALLGÖWER (1961), MÜLLER (1961), and others were convinced of this method.

Well placed screws can hold a reduced fracture rigidly without wide exposure and with little foreign material. Early joint movement is then possible after operation, though weight bearing is not allowed until the fracture is consolidated. Unlike a medullary nail, a screw is not a weight bearing device, but it allows early and comfortable mobilization to be carried out with safety.

It is clear from the literature that besides the fractures mentioned above, most authors recommend the use of screws in fractures in and around joints[1]. The main function of the screw is to compress bone fragments together (DANIS 1947, DECOULX and RAZEMON 1956). The threads of most types of AOI screws therefore do not extend as far as the

---

[1] Among these are fractures in the region of the neck of the femur and pertrochanteric fractures (PUTTI, 1942; REIMERS, 1951; MANCINI, 1952; SCHULTZ, 1953; DICKSON, 1953; WASSNER, 1955; BLÜMEL, 1955; SCHUMPELIK, 1955; BERENTEY, 1956; CLAWSON, 1957; MARWEGE, 1957; WADE, 1959); malleolar fractures (HACHEZ-LEBLANC, 1950; FÜRMAIER, 1951; SIGEL, 1951; DESENFANS and EVRARD, 1952; TROJAN, 1953; FACKERT, 1954; BUCK-GRAMCKO, 1955; RIESS, 1955; MAYER, 1956; FREDENHAGEN, 1957; BRAUNSTEIN, 1959; WADE, 1959; BRAUN, 1960); and fractures of the upper end of the tibia (PALMER, 1951; KNOBLAUCH, 1953; SLEE, 1955; WASSNER, 1955). Some authors recommend the use of the screw in acromioclavicular dislocation (DOHN, 1956; BOSWORTH, KUCHENREUTER, 1956; PETROKOV, 1959), whereas BAUMANN (1960) uses it chiefly in the elbow.

head. The exception is the cortex screw which requires a wider hole in the proximal cortex if its threads are to grip the distal cortex and exert compression.

For cortical use we abandoned the screw which originally had a thread in its distal part only. This screw, similar to BAUMANN's, was difficult to remove from a shaft fracture, as it then had to cut its own thread from behind in the proximal cortex. When the cortex was too thick or too hard, the screw would break before it could be extracted. For plate fixation, however, we need a fully threaded screw in order to obtain a grip on both cortices. Since enlarging the hole in the proximal cortex will allow the screw to exert compression it was unnessary to produce a different type of screw.

The main difference between the screws commonly available and the AOI screws is that the latter are not self-tapping. Before screws are inserted, threads must therefore be tapped in the holes following the technique described by DANIS in 1949.

As cancellous and cortex screws require threads of different width we have had to develop two types of screws. We have also needed smaller versions for bones like the fibula, the scaphoid and the phalanges.

Cortex and cancellous screws have a round head with a hexagonal socket, while scaphoid screws have a Philips head. The hexagonal hole in the screw head allows it to fit onto the screwdriver without any special holding device. The three types of screws are the *cortex*, *cancellous*, and *scaphoid* screws.

The cortex screw (Fig. 38) has a saw-like profile to its threads which are separated by rounded spaces so that there can be only minimal tension between each pair of threads. The shank of the screw measures 3 mm. in diameter, the over-all width of the threads is 4.5 mm. and the distance between threads is 1.8 mm. Where the thread is exerting its main compression force it is nearly perpendicular to the axis of the screw (87°).

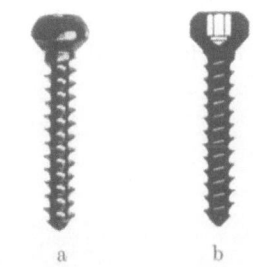

Fig. 38a and b. Cortex screw.
a Side view. b Longitudinal section

The point of the screw is obtuse. The head of the screw meets the shaft in a conical manner matching the countersunk hole in the plate. The hexagonal socket has a diameter of 3.5 mm. (Fig. 39).

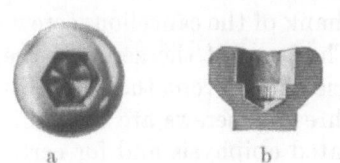

Fig. 39a and b. Screw head.
a From above.   b Vertical section

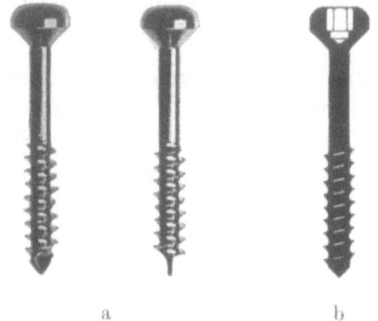

Fig. 40 a and b. Malleolar screw.
a Side view from 2 angles
b Longitudinal section

As we often need smaller screws than the cancellous ones for the fixation of smaller fragments in cancellous bone, we have developed an adaptation of the cortex screw, known as the *malleolar screw* (Fig. 40). These are only partly threaded but like LAMBOTTE's screw are self-tapping. The heat produced by self-tapping in cancellous bone is not significant.

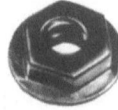

Fig. 41. Nut for use with a cortex screw

Should the cortex be so thin or so porotic that when a cortical screw is tightened up it gives way, a nut (Fig. 41) has been designed with an internal thread to match that of the screw. It is tightened with a wrench and together with the screw it then has the effect of a nut and bolt.

The threads on the *cancellous screw* (Fig. 42) are designed on the lag screw principle and are wider and further apart, being set on the screw in its distal 16 or 32 mm. The shank of the cancellous screw measures 3.5 mm. The threaded part is 6.5 mm. in diameter. The head of the screw is the same as that of the cortex screw. Small washers may be used to prevent the head of the screw from sinking into soft cancellous bone. The short threaded screws are used chiefly for fractures of the femoral neck in adolescents, in separated epiphysis and for certain fractures of the tibial plateau. In most fractures around joints we prefer the longer threads. To exert compression the threads are engaged only in the distal fragment.

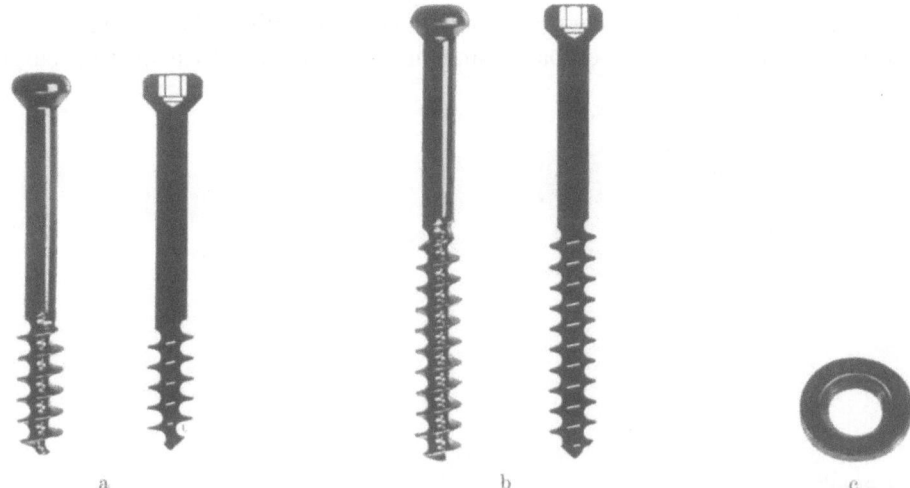

Fig. 42a—c. Cancellous screw: a Standard screw in side view and section. b The long screw in side view and section. c Washer

The *scaphoid screw (navicular)* (Fig. 43) needed a head small enough to avoid distortion of tissue when the screw is used in an oblique position. It is therefore only 6 mm. wide. The small size of the head ruled out a hexagonal socket and so the cross-slot of the Philips type was chosen with the special screwdriver it needed. The threads of the screw are of the same pattern as those of the cortex screw, but its diameter is only 3.5 mm. over all with a shank diameter of 2.0 mm.

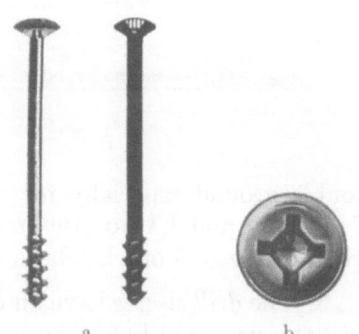

Fig. 43a and b. Scaphoid (Navicular) screw: a Side view and section. b The screw head seen from above

Additional tools were developed to allow routine screwing of long spiral and oblique fractures of the tibia:

1. The *screw driver* has a hexagonal point of 3.5 mm. that fits accurately into the recessed head of the screws (Fig. 44). It obtains a tight enough fit to allow easy extraction

of the screw without slipping. Patients who may have the screws removed by a different surgeon are provided before discharge with a smaller simplified hexagonal wrench with the same cross-section to avoid embarrassing moments for an unsuspecting surgeon.

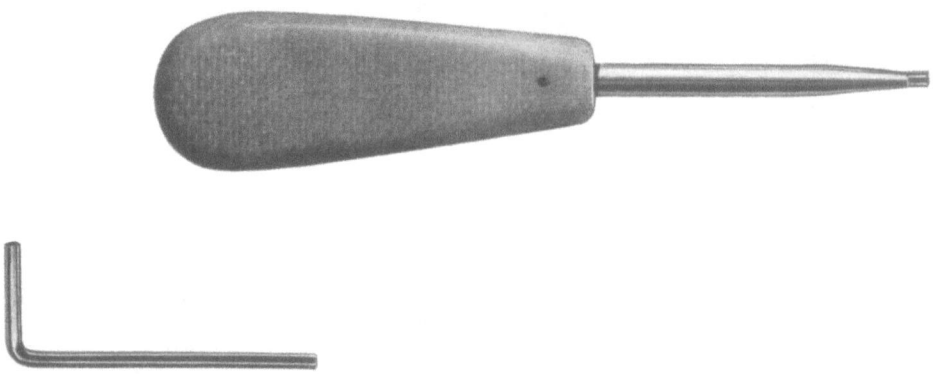

2. The *2 standard drills* have a diameter of 3.2 and 4.5 mm. respectively. A variant of each of these is fitted with an arresting device so that it cannot suddenly plunge in too deeply beyond the second cortex. This device stops further movement of the drill when it comes to lie up against the end of the drill sleeve. The tips of the drills have been

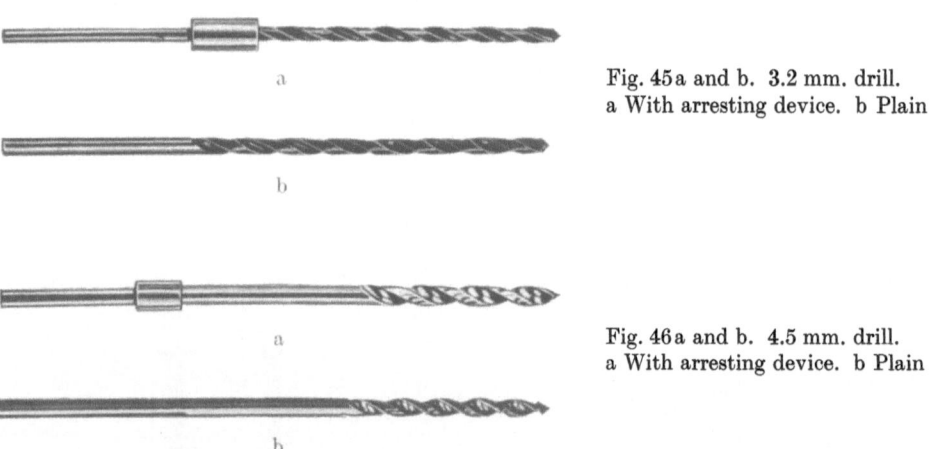

Fig. 45a and b. 3.2 mm. drill.
a With arresting device. b Plain

Fig. 46a and b. 4.5 mm. drill.
a With arresting device. b Plain

double ground especially for use in bone, according to the specifications of BECHTOL, FERGUSON and LAING (1959), so that they neither tear the cortex nor become too hot when the second one has been perforated.

3. The *drill sleeves* have an outer diameter of 4.5 mm with a bore of 3.2 mm. Inserted into the proximal hole they ensure that the drilling of the hole in the distal cortex will be in true alignment. When drilling diagonally they protect the drill against breakage. The tip of the 3.2 mm. diameter drill with the arresting device (Fig. 47) protrudes 13 mm. from the 48 mm. sleeve and for only 8 mm. from the 53 mm. sleeve. The short or long sleeve is selected depending on the thickness of the cortex and the direction of the drill hole.

4. The *drill guide* (Fig. 48) was developed to prevent a drill hole being sunk too close to a poorly visualized posterior fracture line. The tip of this guide is firmly hooked into the bone at least 5 mm. from a fracture line. Most screws are inserted from the medial or lateral borders of the tibia so that their points of entrance or exit lie on one of these

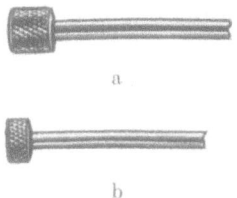

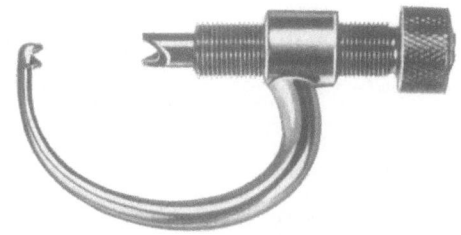

Fig. 47 a and b. Sleeves for use with drills.
a Long: 53 mm.   b Short: 48 mm.

Fig. 48. Drill guide for 4.5 mm. drill with
arresting device

borders or less often on the posterior border of the tibia; the points of the drill guide usually stradlde one of the bone edges. Before drilling through the first cortex the drill guide is tightened up so as to compress the fragments together.

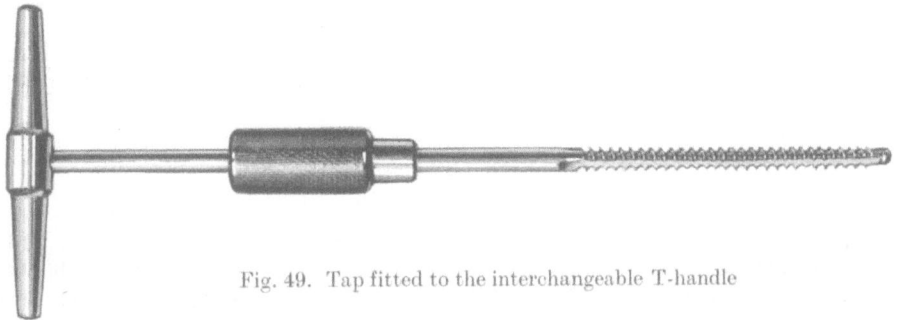

Fig. 49. Tap fitted to the interchangeable T-handle

5. The *tap* is a precision instrument that must be held carefully between thumb and index finger tip and not by the whole hand. When the sharp instrument can no longer be turned easily, it should be reversed a quarter turn to let impacted chips of

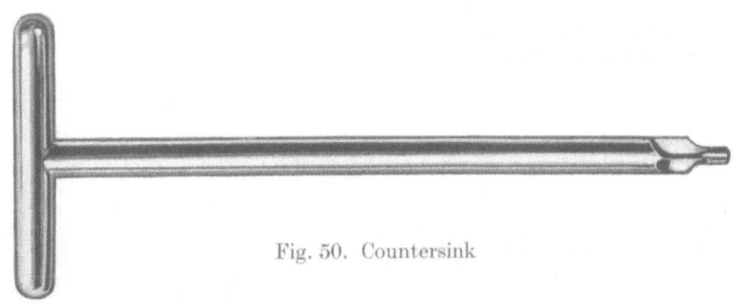

Fig. 50. Countersink

bone fall into the groove of the tap. This instrument should always be kept in its protective sheath to avoid damage to the cutting edges. It may be re-ground two or three times without loss in thickness (Fig. 49). A universal T-handle is available for these taps so that only the cutting part needs to be changed.

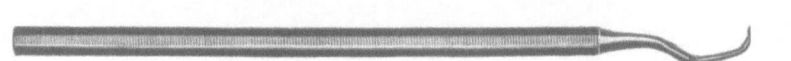

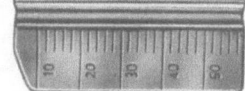

Fig. 51. Small sharp hook

Fig. 52. Measuring scale for screws

6. The *countersink* is designed to drill a conical depression to receive the screw head. This countersunk hole should not be deeper than 2 mm. and must never perforate the whole cortex.

7. The small *sharp hook* is used very often for the reduction of small fragments or to assess the accuracy of a reduction or to remove small splinters. It can also be used to clear ingrown soft tissue from the hexagonal socket head before removal of the screw.

8. The *measuring scale* serves to measure the length of the screw including its head. The length is read at the tip of the screw.

Technique of Screw Fixation

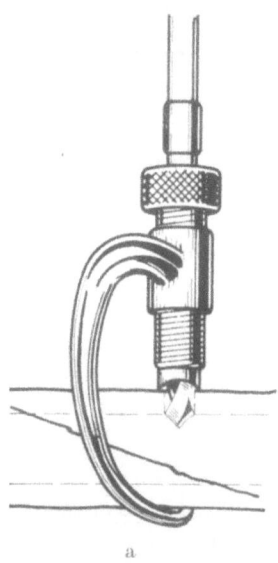

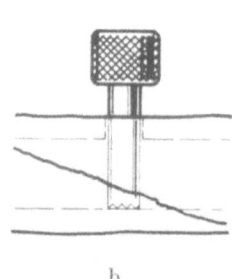

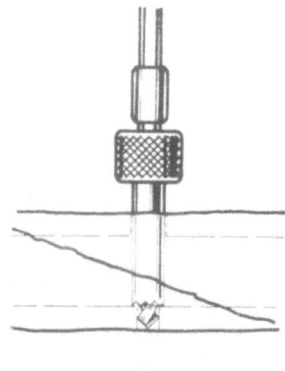

a

The drill guide is placed so that its tip is at least 5 mm. from the fracture line and is then tightened up. The proximal cortex is drilled with a 4.5 mm. drill fitted with an arresting device.

b

The long drill sleeve is used for a transverse hole and the shorter one for oblique drilling.

c

The far cortex is drilled with a 3.2 mm. bit fitted with an arresting device.

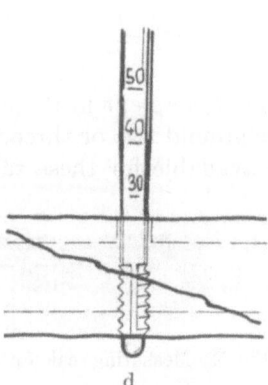

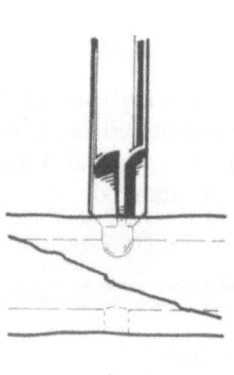

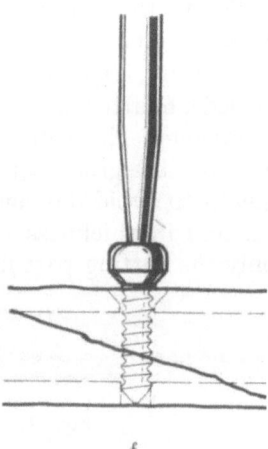

d

The hole in the far cortex is now tapped and the length of the screw estimated.

e

A hole for the screw head is countersunk in the near cortex using the countersink tool.

f

The AOI cortex screw is inserted with a screw driver. The screw is first tightened slightly. Only after all the screws have been inserted, they are tightened up in series.

Fig. 53 a—f.

Rationale of Screw Placement

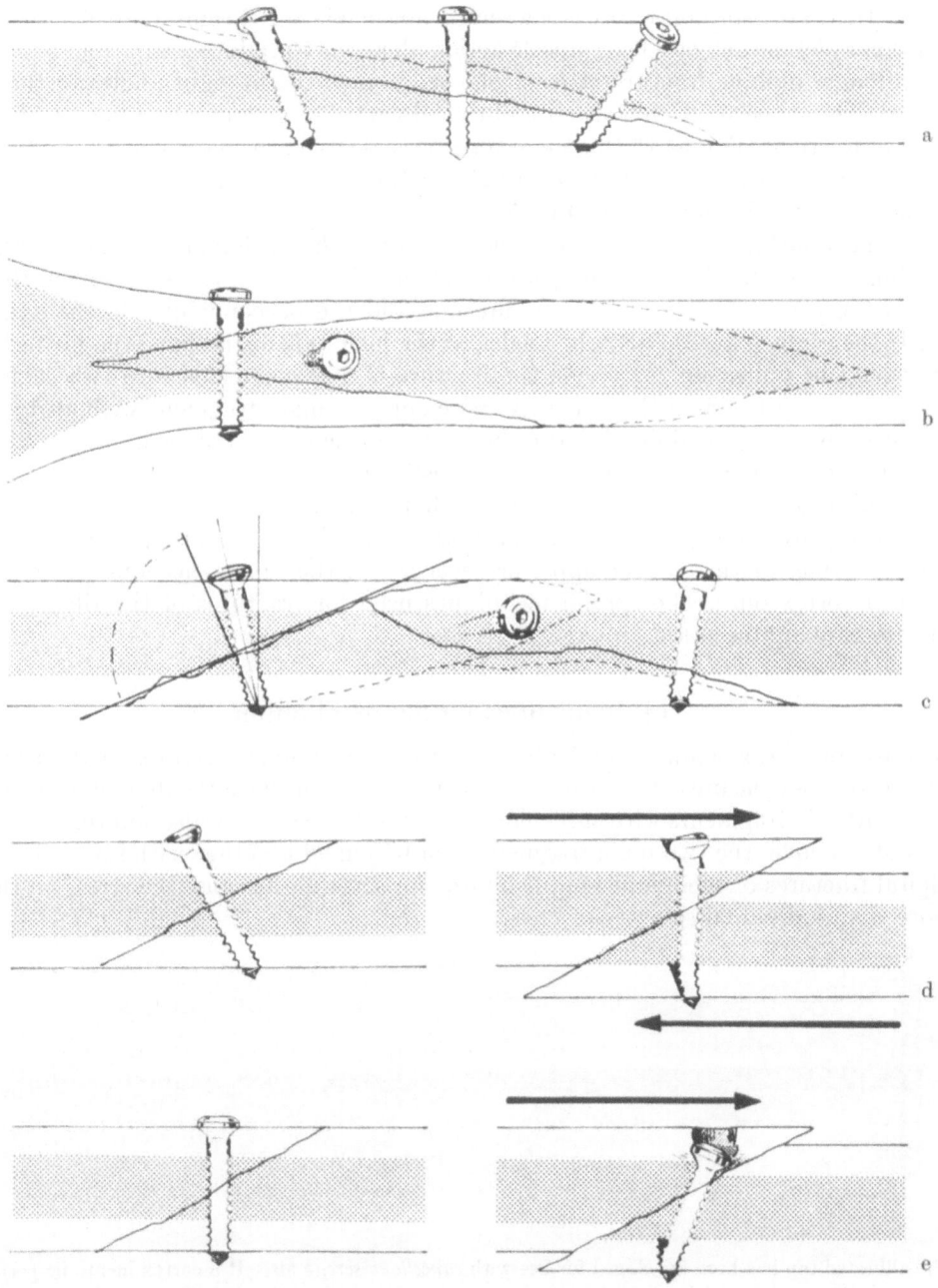

Fig. 54a—e. a Simple spiral or long oblique fracture in which one screw is placed at a right angle to the shaft. b The narrow end of a triangular fragment can be gripped under compression when a screw is inserted through the main fragment only. c Simple butterfly fragment: one screw transfixes both main fragments, the other screws are inserted to bisect the angle between lines drawn at right angles to the axis of the shaft and to the fracture line itself. d A screw inserted at a right angle to the fracture line will not prevent overriding of the fragments when pressure in the long axis is applied. e When the screw is inserted at a right angle to the axis of the shaft of the bone, overriding of the fragments only occurs if the head of the screw penetrates the whole cortex or if the threads tapped in the bone are disrupted

a) Technique of Screw Fixation

The method by which some of the instruments are used is shown in diagram form in Figs. 53 and 54. Perfect reduction is required together with minimal exposure of the fracture, but the correct placing of the screws is also of primary importance in obtaining rigid fixation. In a short spiral fracture screws must not be placed at right angles to the fracture line nor parallel to each other, or muscle action alone may produce a slip (Fig. 54, a and c).

In a longer oblique fracture at least one screw must lie at right angles to the axis of the shaft. The safest fixation is usually obtained with 3 or 4 screws in different planes and different directions (Fig. 54a). It is sometimes possible to fix the narrow apex of a triangular fragment by placing the screw transversely in the main fragment only, the apex being then held by lateral compression (Fig. 54b).

In fixing a butterfly fragment one screw should transfix both main fragments (Fig. 54c). According to DANIS the remaining screws should be placed so as to bisect the angle between the perpendicular to the fracture line and the perpendicular to the axis of the bone. If the screw is placed at right angles to the long axis of the bone the butterfly fragment would be pulled up. As a rule the fracture is first converted into two components only by temporarily fixing the butterfly fragment to a main fragment without tightening this first screw. The remaining fracture line is then accurately reduced.

If the two main fragments cannot be transfixed with a screw a plate will usually be needed unless both fracture lines are longer than twice the diameter of the shaft. Where there is a longitudinal split in the distal fragment of the tibia, this split is screwed first.

For screwing fractures of the upper or lower end of the tibia cancellous screws are used instead of cortex ones. The special techniques used for fractures of the tibia as well as their aftercare are discussed on page 77 et. seq.

b) Indications for Screw Fixation

The use of cortex screws is indicated in spiral and oblique fractures of the tibia when the fracture line measures at least 6 cm., that is more than twice the diameter of the shaft. Simple butterfly fragments with sufficiently long fracture lines are also suitable for screwing if, as stated above, the two main fragments can be joined together with screws (Fig. 54c).

Spiral fractures of the femur are unsuitable for screwing because the stress on the bone is more than individual screws can resist.

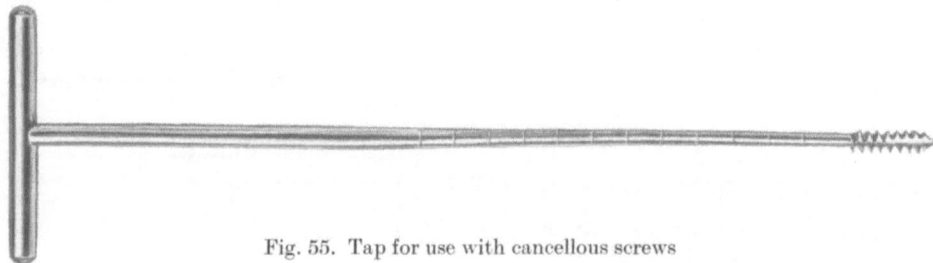

Fig. 55. Tap for use with cancellous screws

A calibrated tap has been developed for use with *cancellous screws* also. If a cortex has to be perforated a 3.75 mm. drill must be used for introducing the cancellous screw but in all other cases the 3.2 mm. drill is adequate. The main indication for using cancellous screws is in fractures near or within a joint when the cortex is thinner than 3.5 mm. Cancellous screws may also be used in the two holes at each end of the AOI compression plate.

For the *scaphoid screw* a drill of 2 mm. diameter, a sleeve to fit it, a Philips-type screw driver and a tap have been developed.

A special *drill sleeve* is fitted with two additional holes into which guiding KIRSCHNER wires can be inserted. This is particularly useful in screwing a pseudarthrosis of the scaphoid, for example, in order to prevent the drill from slipping off the small distal fragment or from getting caught in the soft tissue.

When using the screw driver with an arresting device, the screw is first gripped with the holder and then the screw driver is fitted into the crossed slots of the screw head.

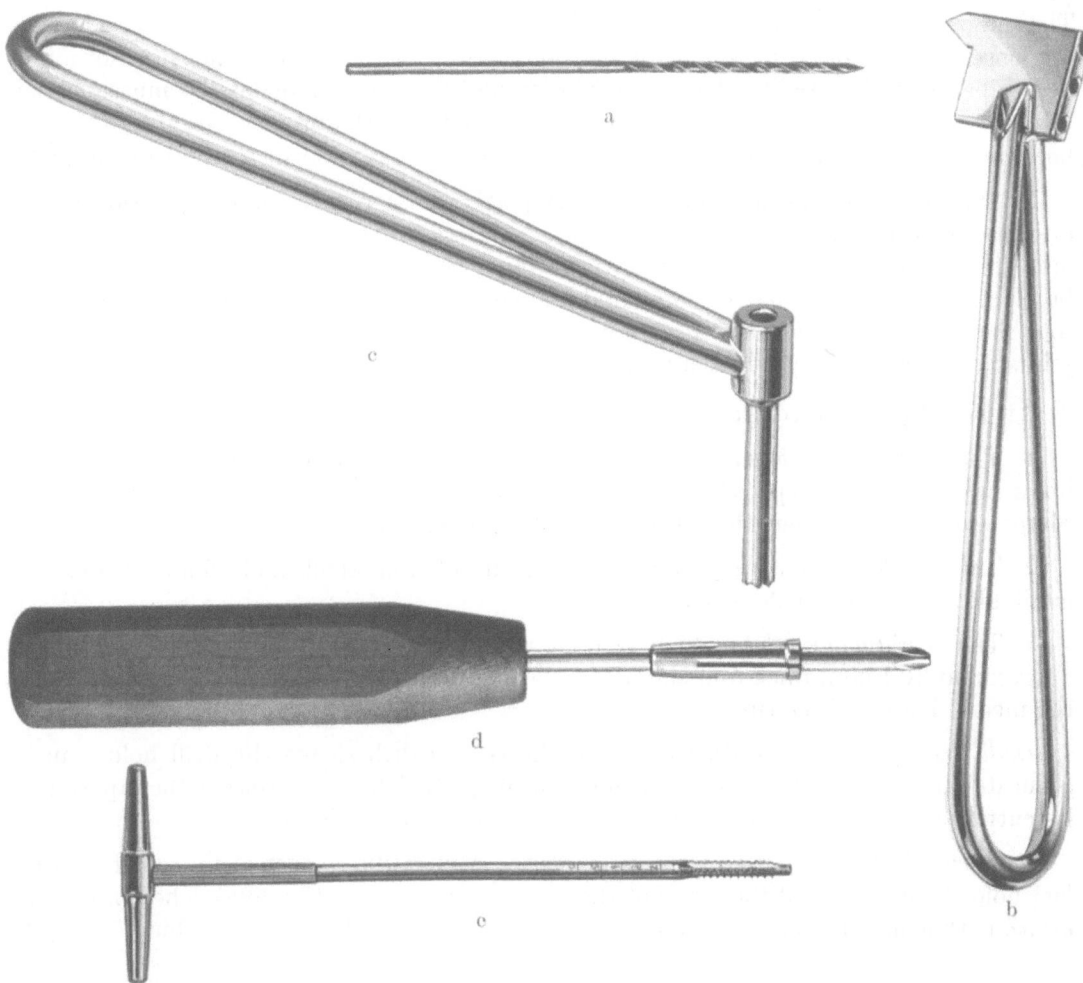

Fig. 56 a—e. Instruments for use with the scaphoid (navicular) screw: a 2 mm. drill. b drill sleeve. c sleeve for the scaphoid tap. d special self-holding screwdriver. e tap, calibrated

The main indications for the scaphoid screw are pseudarthroses of the scaphoid, oblique fractures of the lateral malleolus, fractures of phalanges, of metatarsals and arthrodesis of the interphalangeal joint of pollex or hallux.

4. Compression Fixation with Plates

The **AOI compression plate** can exert considerable pressure to the bone ends at the fracture line thus providing much more rigid fixation. One plate is sufficient in the arm, but in the femur two plates should be applied if possible. In oblique fractures of the tibia, even with more than two fragments, one plate with some additional screws at right angles to it may give adequate rigidity.

DANIS's plate with its built-in compression, DESENFANS's sliding plate, EGGER's slotted plate and BICKEL's plate with oval holes are well known. All of these plates have the disadvantage that the amount of pressure cannot be controlled. Additional fittings, such as tightening screws, slides, etc., increase the possibility of corrosion and make the plates weaker. In DANIS's compression plate especially there is increased danger of corrosion. The screw fixing the compression device often breaks, resulting in the other screws becoming loose. EGGER's plate gives inadequate rigidity from the beginning, since it is not intended to be screwed on tightly. The approximation of the bony fragments by muscle action has proved to be wishful thinking. The long slot soon fills with fibrous tissue and the screws become impacted so that their position can no longer be altered in relation to the plate.

In 1958 we therefore developed the AOI plate with a removable compression device intended to be used during the operation only. All straight AOI plates have a small hole in the long axis of the plate at each extremity into which the hook of the compression device can be placed (Fig. 57a and b). All angulated and condylar plates are provided with this hole too. The two end holes of any plate may be used for cancellous screws in fractures near joints and in other cases where a cortex screw fails to bite.

3 types of plates have proved useful (Fig. 57):

1. The *narrow plate* is slightly cambered, 3.5 mm. thick and 11 mm. wide. The screw holes have a conical depression to match the shape of the screw heads. These narrow plates are available in lengths containing from 2 to 16 holes.

2. The *broader plate* is also slightly cambered, 4.5 mm. thick and 16 mm. wide. It is available with 5 to 20 holes each.

3. The *semi-tubular plate* which is used mainly for tibial and forearm fractures is approximately 1 mm. thick and slightly malleable. It is especially useful when placed on the medial border of the tibia.

Drill sleeve for plates. With the aid of the special drill sleeve the drill holes can be accurately placed in the middle of the holes in the plate. This also protects the tap, so that its cutting edges do not come into contact with the plate during use.

A special drill sleeve for the compression device ensures the correct distance between the last hole of the plate and the screw of the compression device (Fig. 58a). The *compression device* is thus held on one side by a screw and on the other by its hook which enters the

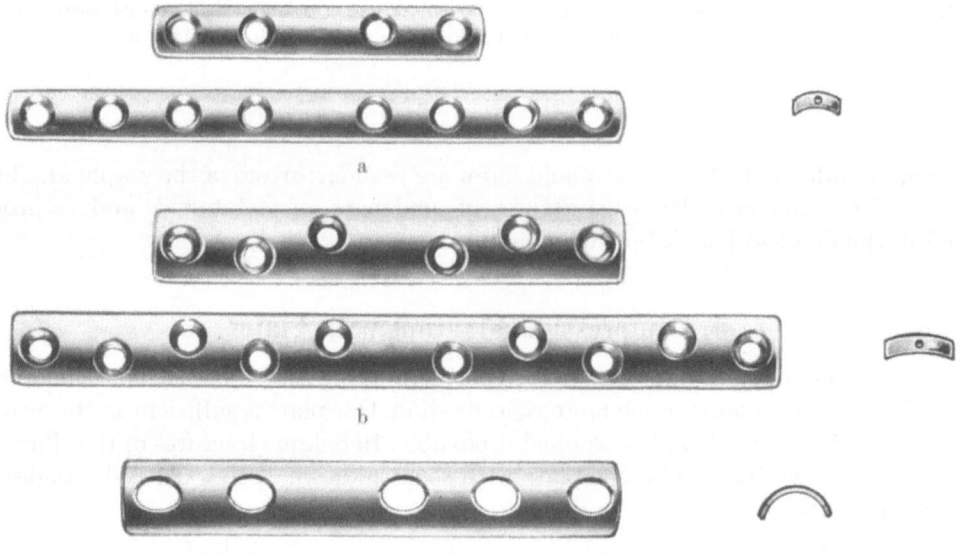

Fig. 57a—c. The AOI compression plates. a narrow plate. b broad plate. c semi-tubular plate with oval holes

last plate hole (Fig. 58b) to engage in this special small hole. The nut of the compression device is tightened with the socket wrench with universal joint, with a small pin wrench or with an open-end wrench. We have found that using the socket wrench the pressure at the fracture site can reach 30 to 40 kg., while using the open-end wrench as much as 60 kg. may be reached. To attempt more than this would either break the compression device or shear off the head of the screw.

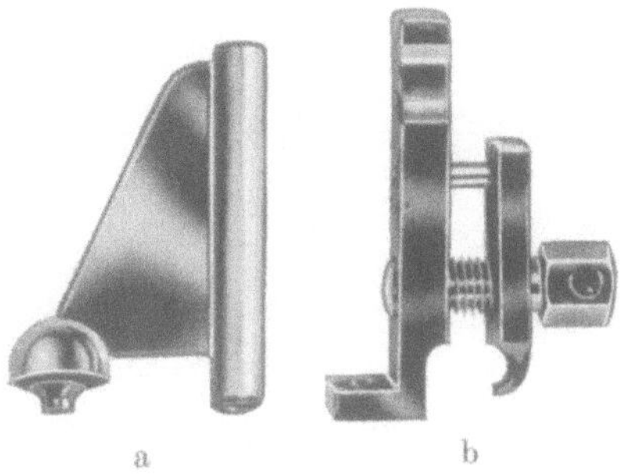

The screw holes must be tapped before the screws can be inserted. The tap itself needs to be longer when used for plate screws since both cortices must be cut. Even when the drill hole is exactly centered, occasional contact between tap and plate is unavoidable.

Fig. 58a and b.
a Drill sleeve for compression device.
b Compression device

The *technique of internal fixation with a compression plate* is shown in Fig. 60. When the plate has been fixed to the shorter fragment with the screw nearest to the fracture line driven home first, the hole for the compression device can be drilled at the right distance from the opposite end of the plate using the special sleeve. This hole must be tapped and the compression device can then be applied. The compressing nut is tightened bringing the fragments into apposition under great pressure. The screws are now inserted into the second fragment and the compression device can be removed.

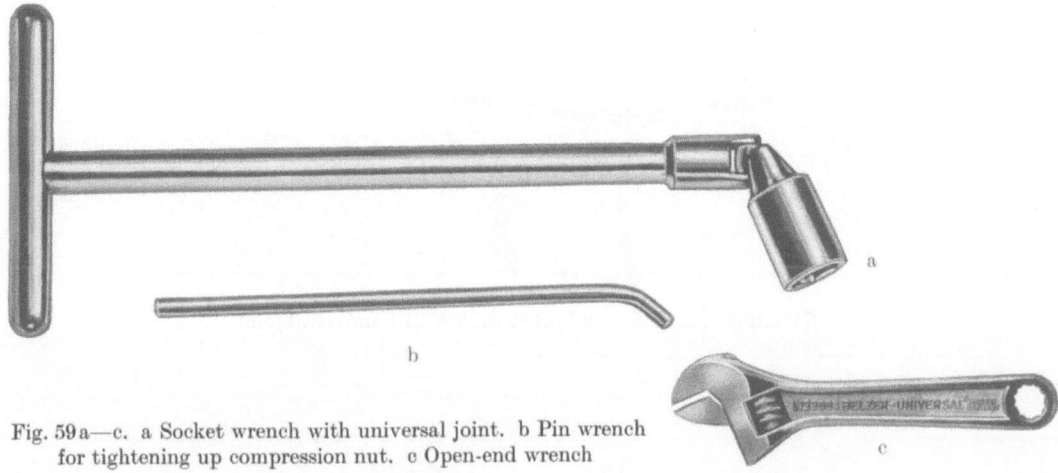

Fig. 59a—c. a Socket wrench with universal joint. b Pin wrench for tightening up compression nut. c Open-end wrench

Indications. In the *upper limb* one plate is usually sufficient. In the forearm it should be be long enough to allow 2 screws to be used on either side, at least 1 cm. from the fracture site. The narrow 4-hole plates are only used with transverse fractures of the radius and ulna, while for oblique or multiple fractures, plates with 5, 6, or more holes are used. The narrow plates give enough support in the forearm, but on the humerus, the broader 6 or 7-hole plates are necessary to stand up to the active mobilization regime.

In the *lower limb* a single plate is not sufficient to give rigid fixation in the absence of such external support as would make early mobilization impossible. For the femur, therefore, we use one broad and one narrow plate at a right angle to each other, thus rendering the leg capable of early weight bearing. Both plates must be tightened simul-

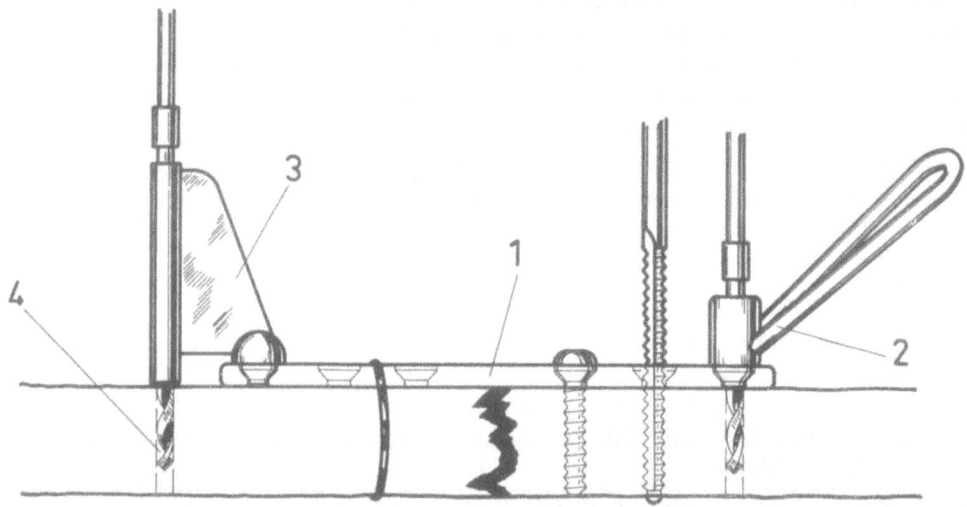

1 Narrow or broad compression plate. 2 Drill sleeve for plate. 3 Drill sleeve for compression device. 4 Drill, cutting the hole for the compression device

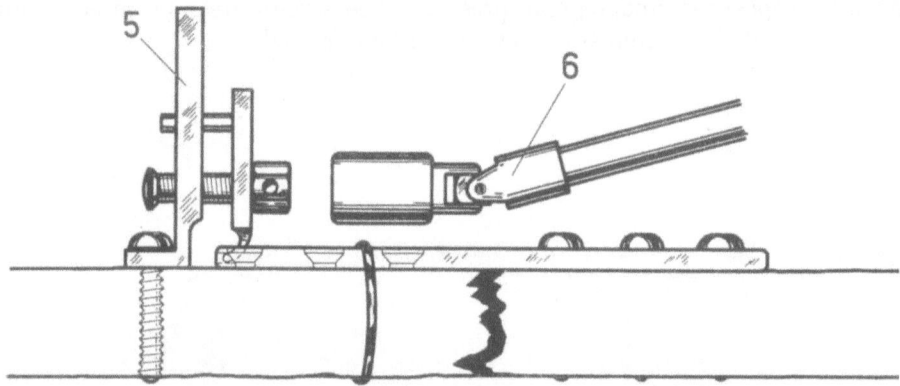

5 Compression device. 6 Socket wrench with universal joint

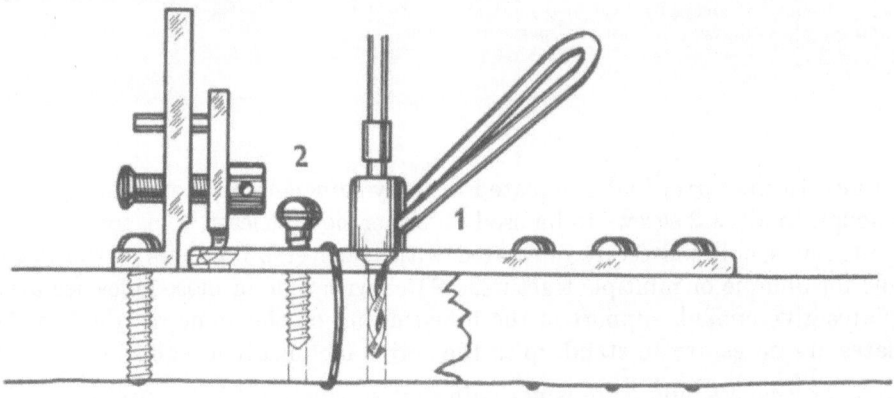

Fig. 60. Technique for internal fixation using the compression plate (see text)

After the fracture surfaces have been apposed the hole is drilled (1) and the screw is inserted (2).
After removing the compression device, the last screw is inserted

taneously; the instrument set therefore contains two compression devices. To attach these two plates, barely half of the circumference of the femur needs to be exposed. In an exceptional case, should only one plate be used on the femur, it is absolutely necessary that this plate be placed in line with the axis of the femoral neck, i.e. over the linea aspera or directly anterior to it. We thereby produce a traction absorbing effect at the site of maximal tension and can place the entire fracture area under compression.

In the tibia, except in transverse fractures, either narrow plates combined with additional screws, placed at right angles to the plate, or narrow plates in combination with semi-tubular plates, must be used if even slight degrees of movement at the fracture site are to be prevented.

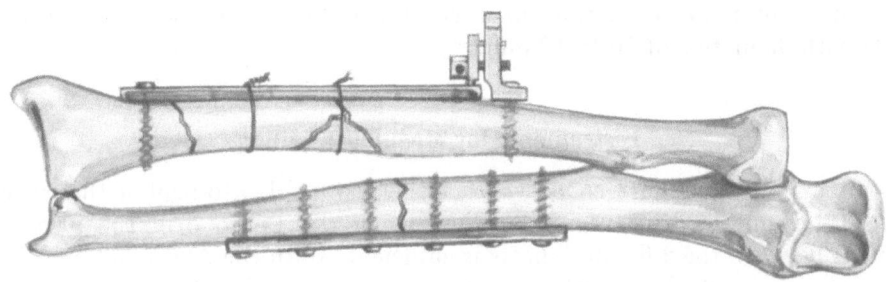

Fig. 61. Segmental fracture of the radius: while the reduction is held by cerclage wires, the fracture is fixed by applying a plate under compression

5. Medullary Nailing

The technique of medullary nailing in which the medullary space is reamed out was described in 1962 by KÜNTSCHER. The instrument set developed by POHL seems to be effective in most situations and we would refer the reader to KÜNTSCHER's book on "Medullary Nailing" which covers all eventualities.

We have abandoned KÜNTSCHER's medullary nail only because we observed certain corrosion symptoms at the point of entry of the nail and because the thick POHL nail was not sufficiently elastic. We felt that a medullary nail should be made in a slotted tubular form, should be flexible, elastic, light and completely corrosion-proof. The curvature of the proximal end of the nail developed by HERZOG has been retained (Fig. 62a).

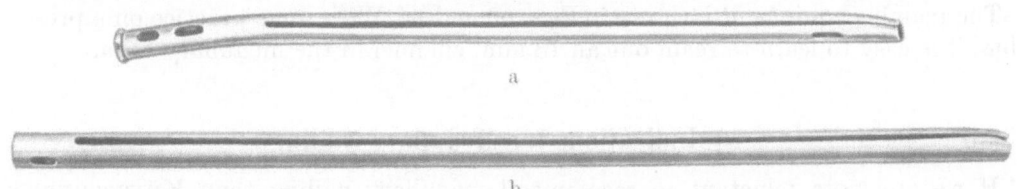

Fig. 62a and b. Medullary nails: a for the tibia; b for the femur

In cooperation with MATHYS and STRAUMANN the AOI nail was developed. It is thin, elastic and polished internally and externally by mechanical, electrical and chemical means. Its elasticity was chosen to be suitable for use in the tibia or the femur. The wall therefore is rather thin for large diameter nails which accounts for some difficulty in the design of an impacting or an extracting device. To make it stronger at the proximal end it has been left tubular here without a slot for a distance of 5 cm. A double hole is placed in the proximal end so that a screw can be passed through it to give improved rotational stability in proximal fractures. The distal end which is almost completely closed, has a slight curve and is provided with two small eyes 3 cm. above its tip. Antirotational wires can be passed through these holes if necessary (Fig. 62). This refinement, which was adopted from HERZOG, might be useful in some uncommon fractures of the distal end of the tibia. The nail ist roughly heart-shaped in section and the slot running up at its length is between 2 and 3 mm. wide.

For the tibia, nails with a diameter of 8 to 16 mm. are available. The AOI femoral nail is slightly curved to match the physiological forward curvature of the femur. The distal end is nearly closed to make it easier to direct. When the nail is correctly placed, the axis between the 2 proximal eyes runs in a ventral-to-dorsal direction. Femoral nails are available with diameters of 10 to 18 mm.

Instruments for Medullary Nailing

To ream out the medullary canal we use either POHLS' Lento-drill or the powerful low-speed AOI pneumatic drill (Fig. 64). When using the Lento drill the insertion of an attachment between the 2 flexible shafts is sufficient. With the AOI machine MATHYS has developed a right-angle drive with a quick-coupling device for the flexible shaft.

The flexible shafts have a diameter of 8 mm. for the tibia and 10 mm. for the femur. Drills of 12.0 mm. or more diameter can be attached to the shaft for use in the femur. These shafts are very elastic in all directions and will not break. An air jet is supplied to allow removal of bone fragments that may have been deposited among the coils of the spring.

The stainless steel drills for reaming are supplied in sizes from 9.5 to 19 mm., and have a small guiding device to keep them properly centered in the medullary canal. Only the 9 mm. drill cuts at the leading end and is firmly mounted on its shaft.

The whole length of the tibial medullary canal is reamed out down to the distal part where the cancellous bone is left intact to provide a firm hold for the nail. The 3 mm. guide rod has a rounded end which prevents its penetrating into the joint and allows a broken drill to be withdrawn. This guide rod would be too weak to drive the nail and so after reaming it is replaced by a 4 mm. rod. To facilitate this exchange a teflon tube is first passed over the original rod which can then be removed leaving the teflon in place. This prevents the dislocation of the fragments during the exchange and allows the medullary canal to be irrigated with saline. Bone chips and powder which might later become sequestra can thus be washed out.

The reaming equipment is shown in Figs. 63 and 64. With some practice on a preserved tibia, it is easy to learn to ream out an 18 mm. channel in the medullary canal.

a) Indications for Medullary Nailing

If we are more reluctant to recommend medullary nailing than KÜNTSCHER, it is because many fractures can be fixed in simpler and less dangerous ways.

Closed medullary nailing does not provide such accurate reduction as screwing, and with distal fractures angulation and rotation occur more easily. Furthermore, in spite of carefully reaming the medullary canal it is seldom possible to obtain such rigid fixation as can be achieved with a compression plate. With nail fixation, therefore, possible rotational deformities must be watched for postoperatively. It is seldom that full weight bearing after medullary nailing can be allowed, and though early mobilization is advocated premature walking is dangerous.

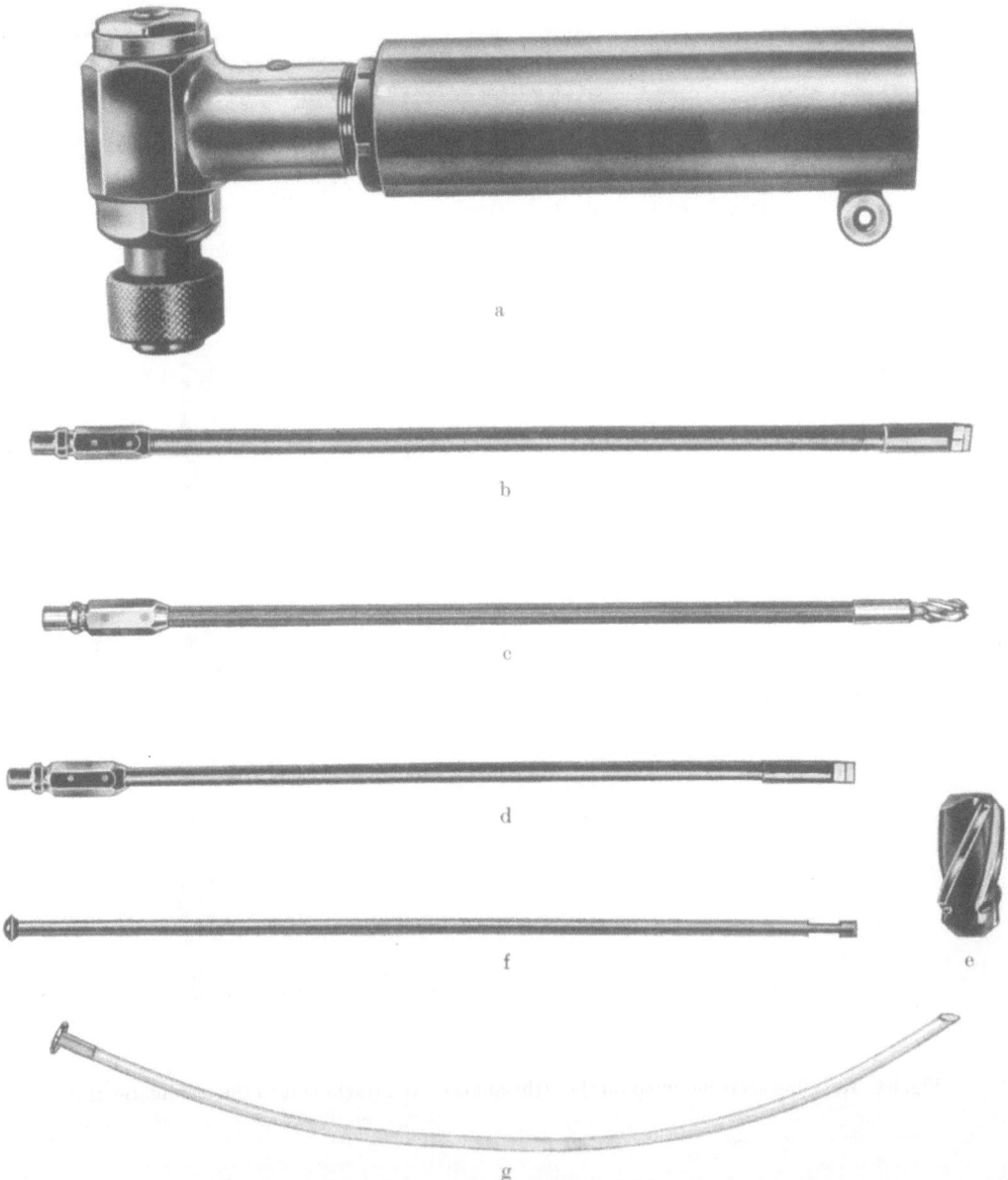

Fig. 63 a—g. Intramedullary reaming instrument set. a Right-angle drive with quick-coupling chuck. b Flexible shaft for use in the femur, diameter 10 mm., length 350 mm., for use with a cutting end of 12 mm. diameter or more. c Flexible shaft for use in the tibia, 8 mm. diameter, 310 mm. length, fitted with a 9 mm. front-cutting head. d Flexible shaft for the tibia, 8 mm. diameter, 310 mm. length for use with larger reamers up to 12.5 mm. diameter. e Stainless steel medullary reamer. f Guide rod of 3 mm. diameter, with ball point, total length 800 mm. g Teflon tube with metal knob

We believe that medullary nailing with a large diameter nail after reaming the canal is indicated for certain fractures of the femur and tibia, and in these it may reduce the time that must elapse before full weight bearing is allowed.

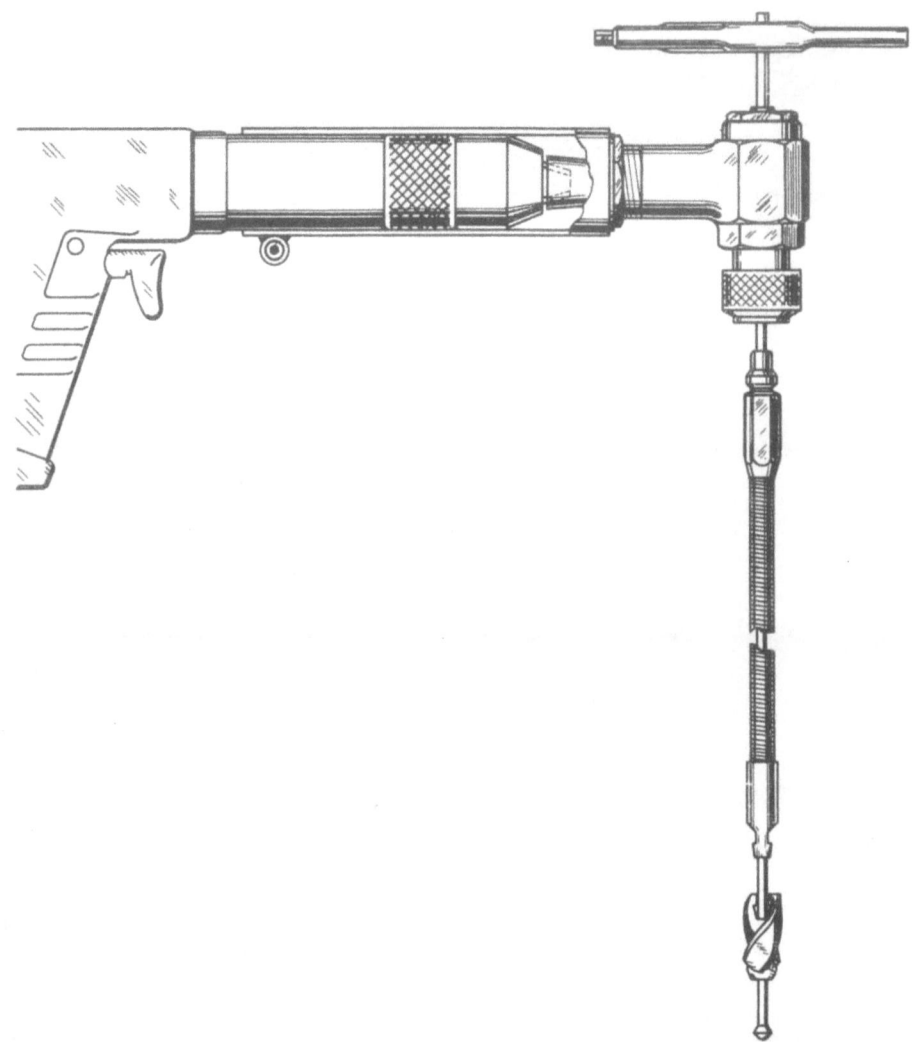

Fig. 64. Reaming shaft mounted on the right-angle drive attachment to the pneumatic drill

Absolute indications

a) For delayed union or pseudarthrosis in the *middle third of the femur or the tibia*, medullary nailing with a wide diameter nail after reaming out the canal is the treatment of choice, provided that rotation has not to be corrected. Slight angular deformities however can be corrected during nailing. In these conditions all other methods are inferior in promoting firm consolidation and quick restoration of function.

b) Short oblique fractures and short spiral fractures in the middle third of the femur can also be safely treated with medullary nails.

Relative indications

In the femur. Comminuted fractures in the middle third of the femur may be treated by medullary nailing combined with cerclage wire fixation of loose fragments. It may be very difficult to preserve the blood supply of the loose fragments.

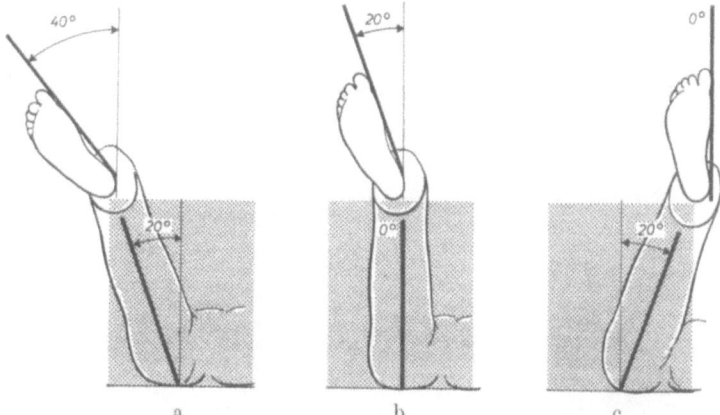

Fig. 65a—c. The physiological position of the foot is in 20⁰ of external rotation. a When the thigh is abducted trough 20⁰, the angle between the axis of the foot and the sagittal plane will be 40⁰. b With the thigh brought perpendicularly to the table the axis of the foot subtends at an angle of 20⁰ to the vertical. c Only when the thigh is adducted through 20⁰ will the foot have a perpendicular axis to the table

In the tibia. Closed fractures of transverse or short oblique type with or without a third fragment, may be treated by medullary nailing in the middle third, even when the skin is in poor condition. Care must be taken if longitudinal fissures are also present.

b) Technique of Medullary Nailing of the Tibia

Open medullary nailing, in which the fracture site is exposed allows accurate reduction and firm fixation. At the same time the fracture hematoma and the bone dust produced by drilling can be sucked out. In comminuted fractures the exposure may endanger the vitality of loose fragments and each case should be judged on its merits.

The small incision required for *blind medullary nailing* provides a smaller risk of infection but accurate reduction especially of any rotational deformity, is difficult particularly when using BÖHLER's extension device (Fig. 65).

Cerclage wiring combined with medullary nailing of the tibia is seldom indicated, but when such wires are used, they should be removed after six weeks.

The medullary cavity is reamed out in each case: for men, 12 mm. nails are usually required, and for women 11 mm. nails. Antirotational wires are only required for distal fractures. During operation, as a rule, the lower leg is placed with the knee flexed between 80 or 90 degrees to prevent the patella from being damaged by the operation or by the nail.

We find some fractures are more suitable for open nailing and others for closed nailing, as follows:

Open medullary nailing is undertaken on fresh fractures where there is undamaged skin, if it can be done within 8 hours, and in pseudarthroses which have rotational or angulation deformities. Careful preparation of the skin is essential. The patient lies on his back on an ordinary table. The fracture is exposed, reduced and fixed with bone holding forceps and cerclage wiring. After this the same procedure is employed as in closed nailing with the lower leg hanging down.

Closed medullary nailing is used in fractures where the skin is damaged or if the 8-hour period has elapsed. We carry this out with the help of a traction device, and the nailing is

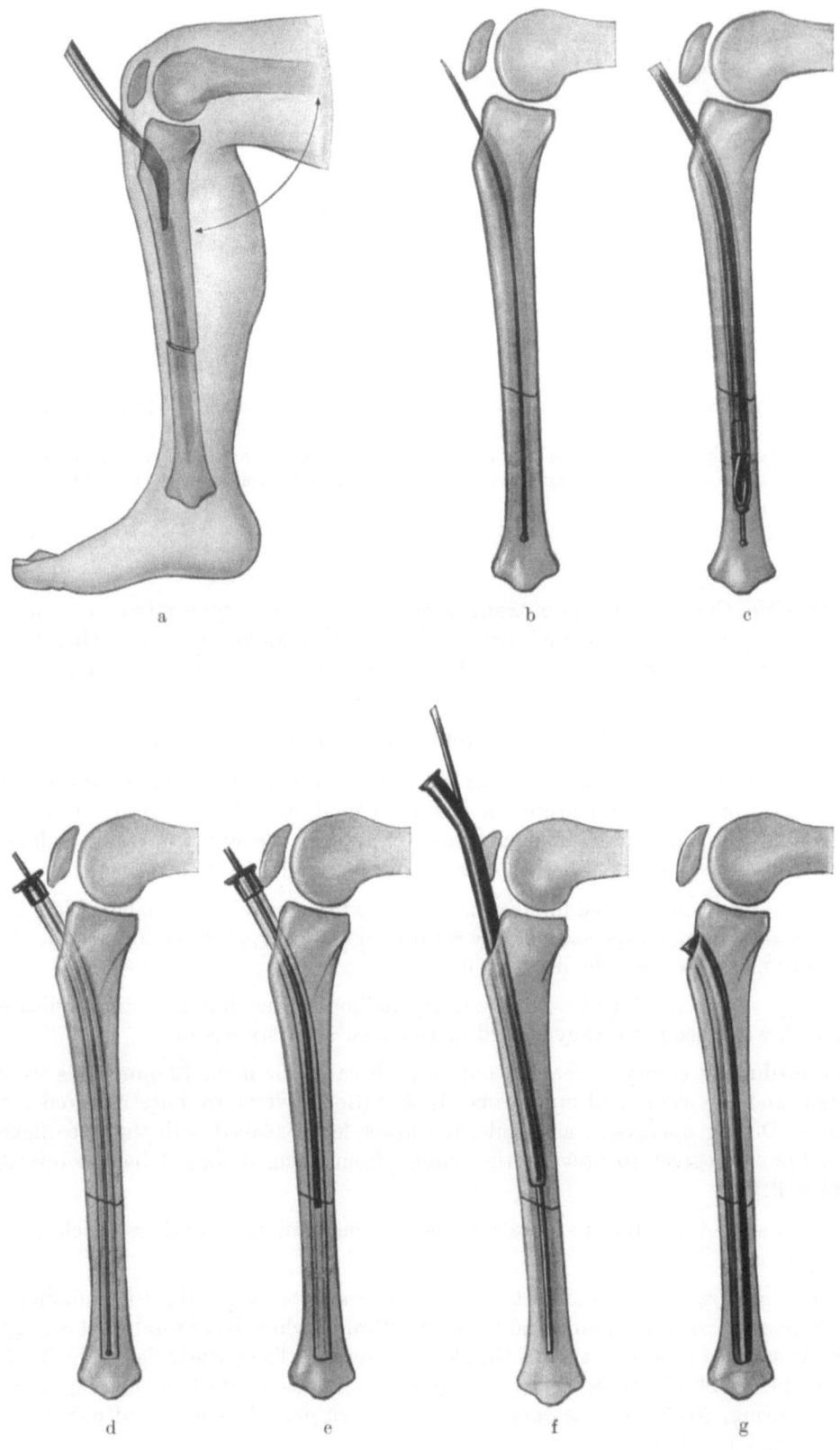

Fig. 66a—g. Technique for medullary nailing (see text)

controlled with the use of an image intensifier. In *pseudarthrosis* of the middle third of the tibia, medullary nailing is performed with the knee flexed at 90° and the lower leg hanging down. Before the 3 mm. guide rod is inserted the medullary canal is reamed out with a hand reamer to a width of 8 mm.

Preparation. To select the right length of the nail the distance from the knee joint to the ankle joint is measured on the uninjured leg and 30 mm. are deducted.

A pneumatic tourniquet is applied and the knee joint flexed to 90°.

General surgical technique for closed medullary nailing of the tibia. A transverse skin incision is made half-way between the tibial tubercle and the lower edge of the patella (Fig. 66a).

A self-retaining retractor is inserted and the patellar tendon incised longitudinally. With an awl a wide hole is made from the tibial tubercle down to the medullary canal. The angle of the awl is altered so that it is pointing parallel with the anterior border of the tibia as soon as the cortex has been perforated.

A 3 mm. guide rod is now introduced into the medullary canal and directed past the fracture towards the ankle joint. An x-ray is taken centered on the ankle joint to confirm that the guide rod is centrally placed and that the estimate of the nail length was correct (Fig. 66b). A metal shield to protect the skin is placed beneath the projecting guide rod.

The medullary canal is now reamed with the 9 mm. instrument and the canal widened half a millimeter at a time until the required diameter has been reached (Fig. 66c). It is important not to damage the soft tissues while using the reamer. An assistant holds the guide rod to prevent rotation.

The reamer is advanced over the guide rod; little force is needed. When it becomes difficult to ream further and the reamer cannot be withdrawn, the guide rod is gripped with a pair of strong pliers. Light blows with a hammer on the pliers will then free the guide rod with the impacted reamer without difficulty. When withdrawing the reamer it should be rotated as slowly as possible and the guide rod kept in place by the assistant. Reaming is complete when the drill can be felt to be cutting cortical bone in the distal fragment. The medullary canal is then irrigated with Ringer solution through a Teflon tube and all debris sucked out. Through the Teflon tube the 3 mm. guide rod is replaced by one of 4 mm.

Nail length is checked by measuring the amount of the guide rod that is projecting, and a nail of suitable diameter is used. As a rule the diameter of the nail for the tibia should be 0.5 mm. (for the femur 1.0 mm.), less than the diameter of the reamer used. The nail is driven in with a hammer over the 4 mm. guide rod, taking care not to damage the soft tissues. If it becomes locked the nail should be withdrawn and the medullary canal reamed out another half mm. It is driven in far enough to allow no more than 5 mm. to project from the tibial tubercle so that it does not interfere with movements of the knee and overlying soft parts (Fig. 66g).

The 4 mm. guide rod should be removed when the nail is still projecting 5 cm. above the tibia. After introducing the nail, a check x-ray may be carried out, again centered on the ankle joint.

To prevent rotation in fractures near the ankle joint, two antirotational wires are driven into the distal cortex through the eyes provided in the nail. The operation is completed by catgut suture of the periosteum, closure of the skin and a compression bandage. The leg is elevated on a foam rubber splint and the wound is usually drained when open reduction has been performed.

Postoperative Treatment. See "Fractures of the Tibia".

Nail Removal. Medullary nails are not removed from the tibia before 12 to 24 months unless they have been causing trouble. For removal of the nail, the leg is allowed to hang free over the end of the table and a 5 kg. weight is attached to the ankle. The upper end of the nail is exposed and the antirotational wires are withdrawn with pliers. Then a hook is inserted through the eye of the nail and the nail is withdrawn with the extraction device. It has proved useful to cut threads inside the upper end of the medullary nail to make its removal, when impacted, easier.

Technique of Re-Nailing. When a nail is found to be too loose so that union is delayed or even prevented, it should be removed and replaced by a thicker one. The canal may be reamed out again, using a 3 mm. guide rod, before introducing the larger diameter nail.

6. Angulated Plates

A modern set of instruments for internal fixation would be incomplete without angulated plates. Their use allows early walking after trochanteric fractures, and the supracondylar fractures of the femur, for instance, can only be firmly fixed with an angulated plate. Active mobilization can then begin a few days after operation.

Many different nails have been designed for fractures of the neck and trochanteric region of the femur. In view of the relatively poor results of nailing femoral neck fractures, REIMERS (1951) and SCHUMPELICK (1955) advocated screw fixation.

We continue to use screw fixation for fractures of the femoral neck only in young patients where the cancellous bone is fairly firm (see chapter on Fractures of the Femoral Neck). In other cases we have sought to develop an angulated plate the shape of which would be suitable for as wide a range of fractures as possible. The H-plate of LAING and O'DONNELL (1961) provides the greatest stability but it is so wide that it cannot always be used. Therefore we have selected a nail with a U-profile which gives almost as good rigidity as that of an H-nail.

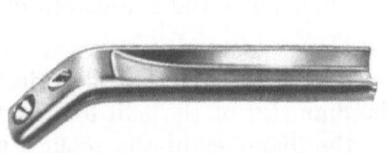 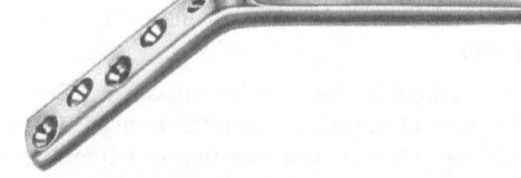

Fig. 67. AOI Blade-plate for the neck of the femur   Fig. 68. Blade-plate for use in trochanteric fractures

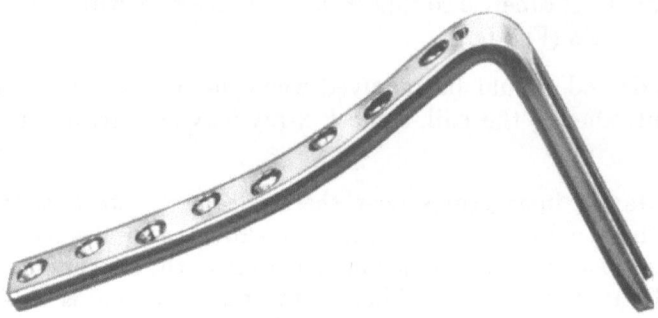

Fig. 69. Condylar plate

The plates are divided in three groups:

Blade-plates for the neck of the femur (Fig. 67).
Blade-plates for trochanteric fractures (Fig. 68).
Angulated plates for condylar fractures (Fig. 69).

a) Blade-plates for the femoral neck. When introduced at an angle of between 120° and 140° the short plate can easily be screwed to the shaft of the femur.

b) Blade-plates for pertrochanteric fractures have a plate of 8 cm. length containing 5 holes, but longer plates can be provided. We have adopted a standard angle of 130° for the following reasons:

The rigidity provided by the 2-piece McLAUGHLIN (1960) nail plate is poor. The corrosion at the site where the nut joins the plate to the nail is greater than in a one piece appliance.

Using the triple drill guide the blade can be inserted at 130° without difficulty, and has proved to be effective. When the angle is more acute, the point of the blade comes to lie too near the weight bearing part of the femoral head. When necrosis of the femoral head occurs later, the acetabulum becomes eroded by the blade and replacement of the dead head with a metal prosthesis would be impossible because of the danger of subluxation.

c) Condylar plates (Fig. 69) are angulated at 95° so that the blade can be inserted parallel to the axis of the knee joint. The angle between the knee joint and the shaft of the femur is 81° (Fig. 70). The shaft is somewhat conical, however, so that when the blade is introduced parallel to the joint line, the plate adapts itself to the cortex of the femur. This slightly alters its application for the tibial condyles where the angle between the tibial plateau and the shaft is normally 90°.

A sharp and specially shaped *chisel* (Fig. 71a) is used to cut a channel for the blade in cancellous bone. This tool is ground so that it cannot become stuck in the cortex either laterally or distally which is useful in nailing the femoral neck. The chisel is loosely held and driven gently forward with light taps of the hammer so that it slips past the calcar femoral to find its way into the center of the neck.

The *blade director* is fixed to the chisel to prevent tilting. The hinge screw is first loosened, then tightened up, after the director has been opened to the desired angle. A *slotted hammer* is used both to remove the chisel and to withdraw the angulated plates when used in conjunction with the driver-extractor. It also helps to control the direction in which the chisel is inserted by preventing any rotation. By applying its end over the trochanter

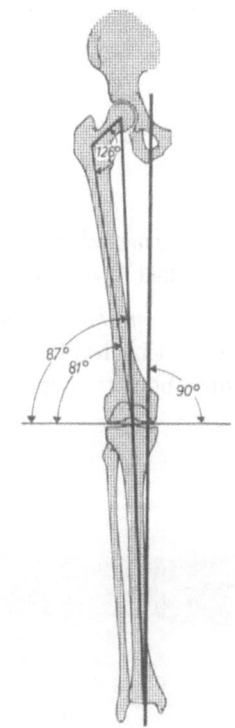

Fig. 70. Normal lines of axis of the knee joint: The angle between the axis of the body and the knee joint is 90°, but between the mechanical axis and the knee joint it is 87°. Between the axis of the shaft of the femur itself and the knee joint the angle is 81° (from MÜLLER, M. E.: Femur osteotomies near the hip. Thieme, Stuttgart 1957)

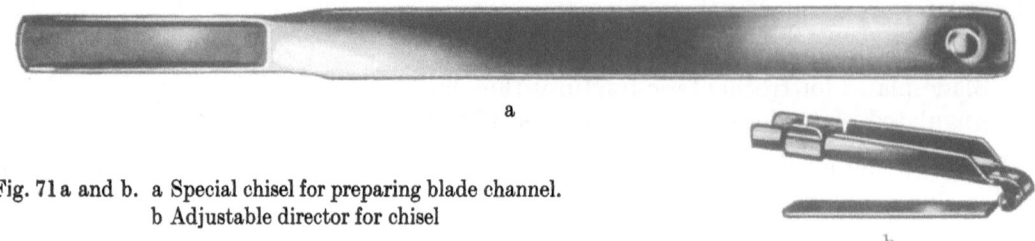

Fig. 71 a and b. a Special chisel for preparing blade channel.
               b Adjustable director for chisel

the fragments can be impacted. The driver-extractor is attached to the plate with the help of a socket wrench with universal joint, an open-end wrench or a STEINMANN pin. With its use the plate can be held at any required angle for insertion, and it can be used also as an extraction device with the help of the slotted hammer.

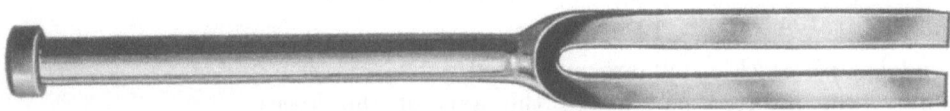

Fig. 72. Slotted hammer

The *pointed impactor* shown in Fig. 74, *with the conical tip* is used for driving the plate in the last few millimeters.

The *long handled drill sleeve* prevents the drill from making eccentric holes and from penetrating too far in the soft tissues after the second cortex has been perforated. It also stops the soft tissues from becoming wrapped around the drill superficially.

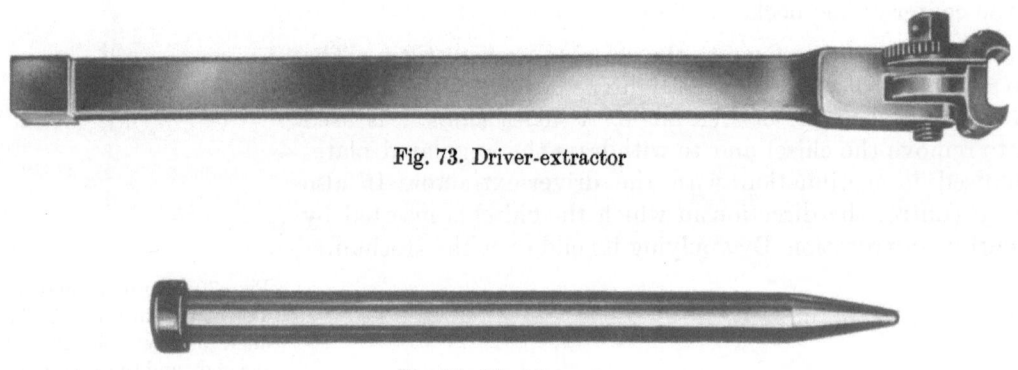

Fig. 73. Driver-extractor

Fig. 74. Final impactor

The *drill guide* (Fig. 76a) to control the angle in which the nail is inserted, keeping it at 130°, was developed at the request of several surgeons. It is applied so that the distance between its upper edge and the promontory of the greater trochanter is 25 mm. A 3.2 mm. drill is inserted into the device as a guide to the direction of the plate in sagittal and coronal planes.

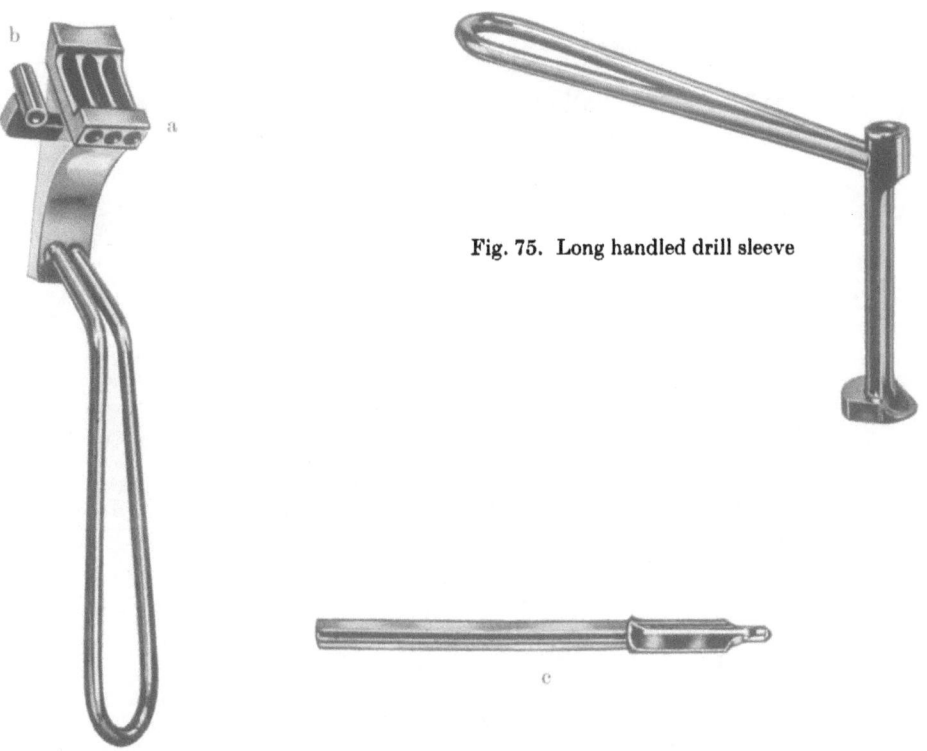

Fig. 75. Long handled drill sleeve

Fig. 76 a—c. a Triple drill guide. b Attachment. c Router

Using the drill guide and a 4.5 mm. drill the slot is cut for the entry of the blade through the cortex of the femoral shaft. The 3 drill holes are joined with a router which cuts a groove on all sides.

The use of these tools in treating a trochanteric fracture is shown in Fig. 77.

Steps in the Use of the Angulated Plate Instrument Set

a) Using the drill guide the slot is first cut for the entry of the blade.

b) The special chisel is driven in 2 to 3 cm. with the help of the adjustable director.

c) The fracture is reduced under direct vision and is temporarily fixed with crossed KIRSCHNER wires at which point a.p. and lateral control x-rays are taken. The chisel is then driven in until its widened shaft reaches the cortex.

d) The selected plate is now fixed in the driver-extractor and the chisel extracted with the slotted hammer. The blade of the blade-plate is placed into the precut canal.

When a condylar plate is used for a supracondylar fracture, the lower fragment is first screwed to the plate. The compression device is then applied at the upper end of the plate, compressing the fracture longitudinally (see chapter on Supracondylar Fractures).

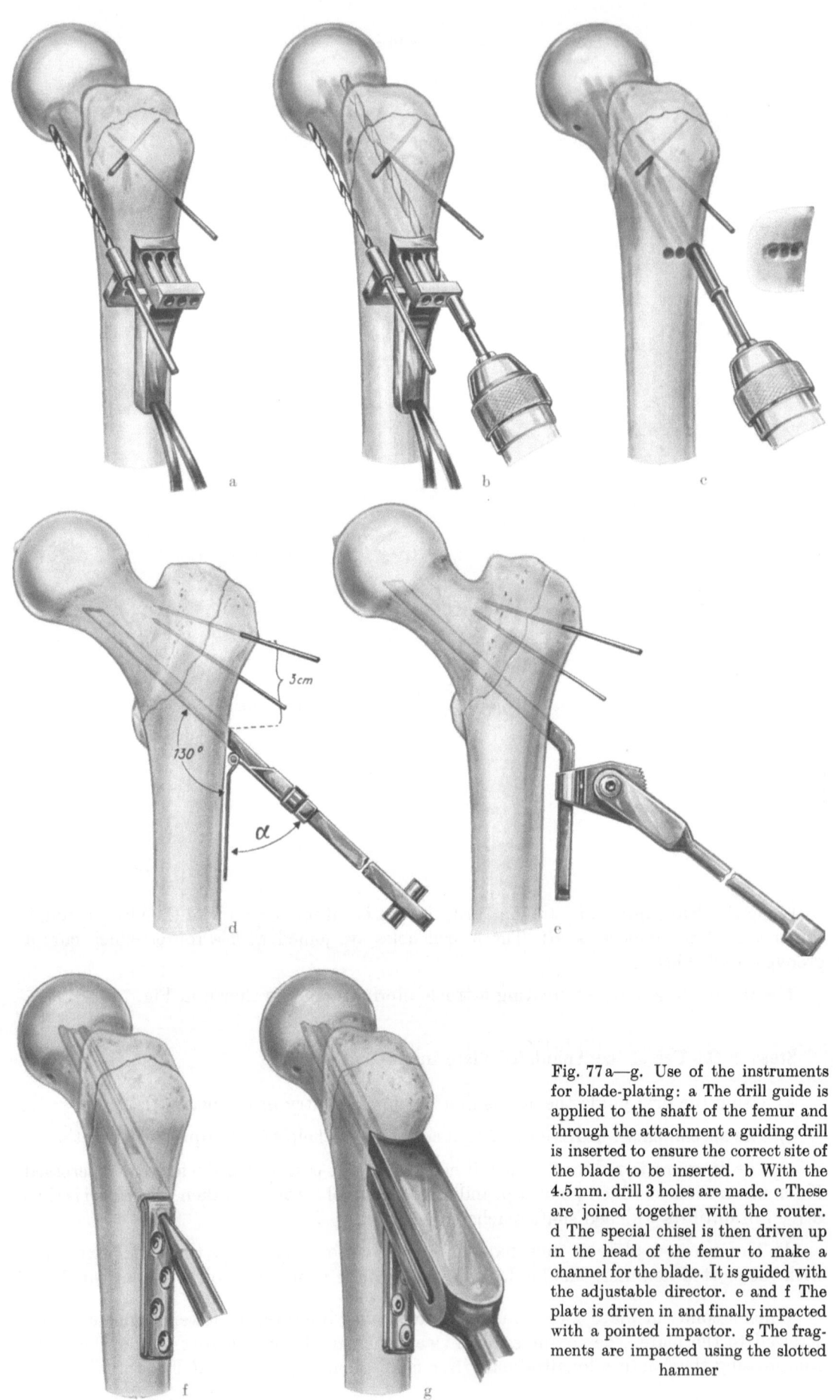

Fig. 77 a—g. Use of the instruments for blade-plating: a The drill guide is applied to the shaft of the femur and through the attachment a guiding drill is inserted to ensure the correct site of the blade to be inserted. b With the 4.5 mm. drill 3 holes are made. c These are joined together with the router. d The special chisel is then driven up in the head of the femur to make a channel for the blade. It is guided with the adjustable director. e and f The plate is driven in and finally impacted with a pointed impactor. g The fragments are impacted using the slotted hammer

7. Compression Fixation with External Compressors

In 1932 KEY of Australia was the first to recognize the advantages of applying external compressors in arthrodesis of the knee joint. But it was CHARNLEY[1] of Manchester who developed the method in 1948 and supported it with experimental studies. By 1954 he was able to report a series of 100 knee arthrodeses of which 80% were consolidated in less than a month. In 69 of these cases the indication for arthrodesis was tuberculosis. In the only 2 operations that failed, the joint condition was the result of syphilis.

CHARNLEY has also used compression clamps for producing arthrodesis of the shoulder and ankle joints. In 1954 MÜLLER advocated a similar method for intertrochanteric derotation osteotomy in childhood and for other operations on the tibia. In 1959, in collaboration with ALLGÖWER, he demonstrated the pros and cons of the method in the treatment of nonunion. Compression arthrodesis with external clamps has proven useful in arthrodesis and osteotomies in cancellous bone.

Using STEINMANN pins and external clamps it is clear that the parallel surfaces of all bones can be pressed together so firmly that any lateral or angulating shift of the fragments is impossible. The lie of the pins projecting outside the limb will draw attention to any adjustments necessary in the cut surfaces of the bone. Bony consolidation of the cancellous surfaces under compression had occurred between four and five weeks as was shown in specimens examined by ÜHLINGER (see MÜLLER). Biopsies taken four weeks after knee arthrodesis for instance showed an area at the site of union of fine mesh cancellous bone within the broader mesh cancellous bone of the femur and tibia.

In German speaking areas GREIFENSTEINER in 1953 and BERGERMANN in 1956 used KIRSCHNER wires stretched on stirrups to provide compression. These stirrups are very large and heavy and the optimal compression force of 50 kg. can not be achieved with them. EXNER reports trouble with broken wires. KIRSCHNER wires often cut through the skin and were shown by BÖHLER and his school to be capable of moving within the bone and to produce infection more commonly than when STEINMANN pins are used.

The AOI external compression clamps are similar to those described by CHARNLEY. These compression clamps can be used both with STEINMANN pins and on SCHANZ screws for compression or traction.

Similar devices (Fig. 78) were developed by HOFFMANN (1955) in Switzerland and by ANDERSON in the U.S.A. for the treatment of diaphyseal fractures and were advocated by ISLER (1951), JOHNSON (1951), CREYSSEL, DE MOURGUES, GOUNOT and BOUCHET (1956), RICKLIN (1957), ILLES (1958) for open fractures. The external compressors are really only a development of LAMBOTTE's fixateur externe (1908). The AOI device combines the advantages of CHARNLEY's and HOFFMANN's methods.

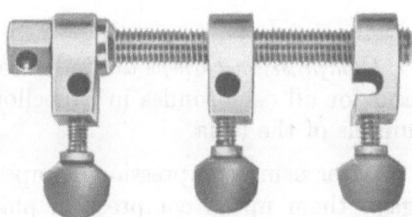

Fig. 78. External compression clamp, showing the slotted end piece

The AOI compression clamps (Fig. 82) are manufactured from stainless steel and are strong, light and easy to handle. They can be dismantled for cleaning by undoing the bolt with an adjustable wrench.

To facilitate the insertion and removal of the innermost pins, as in an intertrochanteric osteotomy, the short compression clamp is provided with an open slot instead of a hole. The clamp can be tightened with a socket wrench, an adjustable wrench or the key for the compression device.

---

[1] Many other workers have reported successful results using CHARNLEY's technique, among them PARISEL of Belgium, POTROT-ROUSSEL of France, GREIFENSTEINER of Austria, MARZ-EXNER and MAXEN of Germany, MORRIS and MOSIMAN of the U.S.A., and H. SKARENBÖRG of Sweden. All emphasize the remarkable speed and security of bone union obtained.

Stainless steel STEINMANN *pins* have a diameter of 4 or 4.5 mm. according to their length and have a trocar-pointed tip. They can be inserted with the universal chuck with T-handle, or into a thick cortex by means of a pneumatic drill. These STEINMANN pins are elastic and break only under a pressure of more than 500 kg.

SCHANZ *screws* are 5 mm. thick and are self-tapping so that drilling with a 3.75 mm. drill is adequate.

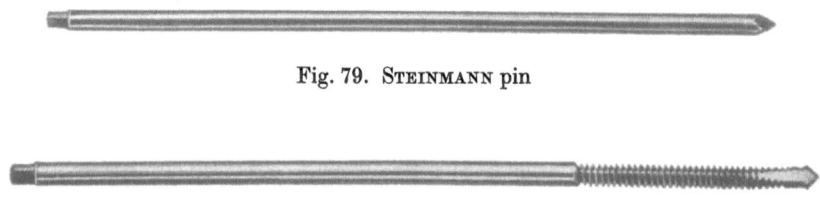

Fig. 79. STEINMANN pin

Fig. 80. SCHANZ screw

The *universal chuck with T-handle* (Fig. 81) can be opened and closed manually without any special key. Newer models can be locked in both directions so that they do not become loose neither when driving nor removing a SCHANZ screw.

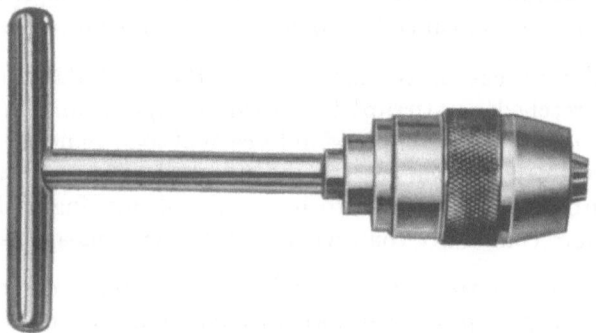

Fig. 81. Universal chuck with T-handle

Compression clamps are indicated for arthrodesis of the knee, ankle or shoulder joints and for all osteotomies in cancellous bone (Fig. 82) and for some types of infected non-unions of the tibia.

After using compression clamps in 28 cases of aseptic nonunion of the tibial shaft we gave them up as compression plates give more rigid fixation and better compression. Medullary nailing combined with reaming replaced compression clamps in other cases.

Nonunion in the presence of infection can be an indication for the use of compression clamps until the fragments are united. Under some conditions fixation of fragments by external pins without compression may be required and in these cases between 4 and 6 STEINMANN pins should be used to prevent angular deformities.

But any use of pins projecting outside the limb establishes a continuity between the atmosphere and the bone providing access for bacteria. The risk of infection from this cause is less with the more firmly seated STEINMANN pins than with rotating KIRSCHNER wires. In any case the skin incision should be the smallest possible, though the surrounding skin must not be so tight that it will necrose. If the small incisions are carefully sutured to fit snugly around the nail at the points of exit and entry the incidence of osteitis can be reduced. It has not occurred in over 300 cases in our series.

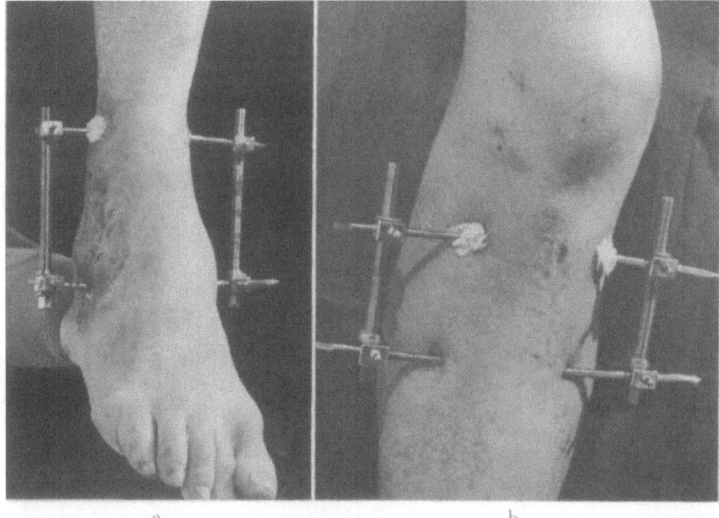

a   b

Fig. 82a and b. External compression clamps used: a For arthrodesis of the ankle. b For a rotation osteotomy of the upper end of the tibia

Fig. 84 illustrates *the technique of compression clamp arthrodesis* of the ankle joint. Early ankle joint arthrodesis can prevent impairments of the circulation and stiffness in the subtalar joint. Primary arthrodesis of the ankle joint is indicated when the articular surfaces are severely damaged and reconstruction proves impossible. Fig. 83 shows an open fracture of the distal end of the tibia in which the proximal bone end was contaminated with dirt and grass, and the surface of the talus largely destroyed. If the subtalar joint is intact, arthrodesis at the correct angle can give the patient years or even decades of comfortable life with a plantigrade foot.

Postoperatively we leave the compression clamps in place for 4 to 5 weeks. After removing the STEINMANN pins a walking plaster is provided for another 5 to 8 weeks.

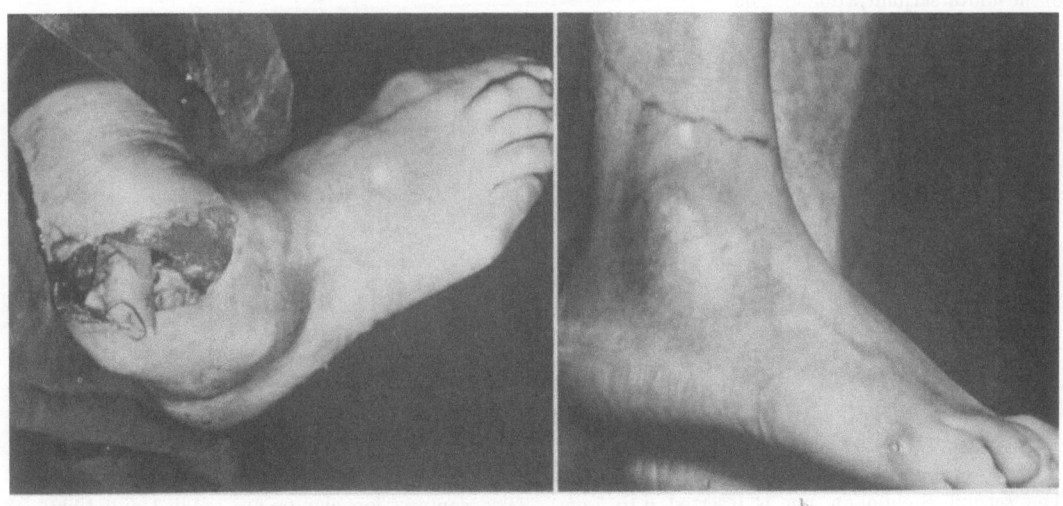

a   b

Fig. 83a and b. a Comminuted compound fracture of the lower end of the tibia and the talus. b Condition of the foot 3 months after primary arthrodesis

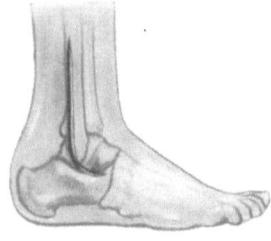
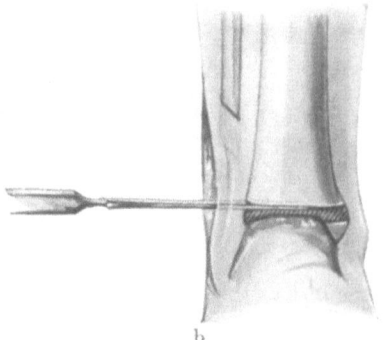

a

b

The tourniquet is applied. Medial and lateral longitudinal incisions are made as shown beginning at
5 cm. above the medial malleolus, 12 cm. above the
lateral malleolus respectively

Oblique resection of the lower 5 cm. of the fibula.
The articular surface of the tibia including part of the
medial malleolus is removed with an osteotome

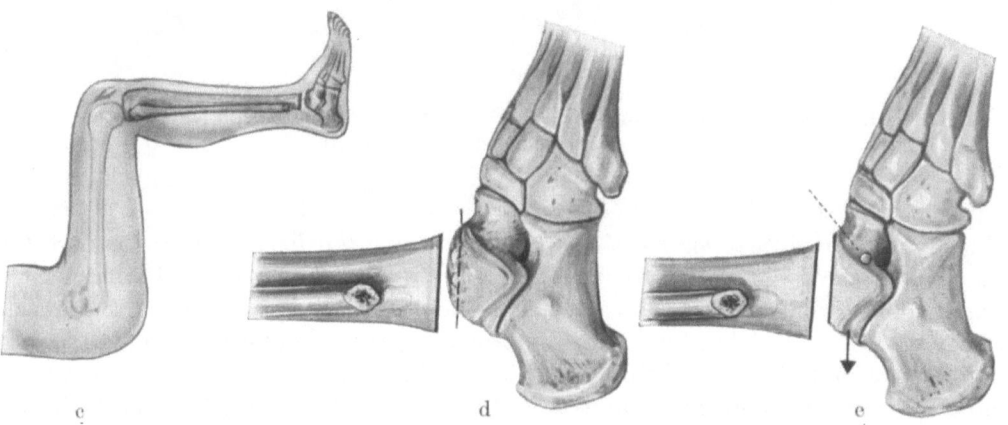

c

d

e

The knee is flexed to 90⁰. The foot
is placed in the same degree of
external rotation as is present in
the normal foot. The forefoot is
dorsiflexed to bring the foot to lie
at an angle of 90⁰ to the axis of the
tibia. In a man, with good mobility
of the midtarsal joint, a dorsiflexion
of 80⁰ gives a good result

The articular surface of the talus
is divided so as to make a flat surface parallel with that on the tibia.

The first Steinmann pin is inserted
parallel to the line of osteotomy of
the talus and 1 cm. distal to it at
a point in line with the anterior border of the tibia. The hole foot is
displaced backwards

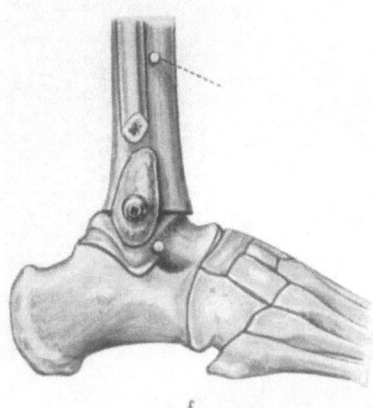
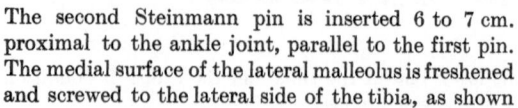
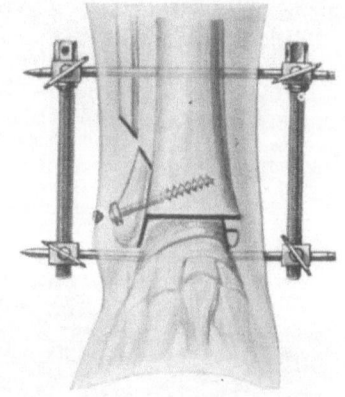

f

g

The second Steinmann pin is inserted 6 to 7 cm.
proximal to the ankle joint, parallel to the first pin.
The medial surface of the lateral malleolus is freshened
and screwed to the lateral side of the tibia, as shown

The compression clamps are applied and tightened
up while checking that the foot is in a plantigrade
position and absolutely firmly held

Fig. 84 a—g. Technique for arthrodesis of the ankle joint using external compression clamps

8. General Instruments

We use either a pneumatic drill or the Lento-drill from the POHL Company of Kiel, for which accessory parts are available.

The pneumatic drill (Fig. 85) has several advantages. Its pistol grip makes it easy to hold and the speed of the motor is controlled by pressure with the index finger. The drill stops instantly when the finger pressure is released, which is not possible with an electric drill. It is geared to give between 350 and 500 revolutions per minute, which is enough for any medullary reaming procedure. Should the reamer get stuck in the medullary canal, the motor can be stopped at once; this is also useful at the moment of penetrating the distal cortex. The disadvantage of a pneumatic drill is the need for a source of compressed air, but cylinders can be used if a compressor is not available. There is an air exhaust at the back of the motor, but the air filter needs regular examination.

In addition to the instruments mentioned above we need for internal fixation HOHMANN levers, raspatories, elevators, hammers, chisels, awls, etc. These should be made of stainless steel.

a) The AOI Set of Instruments

A complete AOI instrument set is stored in 6 individual aluminum boxes which may be sterilized intact. Each instrument has its individual place in the box and boxes are classified according to their contents, as cortical bone set, cancellous bone set, compression plate set, general hip instrument set, medullary reaming instrument set and medullary nail impaction and extraction set. For easy identification the boxes have been anodized in different colors. For use the instruments are removed from their aluminum box and laid out on the instrument table.

Although we realize that instruments for internal fixation may need modification at intervals, photographs of the various standard sets will be shown so that both doctors and nurses can identify them.

We have arranged the instruments in sets so that the surgeon has the full range available for any particular operation, as we have found that without this the very instrument that is most urgently needed has been omitted in laying up. We have also found that surgeons who order instruments independently may leave out one item that they thought dispensable. But for really efficient internal fixation a complete instrument set should be regarded as indispensable.

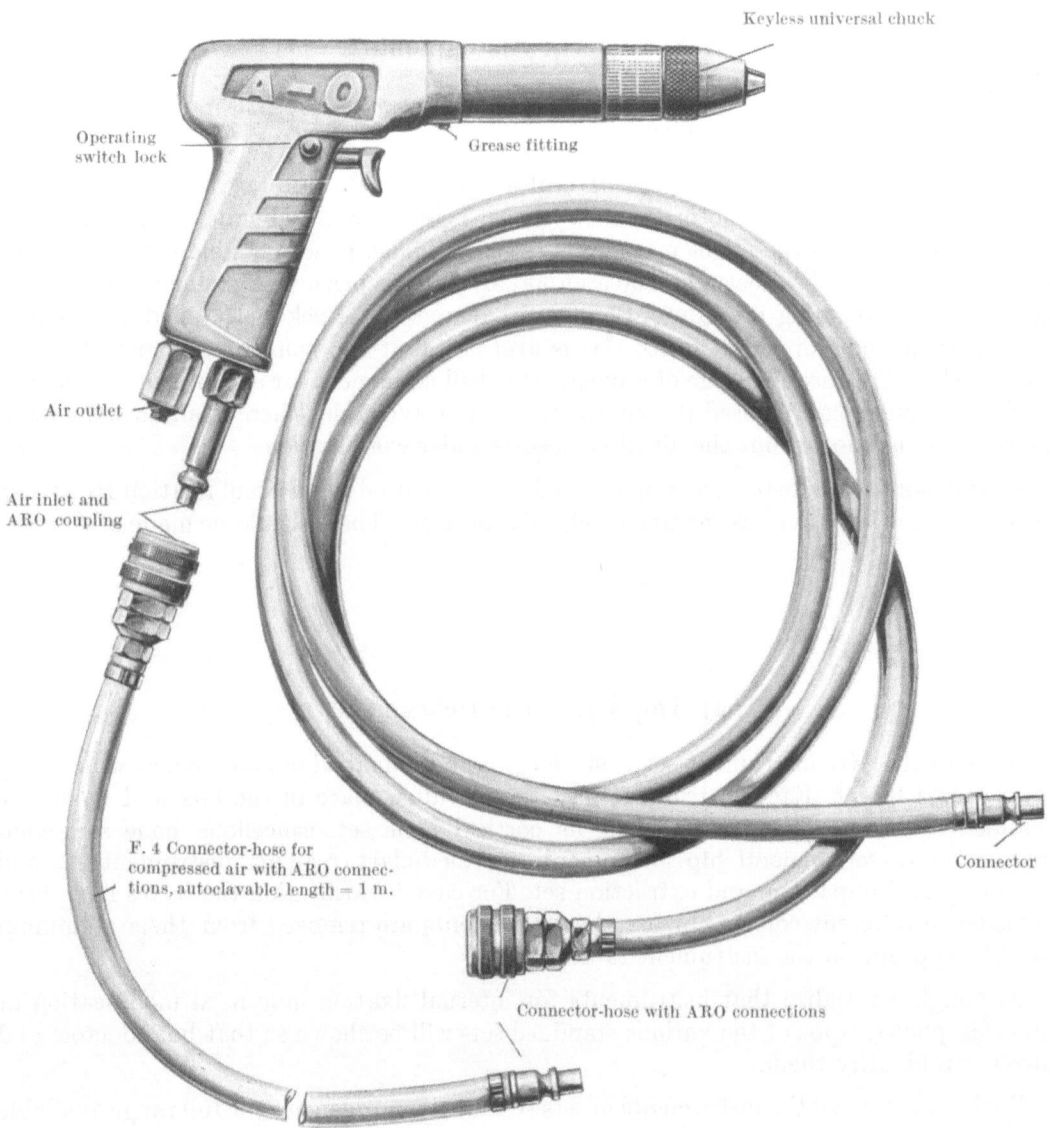

Keyless universal chuck

Operating
switch lock

Grease fitting

Air outlet

Air inlet and
ARO coupling

F. 4 Connector-hose for
compressed air with ARO connections, autoclavable, length = 1 m.

Connector

Connector-hose with ARO connections

Fig. 85. Pneumatic drill with speed reduction gear

b) Cortical Bone Set

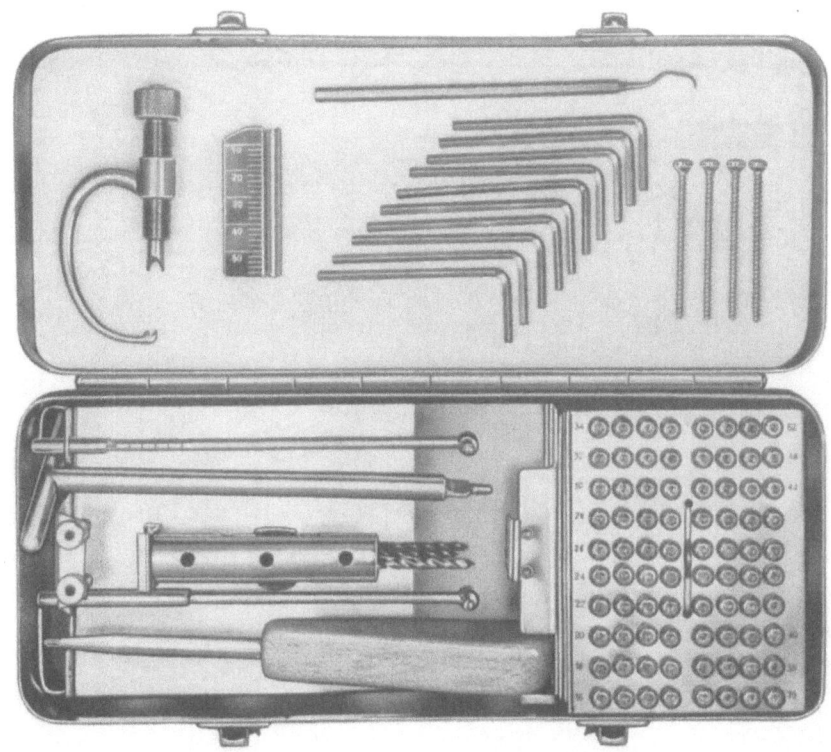

Fig. 86. Cortical bone set, standard set

A-1	Aluminum case, red, with 2 trays
A-2	Cortex screws, ⌀ 4.5 mm.
	lengths: 16 – 18 – 20 – 22 – 24 – 26 – 28 – 30
	32 – 34 – 36 – 38 – 40 – 44 – 48 – 52
	60 mm. total 84 pieces
	(26 – 28 – 30 – 32 8 each)
	(other sizes 4 each)
A-3/0	Handle for cortex screw taps
A-3/1	Cortex screw tap, short 2 pieces
A-3/2	Cortex screw tap, long 2 pieces
A-4	Countersink
A-5/1	Screw driver for screw with hexagonal socket heads
A-7/1	Drill sleeve for 3.2 mm. drills, 53 mm. long, for perpendicular drilling
A-7/2	Drill sleeve for 3.2 mm. drills, 48 mm. long, for oblique drilling
A-8/1	Drill bit, ⌀ 4.5 mm.
A-8/2	Drill bit, ⌀ 4.5 mm., with stop
A-8/3	Drill bit, ⌀ 3.2 mm. 2 pieces
A-8/4	Drill bit, ⌀ 3.2 mm., with stop
A-9/1	C-clamp drill guide
A-13	Measuring scale for screws
A-15	Small hexagonal wrench (to give to patients) 10 pieces
A-18	Small sharp hook for checking alignment of fracture ends and for removal of ingrown tissue from screw head
A-19	Screw holding forceps

Supplementary Instruments

A-5/2	Screw driver for screws with hexagonal socket heads, long type
A-6	Screw driver with metal T-handle for removal of screws
A-7/4	Sleeve for tap A-3/2, to protect tissue
A-9/2	Pointed drill guide
A-10	Simple wire tightener
A-11	Wire cerclage instrument
A-12/1	Wire with eye, ⌀ 1.2 mm., hard
A-12/2	Wire with eye, ⌀ 1.0 mm., soft
A-14	Wire cutter
A-16/1	Coil of wire, ⌀ 1.2 mm., hard, length 10 m.
A-16/2	Coil of wire, ⌀ 1.0 mm., soft, length 10 m.
A-17	Cortex screw nut
B-9	Open-end wrench for Nut A-17
A-20	Universal chuck for "Lento drill"
A-21/1	Kirschner wire, ⌀ 1.0 mm., length 150 mm. (triangular point)
A-22/1	Kirschner wire, ⌀ 1.4 mm., length 150 mm. (triangular point)
A-22/2	Kirschner wire, ⌀ 1.4 mm., length 300 mm. (flat point, for drilling)
A-23/1	Kirschner wire, ⌀ 2.0 mm., length 150 mm. (triangular point)
A-23/2	Kirschner wire, ⌀ 2.0 mm., length 300 mm. (flat point, for drilling)
A-24/1	Kirschner wire, ⌀ 2.5 mm., length 150 mm. (triangular point)
A-24/2	Kirschner wire, ⌀ 2.5 mm., length 300 mm. (flat point, for drilling)

c) Cancellous Bone Set

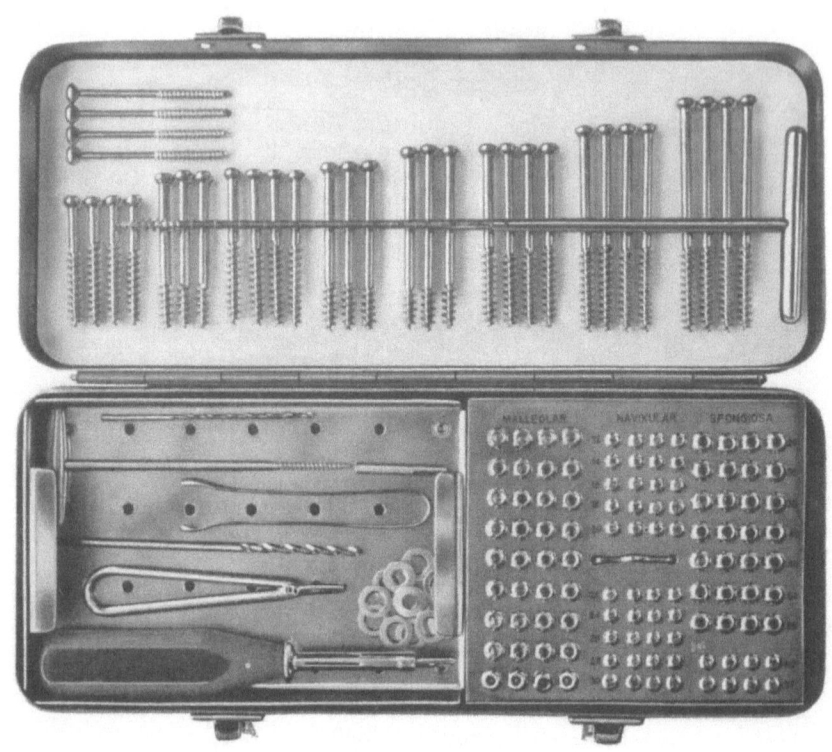

Fig. 87. Cancellous bone set, standard set

B-1/1   Aluminum case, yellow, with red lid, with 3 trays

B-2   Cancellous screws, ⌀ 6.5 mm., length of thread 16 mm.

        lengths: 25 – 30 – 35 – 40 – 45 – 50 – 55
                60 – 65 – 70 mm. (4 each size)
                                40 pieces

B-3   Cancellous screws, ⌀ 6.5 mm., thread length 32 mm.

        lengths: 50 – 60 – 70 – 80 – 90 mm.
        (4 each size)   20 pieces

B-4   Malleolar screws, ⌀ 4.5 mm., shaft, ⌀ 3.0 mm.

        lengths: 25 – 30 – 35 – 40 – 45 – 50 – 55
                60 – 65 – 70 mm. (4 each size)
                                 40 pieces

B-5   Scaphoid (Navicular) screws, ⌀ 3.5 mm., shaft, ⌀ 2.0 mm.

        lengths: 12 – 14 – 16 – 18 – 20 – 22 – 24 – 26
                28 – 30 – 35 – 40 mm. (4 each size)
                                 48 pieces

B-7   Tap for cancellous screws, ⌀ 6.5 mm.

B-10   Screw driver for Scaphoid (navicular) screws

B-14   Washers   12 pieces

B-15   Tap for Scaphoid (Navicular) screws, ⌀ 3.5 mm.

A-7/3   Drill sleeve for 2 mm. drill [Scaphoid (Navicular) screw thread]

A-8/5   Drill bit, ⌀ 3.75 mm. (cancellous thread)

A-8/6   Drill bit, ⌀ 2.0 mm. [Scaphoid (Navicular) thread]   2 pieces

A-19   Screw holding forceps

Supplementary Instruments

B-2   Cancellous screws, ⌀ 6.5 mm., thread length 16 mm.

        lengths: 75 – 80 – 85 – 90 – 95 – 100 – 105
                110 mm.

B-6   Screws for epiphysiolysis, ⌀ 6.5 mm., thread length 16 mm., with stop and small head

        lengths: 50 – 60 – 70 – 80 – 90 mm

B-8/1   Threaded bolt, ⌀ 3 mm., with two nuts

        lengths: 70 – 100 – 120 mm.

B-8/2   Nut for threaded bolt

B-9   Open-end wrench for nut B-8/2

B-16   Sleeve for tap B-15, to protect tissue

d) Compression Plate Set

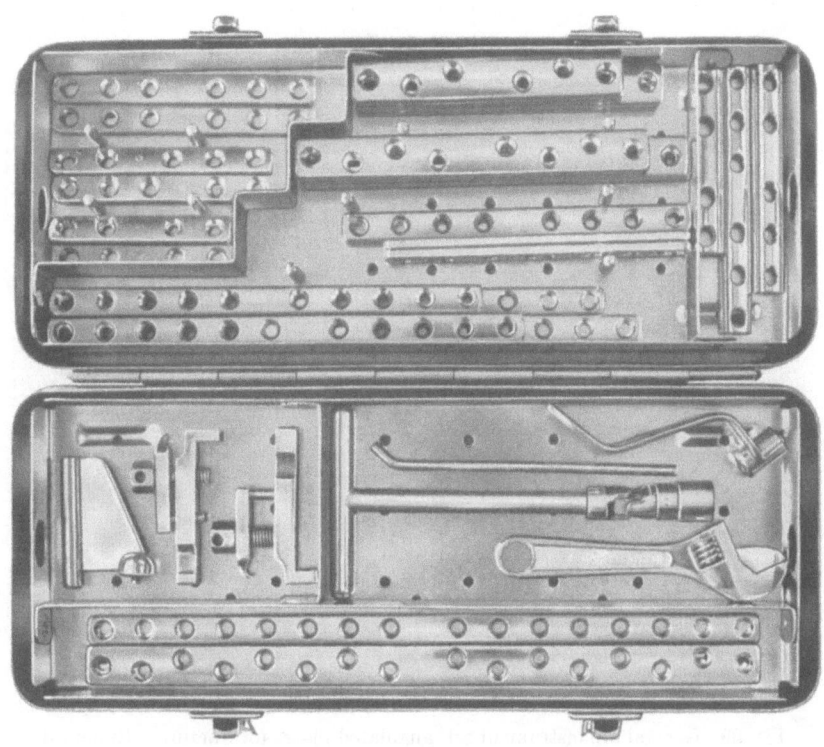

Fig. 88. Compression plate set, standard set

C-1/2	Aluminum case, yellow, with 2 trays		
C-5	Drill sleeve for compression device, matches C-6/1		
C-6/1	Compression device, span 8 mm.		
C-6/2	Compression device, span 16 mm.		
C-7	Socket wrench with universal joint		
C-8	Drill sleeve for plates, long, for 3.2 mm. drill		
C-11	Pin wrench for compression device		
C-16	Open-end wrench for compression device		
C-2/3	Narrow plate (3 holes)	1 each	
C-2/4	Narrow plate (4 holes	4 each	
C-2/5	Narrow plate (5 holes)	2 each	
C-2/6	Narrow plate (6 holes)	2 each	
C-2/7	Narrow plate (7 holes)	2 each	
C-2/8	Narrow plate (8 holes)	2 each	
C-2/9	Narrow plate (9 holes)	1 each	
C-2/10	Narrow plate (10 holes)	1 each	
C-2/12	Narrow plate (12 holes)	1 each	
C-2/14	Narrow plate (14 holes)	1 each	
C-2/16	Narrow plate (16 holes)	1 each	
C-3/6	Broad plate (6 holes)	2 each	

C-3/7	Broad plate (7 holes)	2 each
C-3/8	Broad plate (8 holes)	2 each
C-3/9	Broad plate (9 holes)	2 each
C-3/10	Broad plate (10 holes)	1 each
C-4/3	Semi-tubular plate (3 holes)	1 each
C-4/4	Semi-tubular plate (4 holes)	1 each
C-4/5	Semi-tubular plate (5 holes)	1 each
C-4/6	Semi-tubular plate (6 holes)	1 each

Supplementary Instruments

C-2	Narrow plate available with 2 – 3 – 4 – 5 – 6 7 – 8 – 9 – 10 – 11 – 12 – 13 – 14 – 15 – 16 holes
C-3	Broad plate available with 5 – 6 – 7 – 8 – 9 10 – 12 – 14 – 16 – 18 holes
C-4	Semi-tubular plate available wir 2 – 3 – 4 – 5 6 – 7 – 8 – 9 – 10 – 11 – 12 holes
C-10	T-plate for humerus and tibia length: 68 mm.
C-12	T-plate for humerus and tibia, length: 98 mm.
C-13	T-plate for humerus and tibia, length: 120 mm.
C-14	Plate-lifter
C-15	Plate-extractor

e) General Hip Instrument Set and Angulated Plates for Fractures

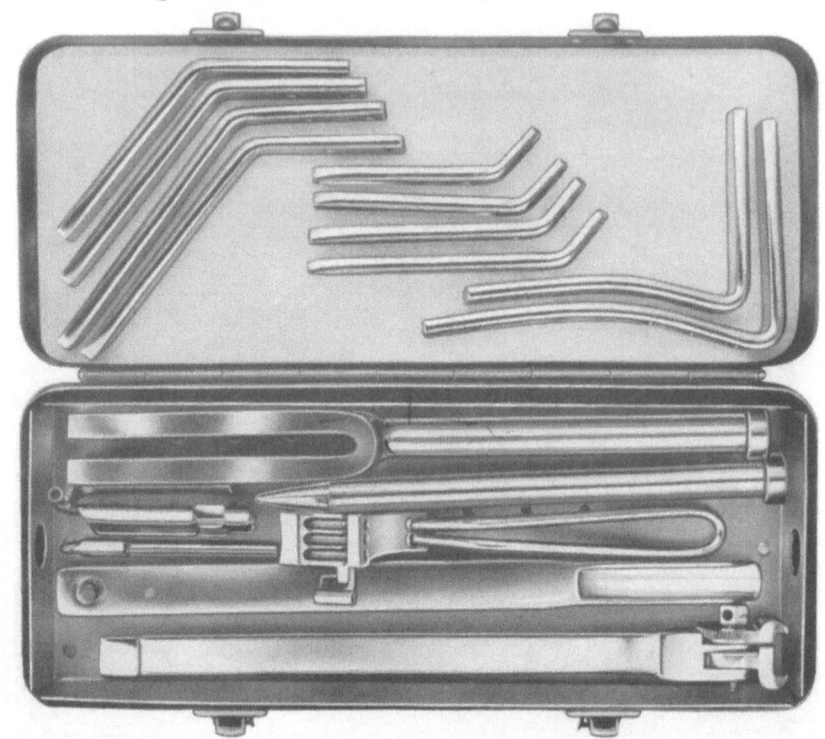

Fig. 89. General hip instrument set, angulated plates for fractures. Standard set

D-1   Aluminum case, dark blue, with tray
D-2/1   Special chisel for preparing blade channel
D-3   Adjustable director for chisel
D-4   Slotted hammer
D-5   Driver-extractor
D-6   Final impactor
D-7   Drill sleeve, long
D-8/1   Triple drill guide for 130° angle
D-8/2   Drill guide attachment
D-8/3   Router
D-23   Pertrochanteric plate, 130°, plate length
          60 mm.
          Blade lengths: 80 – 90 – 100 – 110 mm.
          (1 each blade length)   4 pieces
D-31   Condylar plate, 95°, plate length 135 mm.,
          blade lengths: 70 – 80 mm. (1 each blade
          length)   2 pieces
D-35   Blade-plate for femoral neck, 130°,
          blade lengths: 70 – 80 – 90 – 100 mm.
          (1 each blade length)   4 pieces

Supplementary Plates for Femoral Neck and Condylar Fractures

D-23   Pertrochanteric plate, 130°, plate length
          60 mm.,
          blade lengths: 70 – 75 – 85 – 95 – 105 mm.
D-24   Pertrochanteric plate, 130°, plate length
          104 mm.,
          blade lengths: 80 – 95 mm.
D-25   Pertrochanteric plate, 130°, plate length
          150 mm.,
          blade lengths: 80 – 95 mm.
D-27   Pertrochanteric plate, 130°, plate length
          200 mm., blade lengths: 80 – 90 – 95 mm.

D-32   Condylar plate, 95°, plate length 210 mm.
          blade lengths: 70 – 80 mm.
D-35   Blade-plate for femoral neck, 130°, blade
          lengths: 75 – 85 – 95 – 105 – 110 mm.

Supplementary Hip Instruments

D-2/2   Special chisel for preparing blade channel
          for children's hip plates
D-12/1   Triangular positioning plate 90°/50°/40°
D-12/2   Triangular positioning plate 80°/70°/30°
D-12/3   Triangular positioning plate 100°/60°/20°
D-13   Quadrangular positioning plate 110°/90°/90°/
          70°

Supplementary Hip Plates

D-41   Angulated plate, 120°, with slide, blade
          lengths 65 – 75 – 85 mm.
D-43   Angulated plate 110°, blade lengths
          65 – 75 mm.
D-44   Double-angulated plate, 100°, blade lengths
          65 – 75 mm.
D-45   Double-angulated plate, 90°, blade lengths
          65 – 75 mm.
D-46   Curved plate, 160°
D-47   Curved plate, 170°, blade length 55 mm.
D-48   Straight plate (180°), blade length 50 mm.
D-49   Curved plate, 190°, blade length 50 mm.
D-50   Curved plate, 200°
D-451   Children's hip plate, double-angulated, 80°,
          blade length 50 mm.
D-452   Children's hip plate, double-angulated, 90°,
          blade length 50 mm.
D-453   Children's hip plate, double-angulated, 100°,
          blade length 50 mm.

f) Intramedullary Reaming Instrument Set

G 1	Aluminum case, green, with tray	G-4/2	Flexible shaft for tibia, ⌀ 8 mm. length 310 mm., for reamers of up to ⌀ 12 mm.
G-2	Right-angle drive with quick-coupling for flexible shafts (fits F-1)	G-10	Flexible shaft, ⌀ 8 mm., with fixed reamer of ⌀ 9 mm., with end cutting
G-7	Tissue protector	G-15	Hand reamer, ⌀ 6 – 7 – 8 – 9 mm. (1 each size) 4 pieces
G-11	Medullary reamers		

G-11 Medullary reamers
⌀ : 9.5 – 10 – 10.5 – 11 – 11.5 – 12
12.5 – 13 – 13.5 – 14 – 14.5 – 15
15.5 – 16 – 16.5 – 17 – 17.5 – 18
18.5 – 19 mm.   20 pieces

G-13 Holder for guide rod
G-14 Awl, heavy
G-17 Air jet for cleaning of flexible shafts
G-18 Air tube, 2 mm. diameter   2 pieces

Supplementary Instruments

G-3/2 Flexible shaft (for femur), ⌀ 10 mm., length 410 mm.

Not packed in the case

G-4/3 Flexible shaft (for tibia), ⌀ 8 mm., length 340 mm.

G-9/1 Guide rod, ⌀ 3 mm., with ball end, 800 mm. long   3 pieces

G-9/2 Guide rod, ⌀ 3 mm., with ball end, length 950 mm.

G-15 Hand reamer, ⌀ 5 – 6 – 7 – 8 – 9 11 mm.

G-3/1 Flexible shaft for the femur, ⌀ 10 mm., length 350 mm., for reamers of ⌀ 12 mm. and more

G-16 Handle with quick-coupling, for flexible shafts

G-20 Connector for Lento-drill with quick-coupling for flexible shafts

g) Medullary Nails

Tibia Nails available with ⌀ of 8 to 15 mm. and lengths from 270 to 380 mm.

Femur Nails available with ⌀ of 10 to 18 mm. and lengths from 360 to 480 mm.

L-20 Antirotational wires

h) Impaction-Extraction Set for Medullary Nails

H-1	Aluminum case, green, with tray	H-12/1	Conical threaded bolt for nails, ⌀ 8 – 12 mm.
H-2/1	Extension rod for ram	H-12/2	Conical threaded bolt for nails, ⌀ 10 – 14 mm.
H-2/2	Guide rod for ram		
H-2/4	Ram	H-12/3	Conical threaded bolt for nails, ⌀ 13 – 18 mm.
H-3/1	Extraction hook for old AOI Nails	H-13	Socket wrench
H-3/2	Extraction hook for Kirschner Nails	H-14	Curved driving piece
H-4	Hooked head	H-15	Driving head
H-6	Flexible grip for guide rod H-2/2	H-16	Guide handle for medullary nails
H-9/1	Guide rod, for impacting, ⌀ 4 mm., length 800 mm.	H-9/2	On request only: guide rod for impaction ⌀ 4 mm. length 950 mm.
H-11	Teflon tube, with knob		

i) External Compression Instruments

E-2/1	Steinmann pins, ⌀ 4.5 mm. lengths: 150 – 180 – 200 mm.	E-4	Adjustable wrench
		E-5	Universal chuck with T-handle
E-2/2	Steinmann pins, ⌀ 5 mm. length: 250 mm.	E-6/1	External compressor 80 mm., 2 clamps closed 1 clamp open
E-3/1	Schanz-screw, flat pointed, ⌀ 5 mm., length 170 200 mm.	E-6/2	External compressor 100 mm., 2 clamps closed
		E-6/3	External compressor 120 mm., 2 clamps closed
E-3/2	Schanz-screw, round ⌀ 5 mm., length 170 mm.	E-7	External compressor 150 mm., with 4 clamps

k) General Instruments

O-2/1	Periosteal Elevator, straight, small	O-4/3	Chisel, blade 40 mm. long, width 25 mm.
O-2/2	Periosteal Elevator, straight, large	O-5	Triangular drill: 110×4 mm., 170×5 mm.,
O-2/3	Periosteal Elevator, curved		110×5 mm., 170×6 mm.

O-2/1   Periosteal Elevator, straight, small
O-2/2   Periosteal Elevator, straight, large
O-2/3   Periosteal Elevator, curved
O-3/1   Hohmann bone lever, width 70 mm., with narrow spade
O-3/2   Hohmann bone lever, width 18 mm., with narrow spade
O-3/3   Hohmann bone lever, width 43 mm., with narrow spade
O-3/4   Hohmann bone lever, width 22 mm., with wide spade
O-3/5   Hohmann bone lever, width 35 mm., with wide spade
O-3/6   Hohmann bone lever, width 24 mm. long, wide spade, for hip surgery
O-3/7   Bone lever for operation on the Hallux
O-4/1   Chisel, blade 40 mm. long, width 10 mm.
O-4/2   Chisel, blade 40 mm. long, width 17.5 mm.

O-4/3   Chisel, blade 40 mm. long, width 25 mm.
O-5   Triangular drill: 110×4 mm., 170×5 mm., 110×5 mm., 170×6 mm.

P-2   Bone holding forceps, Verbrugge model: 3 sizes
         No. 1 small, No. 2 medium, No. 3 large
P-3/1   Spare aluminum case
P-3/2   Wooden tray for cortex screws
P-3/3   Wooden tray for cancellous screws and straight plates
P-4   Plastic sheet, width 40 cm., length approx. 100 m.
P-5   Plastic below knee walking caliper, 4 sizes
         No. 1: small, left or right
         No. 2: normal, left or right
         No. 3: large, left or right
         No. 4: extra large, left or right

Special Fractures

I. Fractures of the Tibia

1. Introduction

In view of the diverse forms these injuries may take it is obvious that no one single technique can be blindly adhered to. Each operation must be carefully planned but during the operation a flexible procedure is necessary as a radiologically invisible fracture line may appear to invalidate the preoperative plan. Basically it may be said that long fracture lines can be adequately fixed by screws driven in alternatively from opposite sides, while short fractures or comminuted ones need to be fixed either with a medullary nail or a compression plate. The more we follow up fractures of the tibia after surgical treatment, the less we support the idea that bone should "be burdened with a minimum of foreign material". We feel rather that the most rigid form of internal fixation should be used that is compatible with preserving the blood supply of the bone and soft tissue.

2. Operative Procedures

The 3 anatomical parts of the tibia present their own problems of treatment and will therefore be discussed separately.

a) Fractures of the Shaft
(second and third quarters of the tibia)

Approach. A pneumatic tourniquet is applied and may be left in place for 2 hours.

Screws and plates. A straight longitudinal incision is made 3 mm. lateral to the anterior border of the tibia (Fig. 90). The attachment of the peroneal muscles and their overlying fascia to the anterior border of the tibia should be left intact. The fracture is approached mainly from the medial surface of the tibia and the lacerated periosteum may be gently pushed back from the fracture lines themselves. After exposure of the medial surface of the tibia, the fragments are carefully pulled apart while the hematoma is removed by suction. Dabbing with gauze swabs should be avoided if possible as bacteria may be transferred in this way. The posterior surface of the tibia is carefully inspected from the front through the fracture lines. One has to look especially carefully to find fracture lines of an incompletely detached butterfly fragment. Only when all fracture lines have been clearly visualized can the right method of fixation be selected.

Medullary nailing. A transverse incision is made between the lower edge of the patella and the tibial tubercle. The upper edge of the wound is retracted and dissected upwards and the patellar tendon divided longitudinally to allow the medullary canal to be entered with a large awl. The guide rod is introduced and the canal reamed out to 11 or 12 mm. in diameter.

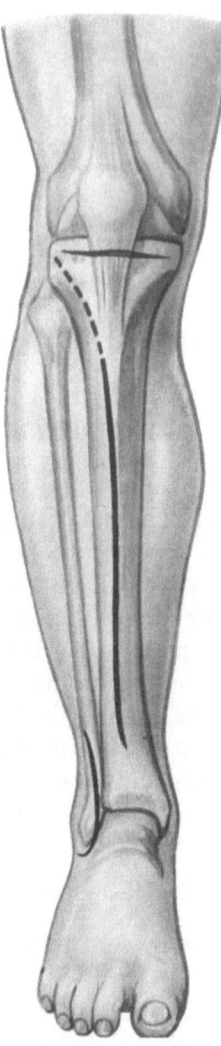

Fig. 90. Skin incisions for fractures of the lower leg. The transverse incision gives good access to the tibial plateau and heals up well with a good cosmetic and functional result. The vertical incision runs a few millimeters lateral to the anterior border of the tibia and crosses the tendon of extensor hallucis longus to expose the medial aspect of the distal tibia. A vertical incision over the tendon hallucis longus must be avoided

Position for nailing. This depends on whether there is a special table available and whether image intensifiers are to be used. It is important to remember the two dangers in nailing, which are rotational deformity and lateral or medial angulation. The axis of the malleoli is usually 25° externally rotated in relation to the axis of the knee joint, but may vary from 10° to 30°.

Open reduction. Approach: See paragraph on screws and plates (page 77).

As open operation can eliminate the two hazards of rotation and angulation we prefer it when the skin and soft tissue allow, and this has been so in the majority of our cases in which nails were used. We begin the operation with the leg flat on the table so that a decision can be made whether or not to use a medullary nail when the actual fracture has been examined visually.

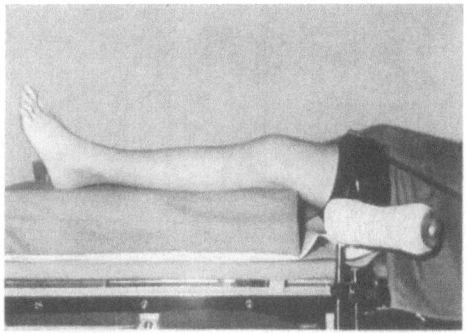

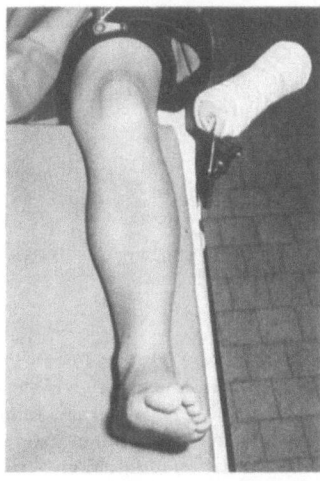
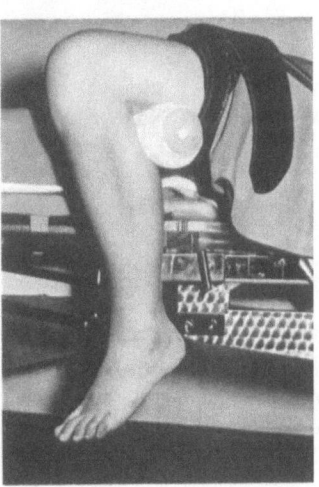

Fig. 91a—c. Attachment fitted to an ordinary operating table for medullary nailing, for closed nailing the leg is allowed to hang over the attachment from the beginning. In open nailing, the fracture is first exposed, reduced and temporarily fixed with the leg horizontal after which it is flexed over the attachment and allowed to hang down. Then the medullary nailing is carried out as with closed nailing

The reduction and alignment of the fragments are done with the patient lying on his back. The reduction is secured with bone-holding forceps or other temporary fixation and the leg is then placed hanging over the edge of the table, supported as shown in Fig. 91 c, after which the medullary canal is approached as described above.

Indications for Different Techniques of Internal Fixation

1. Simple Spiral Fractures

These represent the ideal indication for fixation with screws alone. However, the length of the fracture must be at least twice that of the diameter of the shaft of the bone (Fig. 92).

2. Long Fractures with Butterfly Fragment

This is a good indication for the use of screws only as long as at least one screw can transfix both main fragments. If the 2 main fragments can only be connected by the

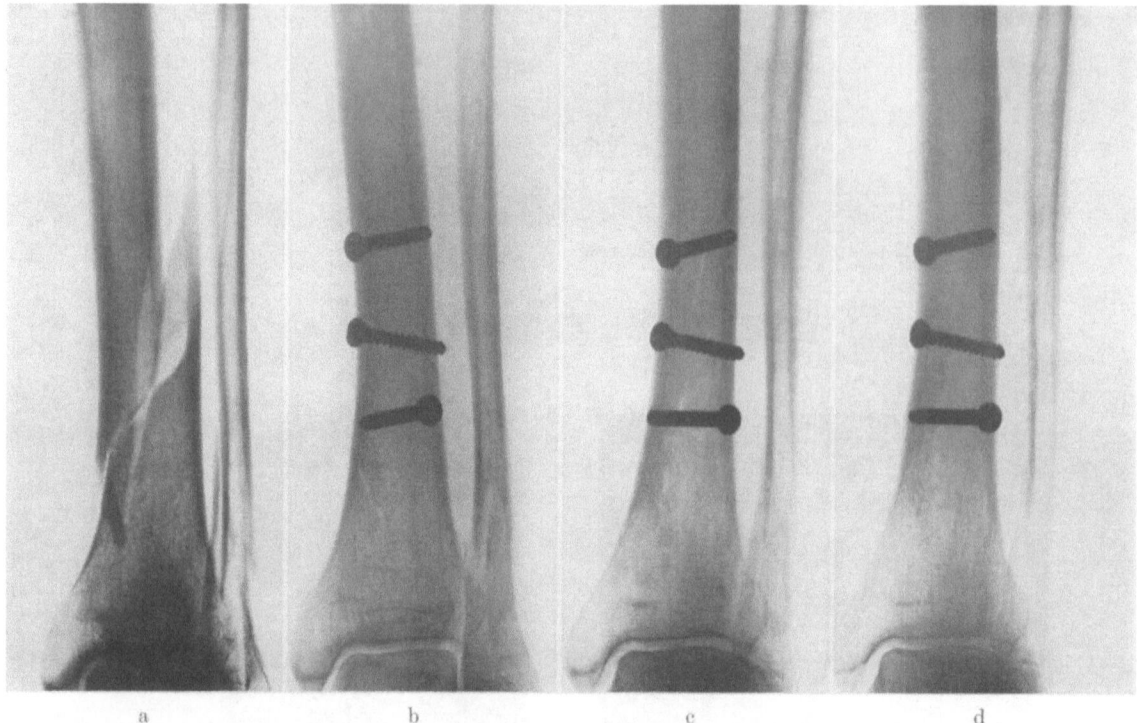

a   b   c   d

Fig. 92a—d. a Simple torsion fracture of lower third of tibia with long fracture line. b Postop. examination: screws placed alternately from opposite directions, clock-wise; fracture line hardly visible. c 15 weeks postop.: slight diffuse bony atrophy distally, fracture line slightly more visible in places than immediately postoperatively. No periosteal reaction whatsoever. d 45 weeks postop: healing with minimal endosteal and periosteal reaction, bony atrophy receding, full restoration of function

= *Long, simple torsion fracture: ideal indication for screw fixation*

butterfly fragment, screwing alone is not indicated, unless the butterfly fragment is in fact almost undisplaced (Fig. 93).

3. Fractures in which the Butterfly Fragment has short oblique fracture lines

and with little contact between the main fragments

In these cases plates and independent screws should be used together. The main function of the plate is to unite the 2 main fragments rigidly (Fig. 94). The technique of plating is dealt with on, page 50.

4. Comminuted Fractures

These can be successfully treated either with compression plates or with medullary nails. We have given increasing preference to plates since they demand accurate reduction and avoid the postoperative sequelae that may occur with medullary nails. Fitting the pieces together, especially a posterior fragment, is often quite difficult but the attempt should always be made. After inspection from the front (see page 77) the fragments should be placed into their proper places. Reduction is usually begun with the posterior fragment as this is the most difficult. Fragments on the medial surface are reduced last. Great force should never be needed. With a little patience and one or more temporary

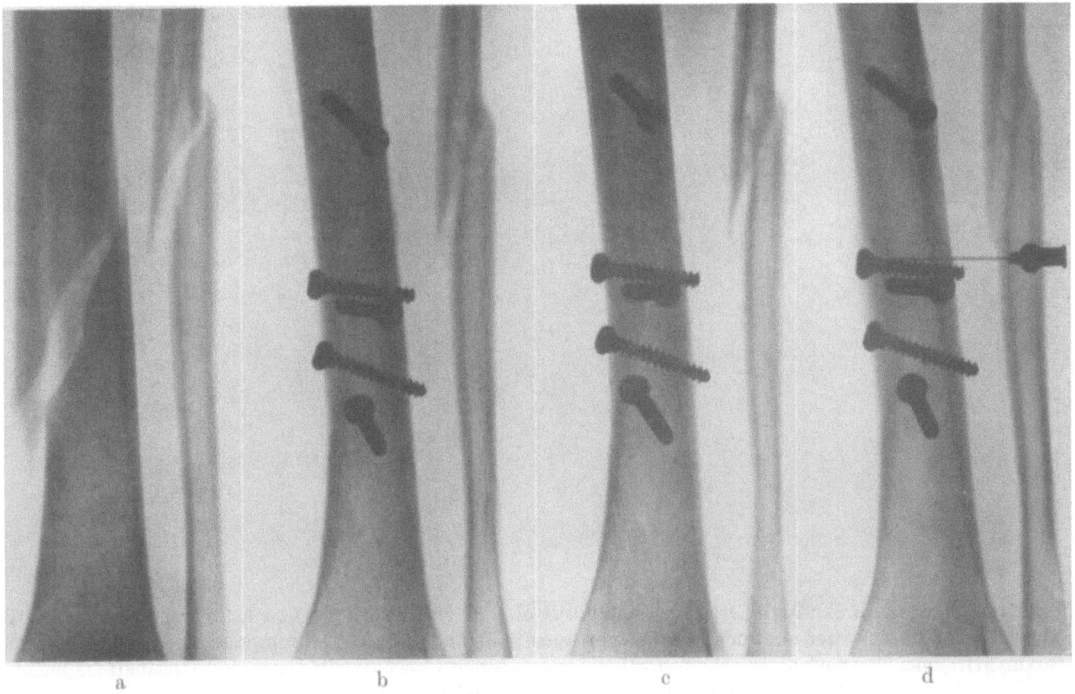

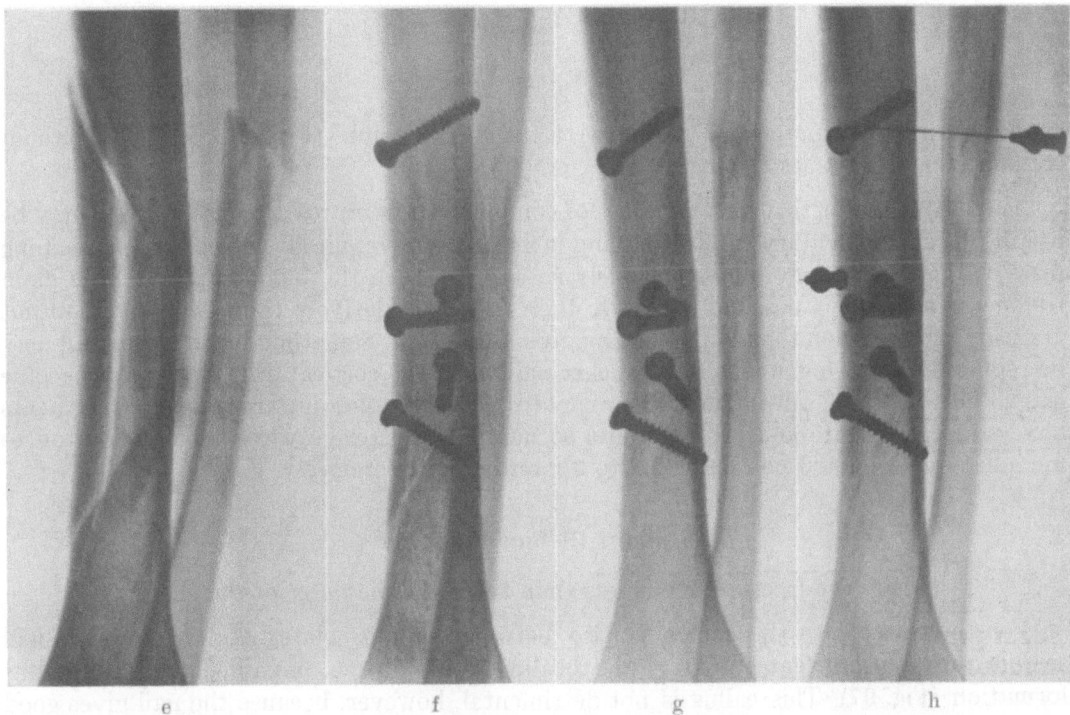

Fig. 93a—h. a and e. Butterfly fracture with good contact between the two main fragments. b and f. 8 weeks postop: fixation performed with 2 screws between the main fragments and 3 screws between butterfly fragment and proximal and distal main fragments. Fracture line still visible in the lateral aspect. c and g. 14 weeks postop: primary bone healing apart from a small cloud of callus proximally. d and h. Condition 26 weeks after the operation when the screws were removed: full restoration of function

= *Butterfly fracture with good contact between the main fragments:* = *good indication for screw fixation*

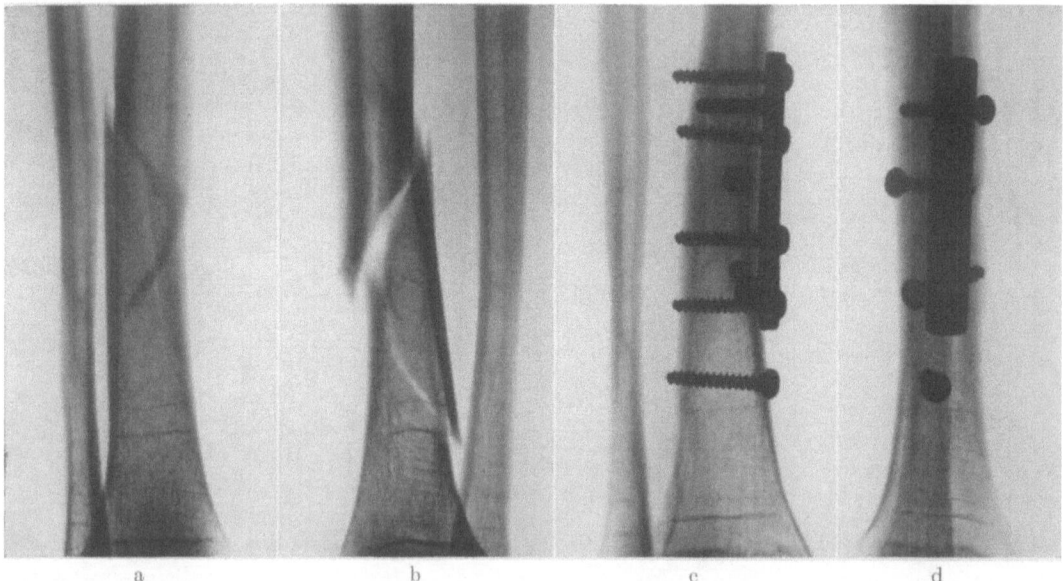

Fig. 94a—d. a and b. Butterfly fracture, small area of contact between the two main fragments. c and d. Appearance 54 weeks after treatment with compression plate and screws. The compression plate connects the two main fragments to one another, the 4 additional screws connect the butterfly fragment to the main fragments. Full restoration of function, uncomplicated course after metal removal

= *Extremely poor indication for screw fixation because of the little contact between the main fragments; good indication for a short plate combined with screws*

cerclage wires an anatomical reduction is usually possible (Figs. 95 and 96) without traumatizing the tissues.

There is no doubt that in some cases of comminuted fractures a medullary nail may be useful but supplementary cerclage wiring is usually also required. In such cases, reaming may be omitted or only done cautiously so as to disturb the blood supply of the main fragments as little as possible. We have then to use a relatively thin medullary nail not granting rigid fixation though preventing gross deformity. Sometimes such a thin nail may be replaced after a few weeks by a thicker nail when the cortical fragments have become less mobile. Reaming out the medullary canal at this time is less hazardous as the fragments have started to unite and are not quite so hard. Any cerclage wires used in additon to medullary nails should be removed 2 to 3 months postoperatively.

5. Short Oblique Fractures

(where the fracture line is less than twice the diameter of the shaft)

For these fractures the choice is also between nails or plates. A nail however will seldom provide sufficient stability, and healing is usually accompanied by much callus formation (Fig. 97). This callus is not detrimental, however, because the nail gives good support across the fracture and the period of postoperative mobilization is not interfered with. In patients where both tibiae are fractured and one is nailed and the other plated or screwed, it is remarkable how much less secure the nailed leg feels to the patient.

When plates are used in the lower leg, any screw that crosses the fracture line should be inserted so that it is exerting a compression force as in simple lag screws. In the upper half of the tibia, two plates should be used whenever possible to make sure of rigid fixation,

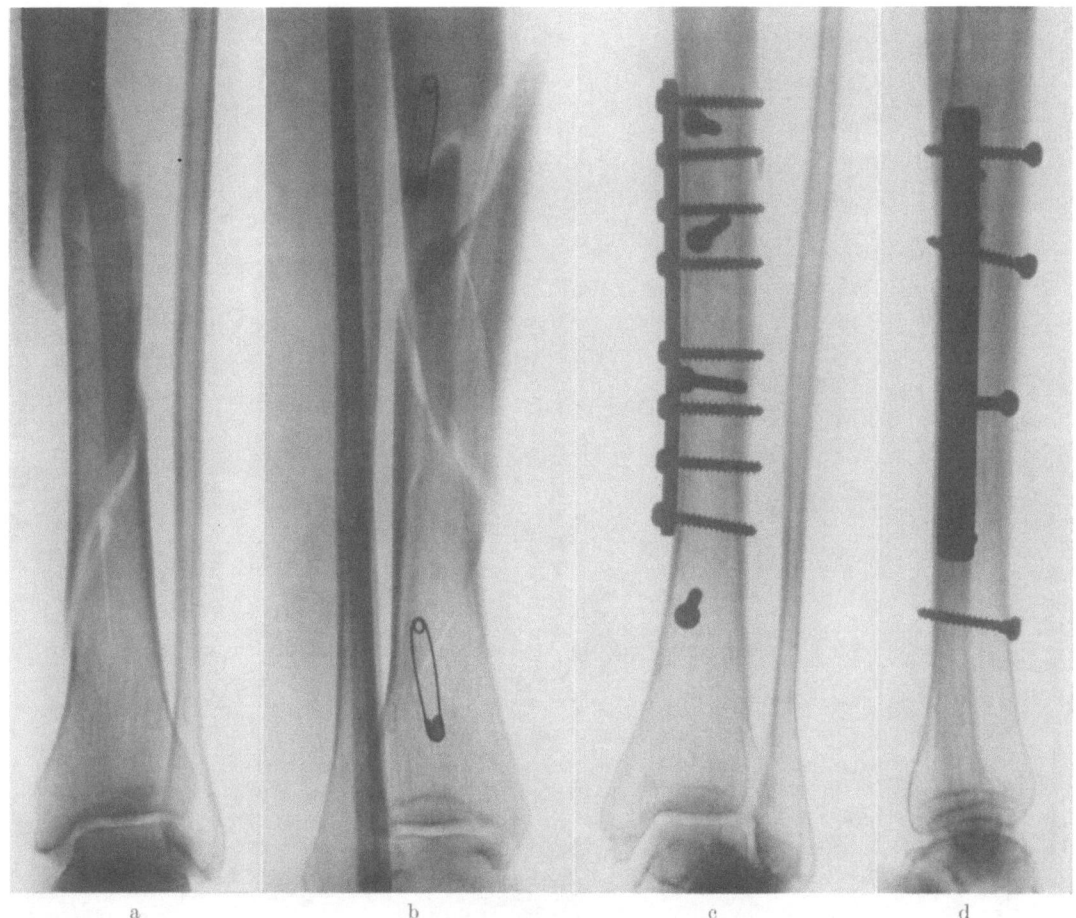

Fig. 95a—d. a and b. Comminuted fracture. c and d. Condition 16 weeks postop: primary bone healing, slight diffuse bony atrophy in the distal fragment. Full restoration of function
= *Indication for long plate with additional screws*

because one plate alone will allow a small degree of movement even during non-weight bearing exercises. In oblique fractures distal to the middle of the tibia the plate is supplemented whenever possible by additional lag screws inserted at a right angle to the plate. Whenever two plates are used, short screws (anchoring in one cortex only) should be alternated with long ones.

b) Fractures of the Lower Quarter of the Tibia

The difficult problems of this region are summarized as follows:

α) A large defect in the cancellous bone may be caused by forward or backward angulation when the bone has been compressed. After reduction the result is a gap (Fig. 98).

β) The articular surface of the lower end of the tibia is often involved in a fracture and needs to be carefully reconstructed. In other cases, fracture lines run as far as the articular surface and then everything must be done to preserve the continuity of the joint itself, so that the tibia remains congruous with the talus.

γ) Fixation of the comminuted lower fragments to the tibial shaft may present a considerable problem.

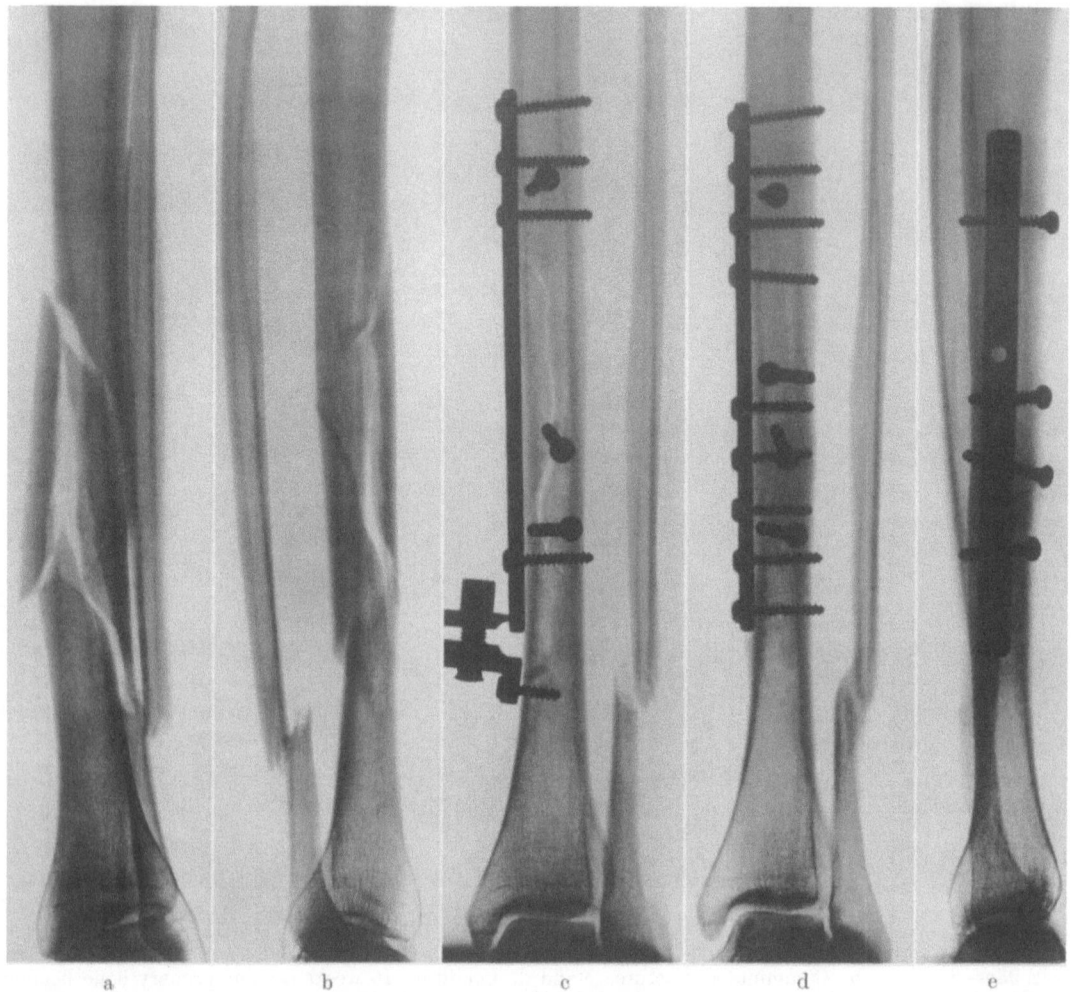

Fig. 96 a—e. a and b. Comminuted fracture. c X-ray during operation: after applying compression with
the compression-device, the plate was fixed distally with one screw. d and e. Condition 31 weeks postop:
bone healing with clear endosteal and slight periosteal reaction, the detached fragments are clearly uniting
with the main fragments. Slight diffuse bony atrophy, full restoration of function

= *Indication for long plate with additional screws*

Surgical approach in fractures of the lower quarter of the tibia. Incisions over the tendon
of extensor hallucis longus are best avoided. The lower end of the incision therefore runs
along the anterior border of the medial malleolus (Fig. 90). The fibula is better approached
from behind and the more posterior it is the larger is, the bridge of skin between the medial
and lateral incisions and the better its blood supply.

Technique. It is important that the subsequent four steps are undertaken consecutively:

1. Primary reconstruction of the Fibula. This should be done as a first step, except in
cases with comminuted fibular fracture. It is often easier than the reconstruction of a
badly shattered tibia. Internal fixation of the fibula often produces better alignment of the
tibial fragments (Figs. 100, 102). The physiological curve of the distal end of the fibula
must be preserved or an overtight ankle mortise and resulting varus deformity may
be produced.

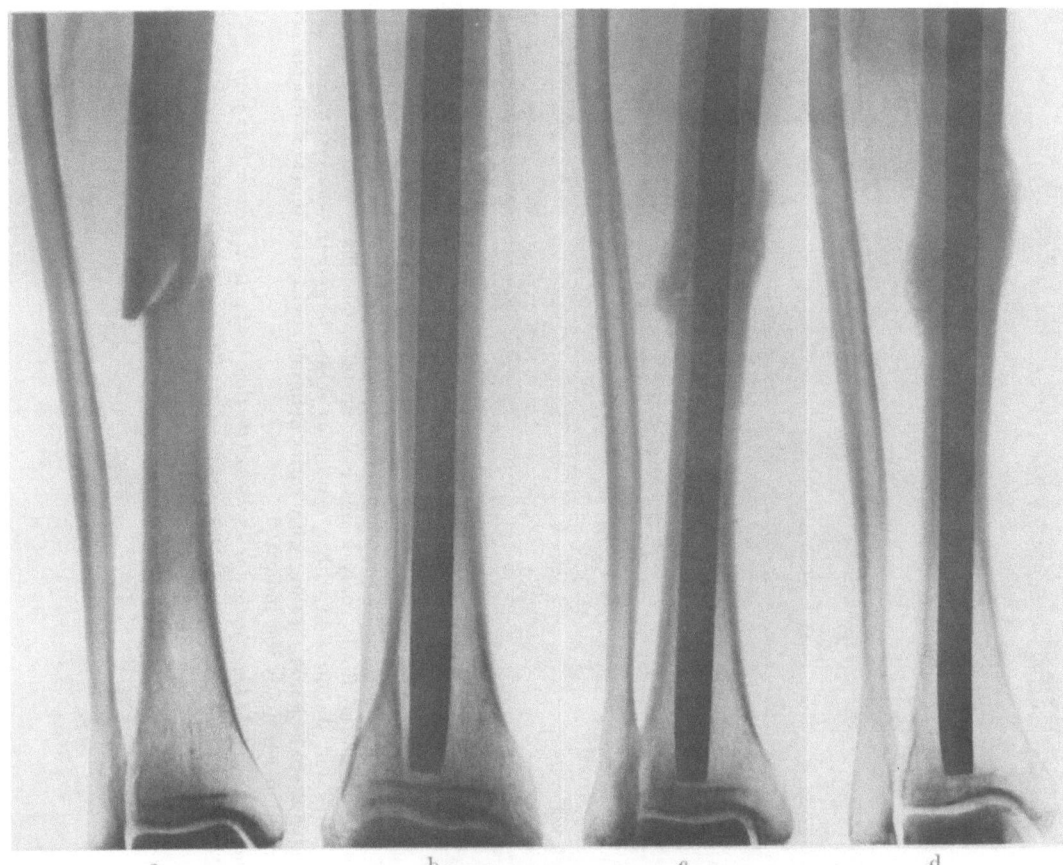

Fig. 97 a—d. a Very short oblique fracture in a very adipose 55-year-old patient with slight cardiac decompensation. b Condition after emergency operation, reaming of the medullary canal and nailing with 12 mm. medullary nail. c 16 weeks postop: good clinical progress, formation of irritation callus as the result of minimal instability in the fracture region. d 32 weeks postop: transformation of the irritation callus into fixation callus. Functionally almost completely back to normal; full restoration of function at 52 weeks
= *Bone Healing with ''fixation callus'' after medullary nailing*

2. *Fixation of the articular surface of the tibia.*

a) Either the articular surface is just fissured or it has become warped. Fissures are often in the sagittal plane as they are usually extensions of vertical fracture lines. These fissures are therefore best fixed by using transverse cancellous screws. Sometimes a cancellous screw may be driven into the fibula from the medial side (Figs. 101, 104), usually in combination with a plate.

b) Primary reconstruction of the lower end of the tibia is required if the articular surface is tilted or if there are gaps between the various fragments (Figs. 98, 105). As most of these fracture lines run in the sagittal plane, reduction can be carried out via an antero medial approach. When satisfactory reduction is obtained, the principles described in 2a may be applied. Temporary KIRSCHNER wires may be used to hold the reduction until the cancellous screws and plates can be applied.

3. *Fixation of the tibia.*
Reconstruction of the fibula by itself cannot always prevent a later varus deformity (Figs. 98, 100). Over the last two years we have usually combined fixation of the fibula with stabilization of the tibia, using a plate applied to its medial surface (Figs. 101 and 105). This additional fixation allows early mobilization, even in these particularly difficult cases.

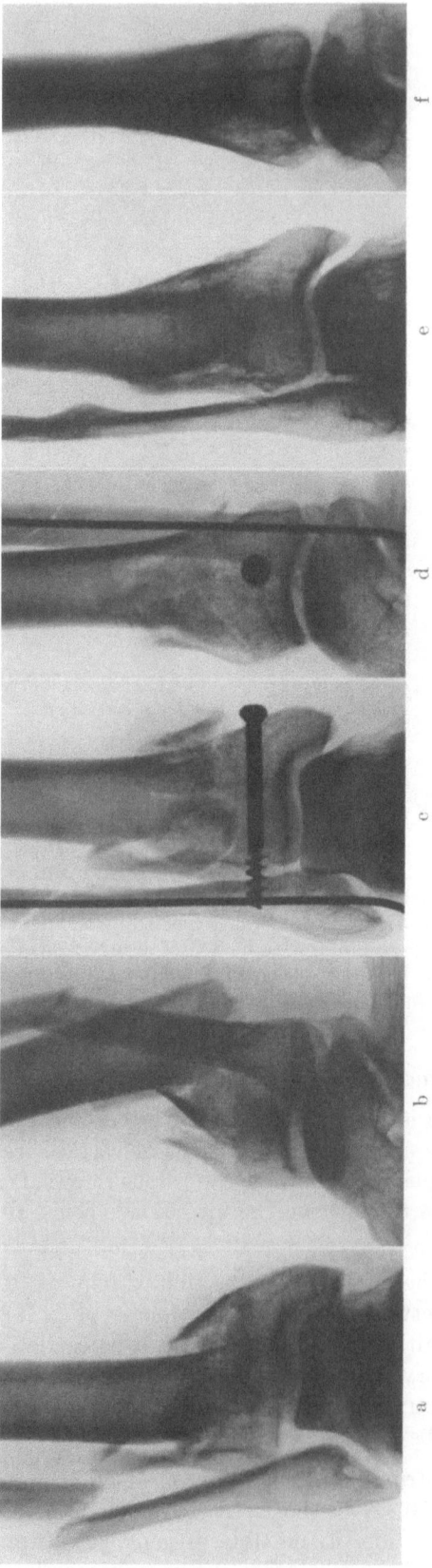

Fig. 98a—f. a and b. Fracture of the lower end of the tibia with destruction of the articular surface and production of a medullary defect at the site of bending. c and d. Condition immediately postop: because of the very narrow medullary cavity of the fibula, only a relatively unstable medullary wire can be inserted. Reduction of the articular surface of the tibia, temporary fixation with Kirschner wires and stabilization with a cancellous screw, large cancellous autograft in the comminuted area. e and f. 70 weeks postop: full restoration of function of tarsal and ankle joints, healing with varus deformity with the onset of discomfort in the subtalar joint so that a correction osteotomy was indicated

= *Important steps in the treatment of this case: fibular reconstruction, reconstruction of the lower articular surface of the tibia and primary cancellous graft*

= *Omission: No medial support resulting in a varus deformity which could easily have been avoided with a small plate applied medially*

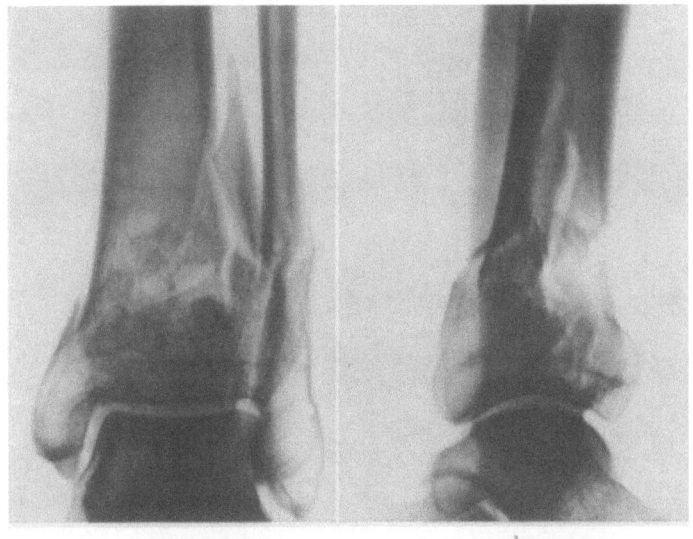

a   b

Fig. 99a and b. Distal comminuted fracture, reduced by splinting, typical anterior cancellous defect, slight varus deformity

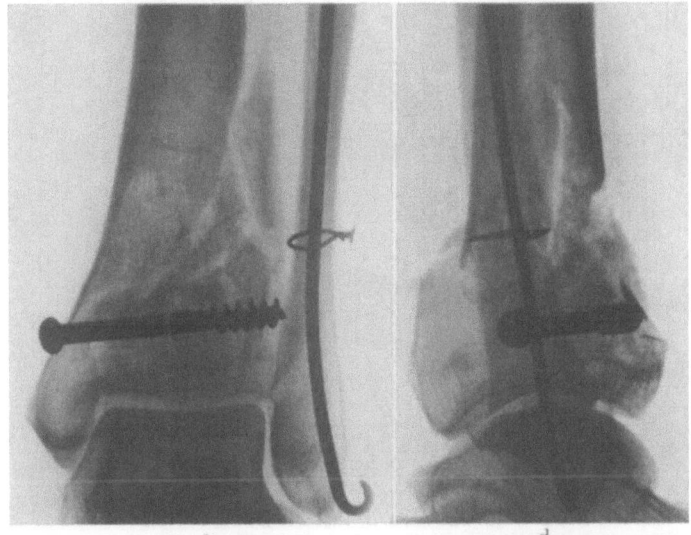

c   d

Fig. 99c and d. Condition after fibular reconstruction, stabilization of the joint surface with a transverse cancellous screw and primary cancellous autograft

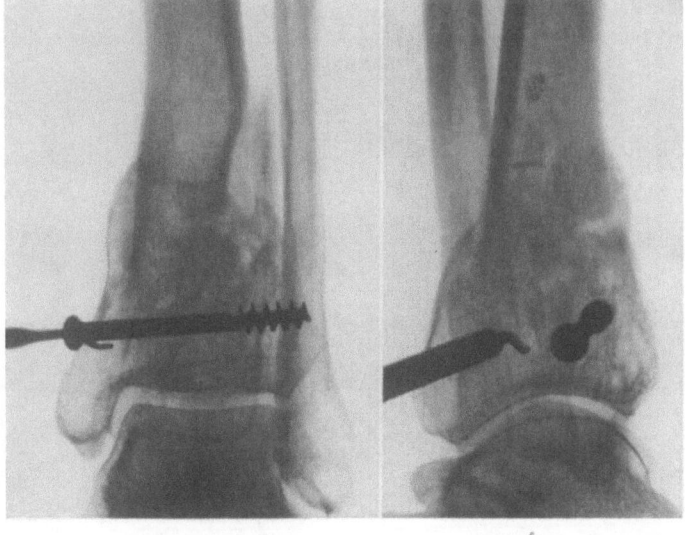

e   f

Fig. 99e and f. Condition at the removal of the metal, 30 weeks postop: functionally almost full recovery. Subjectively without discomfort. (The slight degree of varus deformity is functionally still insignificant, but shows the danger of omitting medial support)

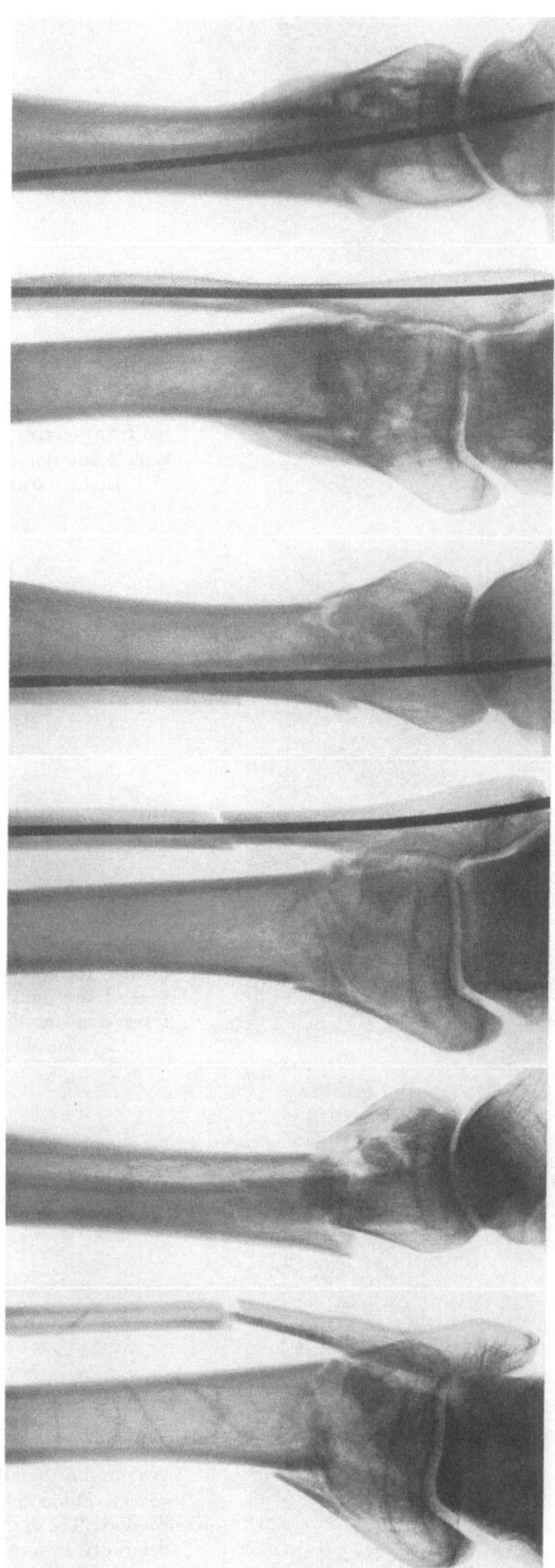

Fig. 100a—f. a and b. Distal comminuted fracture. In Fig. 100b the impacted cortical fragments and the rarefaction of the cancellous bone on the anterior aspect are well visible. As expected, reduction resulted in a large anterior cancellous defect. c and d. Condition immediately after fibular reconstruction and introduction of an extensive cancellous graft. e and f. 33 weeks postop: consolidation with slight varus and backward deformity, full functional recovery of ankle and tarsal joints

= *This case illustrates the two principles of primary fibular reconstruction and primary cancellous grafting. Omission of medial stabilization resulted in secondary varus deformity*

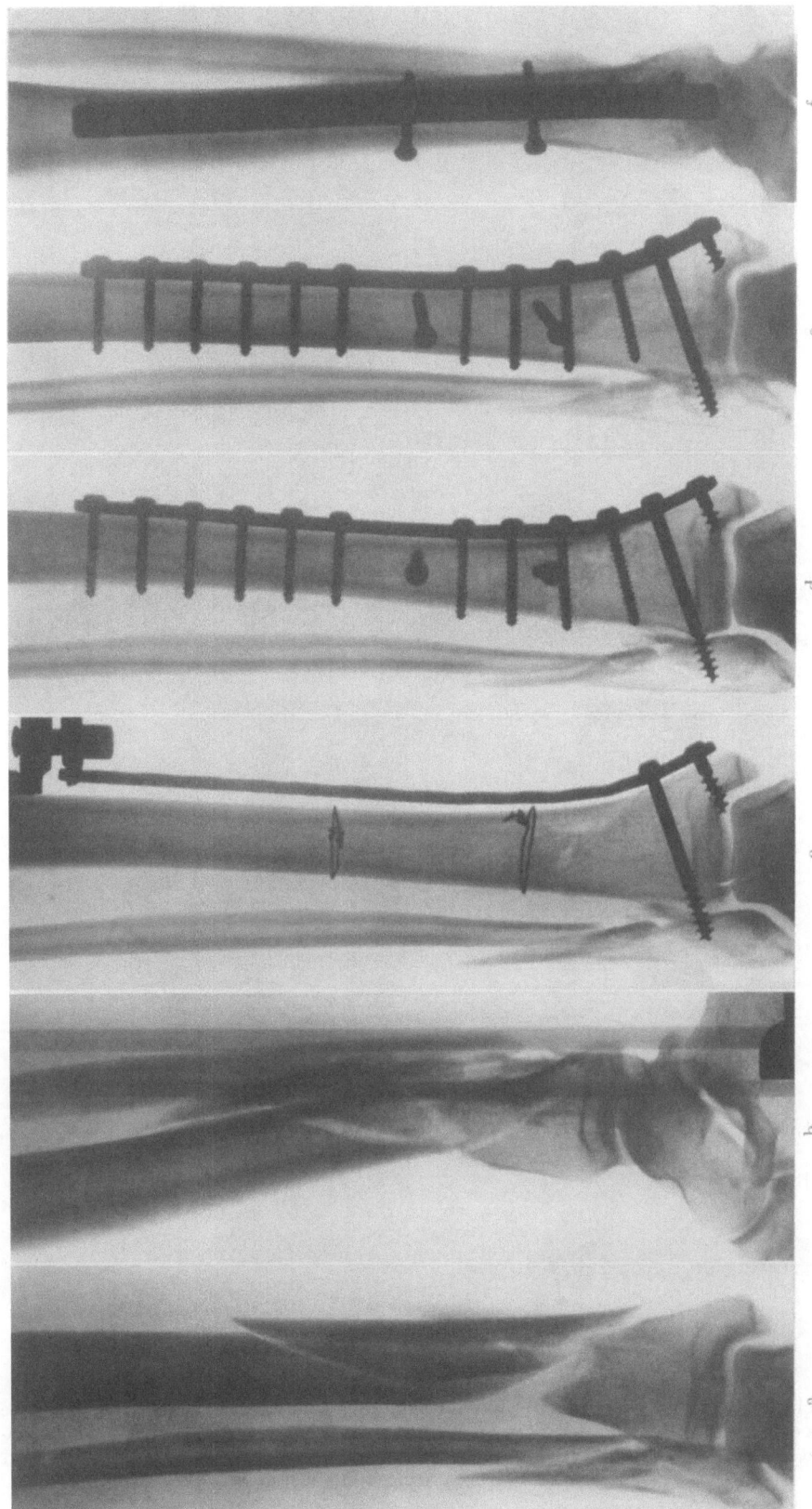

Fig. 101a—f. a and b. Comminuted fracture of lower end of the tibia, fracture lines extending into the joint surface. c Condition after preliminary reduction and insertion of the cancellous graft. Compression of the fracture by long, bent plate. d 1 week postop: Because of the extensive incision medially reconstruction of the fibular fracture was foregone, the lower fibular fragment was partly held by a screw across the tibiofibular joint. e and f. 16 weeks postop: slight diffuse bony atrophy distally, functionally almost back to normal

= For this low tibial fracture, extensive exposure of the medial aspect was considered necessary for the reconstruction and stabilization of the joint surface; as an exception from the rule, the mortise was stabilized from the medial side, primary cancellous graft

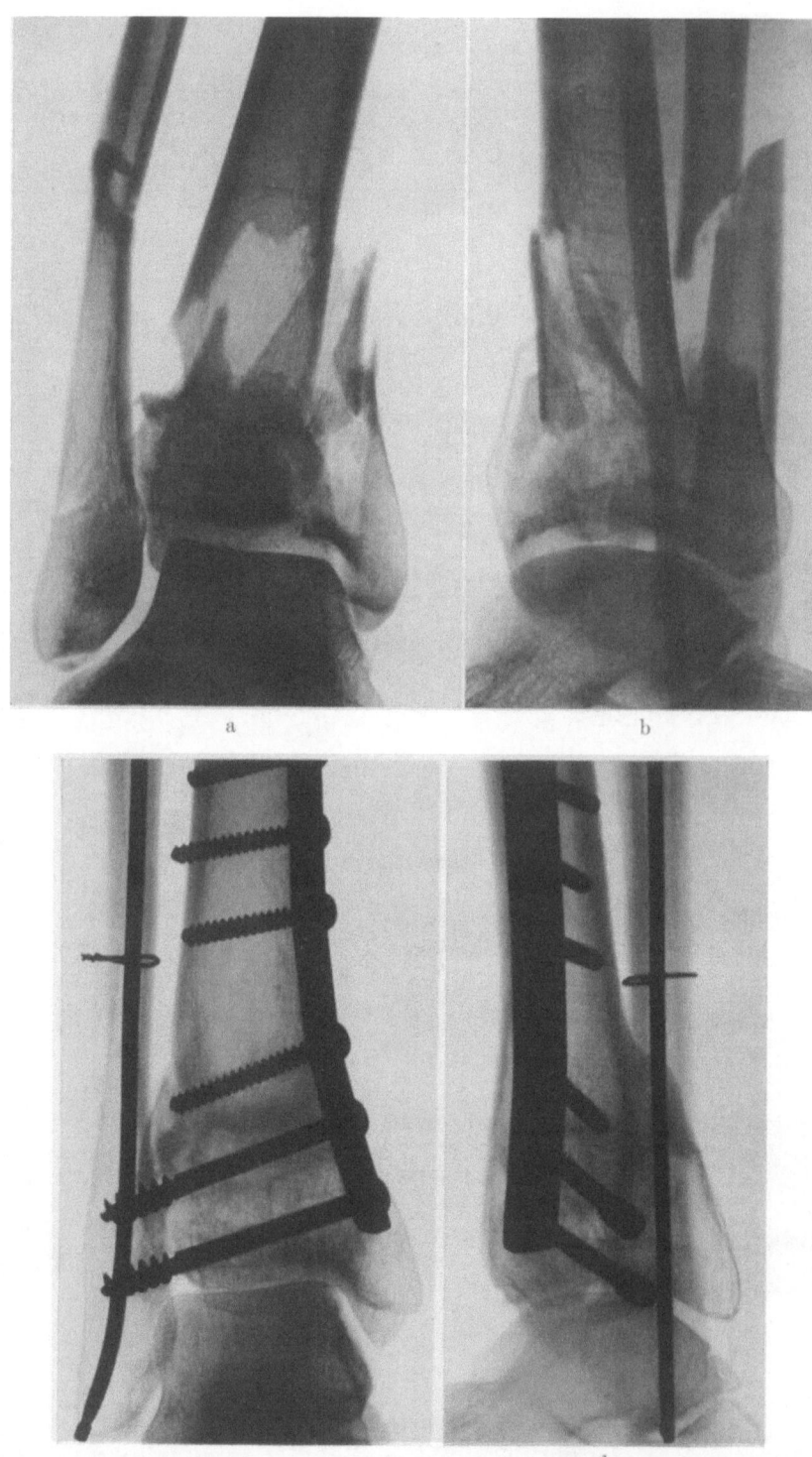

Fig. 102a—d. a and b. Severe comminuted fracture of lower end of tibia with involvement of the joint surface and large cancellous defect. c and d. Condition 28 weeks postop. after primary fixation of the fibula, reconstruction of the joint surface, stabilization from the medial side making use of the fibula, as the tibia offers practically no hold, and extensive primary cancellous graft

= *In spite of minor varus deformity, good result due to the application of the 4 principles of primary fibular reconstruction, reconstruction of the joint surface, medial stabilization, and primary cancellous grafting*

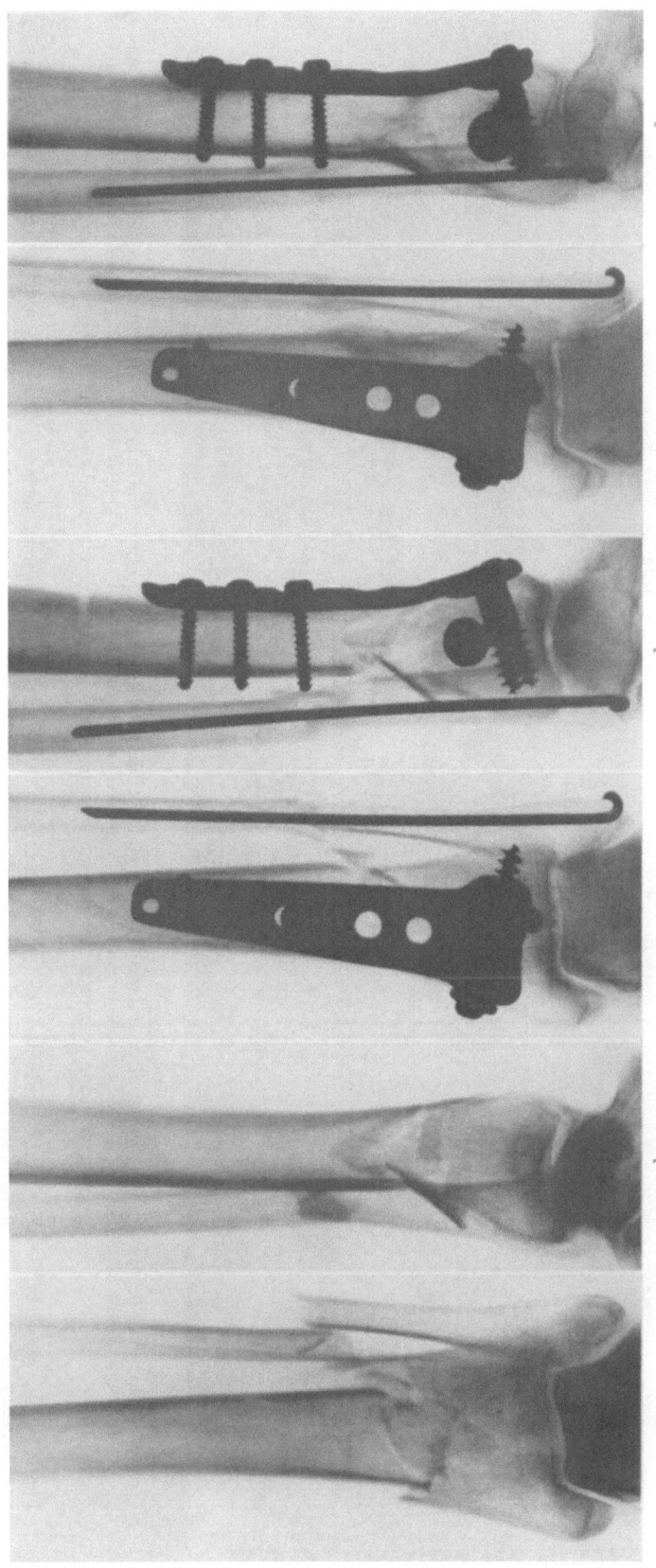

Fig. 103a—f. a and b. Distal transverse fracture of the tibia extending into the joint surface. c and d. Condition immediately after fixation with special T-plate from in front, joint surface successfully stabilized with medial cancellous screws. The T-plate fixes the lower fragment with 2 cancellous screws and thus provides very good stability. Prior fixation of the fibula allows a good reduction of the shortened tibia to be obtained. e and f. 27 weeks postop.: full restoration of function

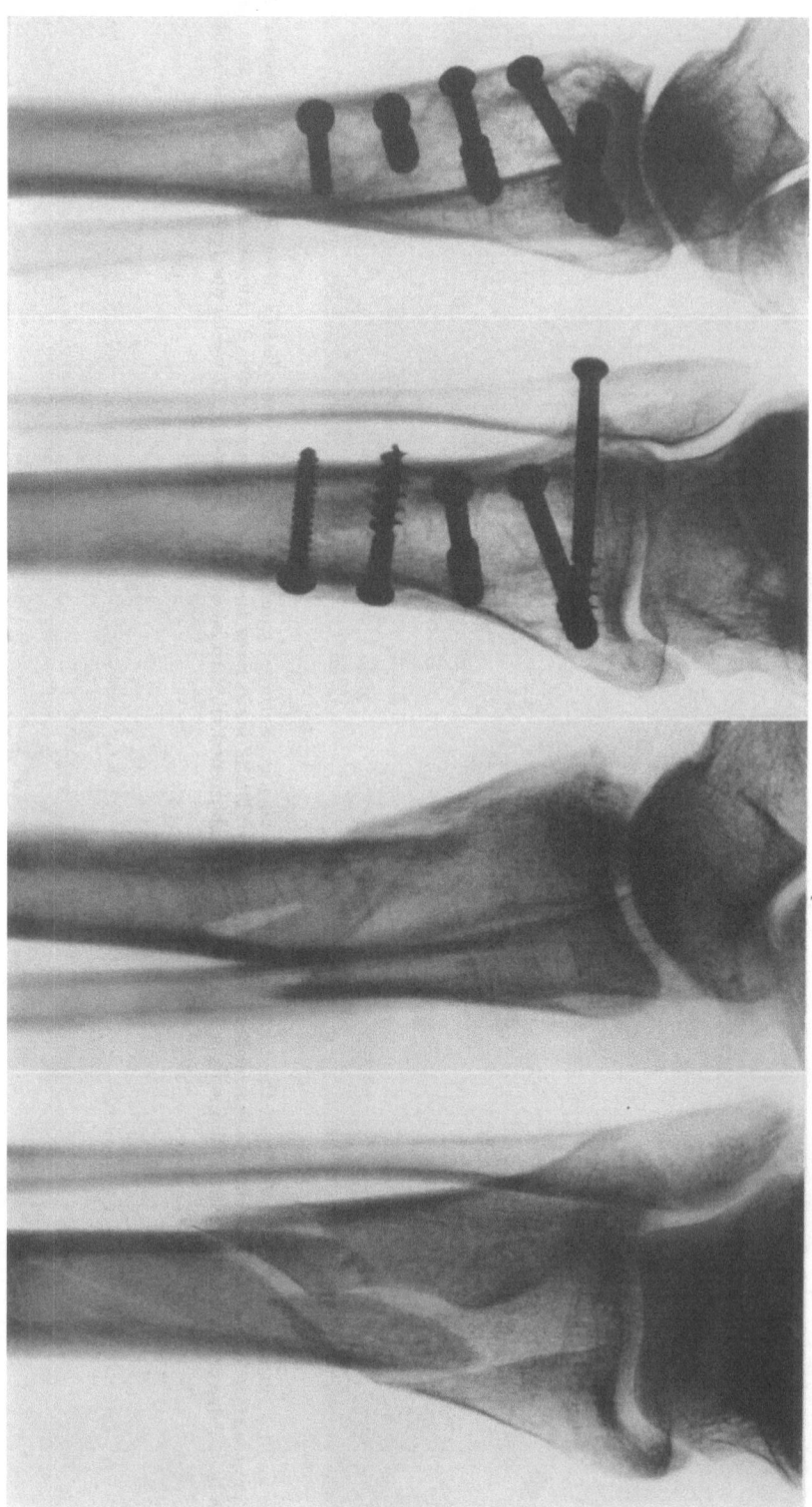

Fig. 104a—d. a and b. Condition 3 weeks after fracture of lower end of tibia with significant gap in the joint surface. c and d. 40 weeks after reconstruction of the distal articular surface by cancellous screws: full restoration of function, condition before screw removal (the screw through the syndesmosis should have been removed 2 months postop. Note area of screw mobility in the fibula)

Fig. 105a—h. a and b. Severe distal comminuted fracture of the tibia with destruction of the joint surface. c and d. Condition immediately postop. after primary fibular reconstruction (because of very narrow medullary cavity, medullary wire only), reconstruction of the joint surface, medial support and cancellous graft. The somewhat inadequate fixation of the medial plate at its upper end is a result of the fact that longer screws gripping the far cortex caused a tilting of the distal joint surface when they were driven home, so that a hemicerclage wire and screw anchoring in one cortex only were used. e and f. 24 weeks postop: severe bony atrophy. The patient could not afford to take care of himself at all, as he was not insured, and while his leg was severely oedematous, he used a walking device and spent hours every day patrolling a mountain district for which he was responsible. g and h. 39 weeks postop: ossification has begun, soft tissues are still somewhat oedematous, but clearly improved, ankle and talar joint still restricted to ²/₃ of their function, improving

= Severe case of fracture of the lower tibia which demonstrates all 4 principles of reconstruction, though with rather little medial support. Jeopardization of the result by very inadequate postoperative treatment due to patient's social condition, as a result of which he continued to work with a severely oedematous leg

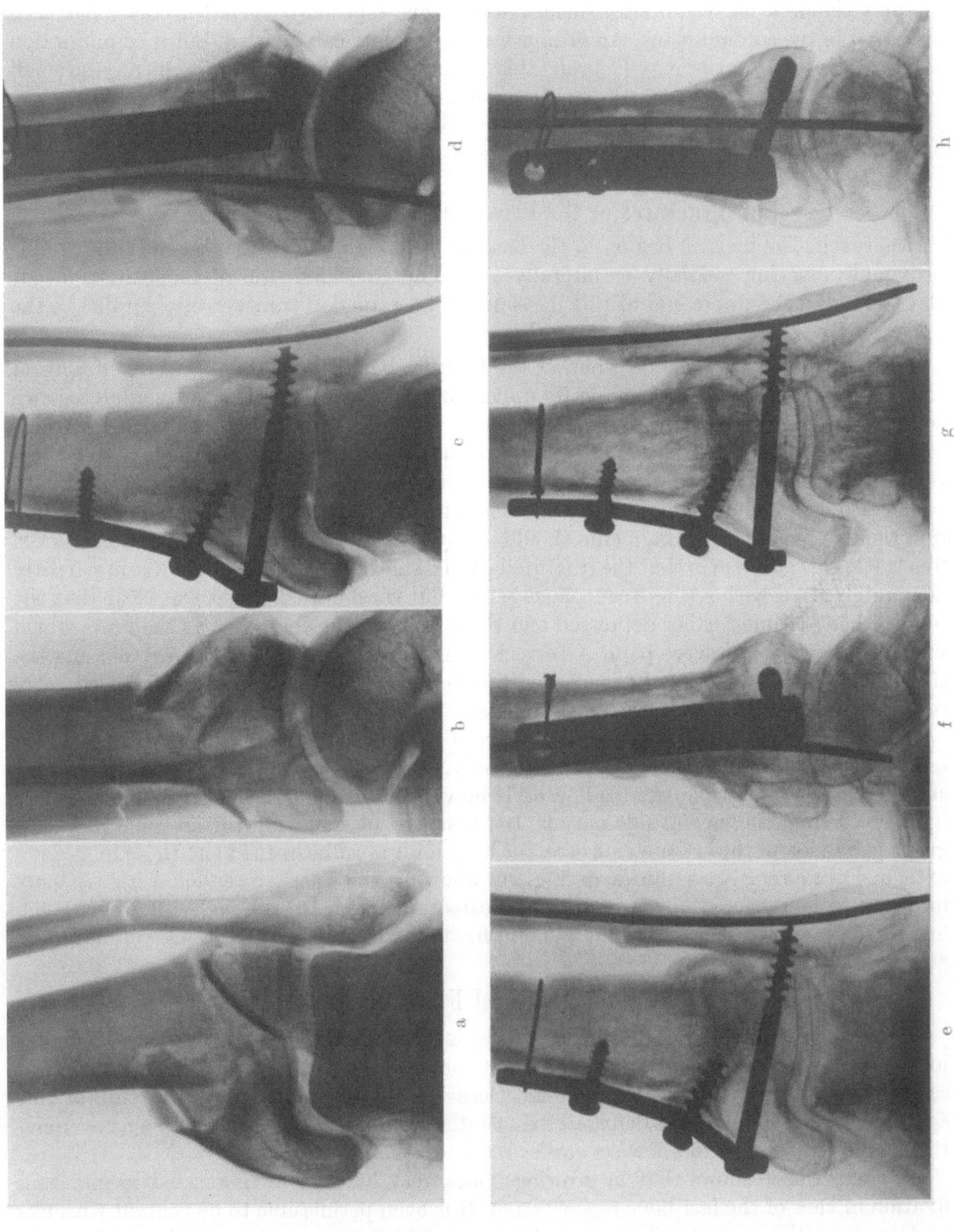

4. Primary autogenous cancellous grafting to fill up the defect in cancellous bone after fracture reduction. When fractures are somewhat above the lower articular surfaces of the tibia it is also useful to pack the medullary canal with cancellous chips taken either from the greater trochanter or from the iliac crest (Figs. 100, 102). Sometimes it may be better to apply the plate on the anterior surface of the tibia, especially where the cortex has been fractured in the coronal plane. An ordinary straight plate can be used, but if comminution is severe a special T-plate may be preferable, especially when the distal fragment is so small that it can only be gripped with one screw of a normal plate (Fig. 103).

Primary arthrodesis of the ankle joint should be reserved for the severest type of case only, most often when there has been associated major damage to the talus.

c) Fractures of the Proximal Quarter of the Tibia

Approach. The incision begins on the crest of the tibia (below the tubercle) and extends proximally curving medially or laterally according to which side of the plateau needs elevating, and the upper end of this incision can be extended transversely, parallel to the upper surface of the tibia if necessary (Fig. 90).

Procedure. This depends on whether the fracture has entered the joint line: Fractures confined to the shaft of the bone in its upper quarter may be dealt with by applying two compression plates, part of the screws anchoring in one cortex only. If the articular surface is involved, problems of fixation are similar to those in the region of the ankle joint. When the tibial plateau is not deformed but simply split or fissured, fixation can be obtained with transverse cancellous screws or sometimes with threaded bolts. To hold the reduction rigidly enough, large fragments should always be fixed at least at two points. Fig. 106 illustrates this problem in that the fractured medial side of the tibial plateau was apparently adequately fixed with a single cancellous screw, but six months later it was clear that the plateau had become further depressed and there was a varus deformity at the knee, which was accompanied by severe pain. A corrective osteotomy was then necessary holding the tibial plateau in a functional position with a massive metal implant. This allowed early restoration of function and removed the pain.

Reconstruction is more difficult when part of the tibial plateau has been depressed and temporary wire pin fixation may be necessary. The aim should be to secure sufficient stability in the rebuilt plateau to allow early movement after operation. An angulated plate introduced from the medial side may be the best way of achieving this in some cases. To give a good view of the articular surface, the knee joint must be opened and the skin incision extended transversely as shown in Fig. 90, allowing the patellar tendon with its bony insertion to be reflected upwards, using an osteotome (Fig. 107). Usually, however, such heroics are not necessary and reduction and fixation with cancellous screws and plates are adequate.

3. Indications for Internal Fixation in Adolescents

Bone healing in a growing lower leg proceeds so rapidly and the danger of permanent joint stiffness after immobilization is so slight that surgery is seldom indicated for medical reasons before the epiphyses have closed. Occasionally an isolated tibial fracture at this age may have so much varus deformity that intervention is advisable, and we have sometimes adopted surgery to allow an earlier return to school.

Our experience shows that in growing bones very little metal is needed to maintain fixation in view of the fast bone regeneration. It is even permissible to be content with less perfect apposition of butterfly fragments than would be accepted in adults, and to use a primary plaster cast. This, however, does not justify using indifferent techniques on growing bone, but it does allow a less than perfect reduction to be accepted since the good blood supply of the periosteum and endosteum will allow early bone regeneration, and callus will often occur so quickly that the rigidity produced by a surgical plate is only needed for a short while.

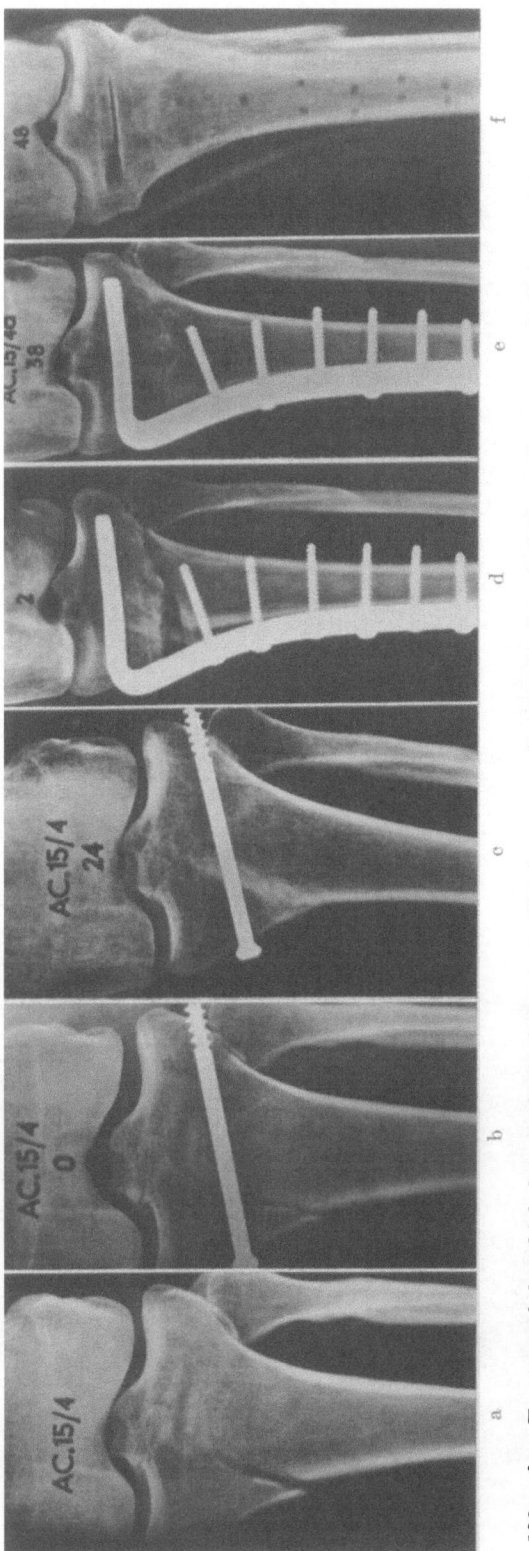

Fig. 106a—f. a Fracture of the tibial plateau. b Condition immediately postop: fixation by one single cancellous screw, slight varus deformity. c 24 weeks postop: significant varus deformity with good bony consolidation and basically satisfactory tibial plateau. Severe pain laterally. d Condition after corrective osteotomy on the medial side (to avoid any loss in length). In spite of massive metal implant, immediate relief of discomfort. e 38 weeks following osteotomy: patient free of pain. f 48 weeks following osteotomy: condition immediately after metal removal, uncomplicated course, patient has no complaints
= *Seemingly "elegant internal fixation using little metal" proves to be inadequate in preventing secondary displacement. A large implant properly applied causes no reaction and results in full functional recovery*

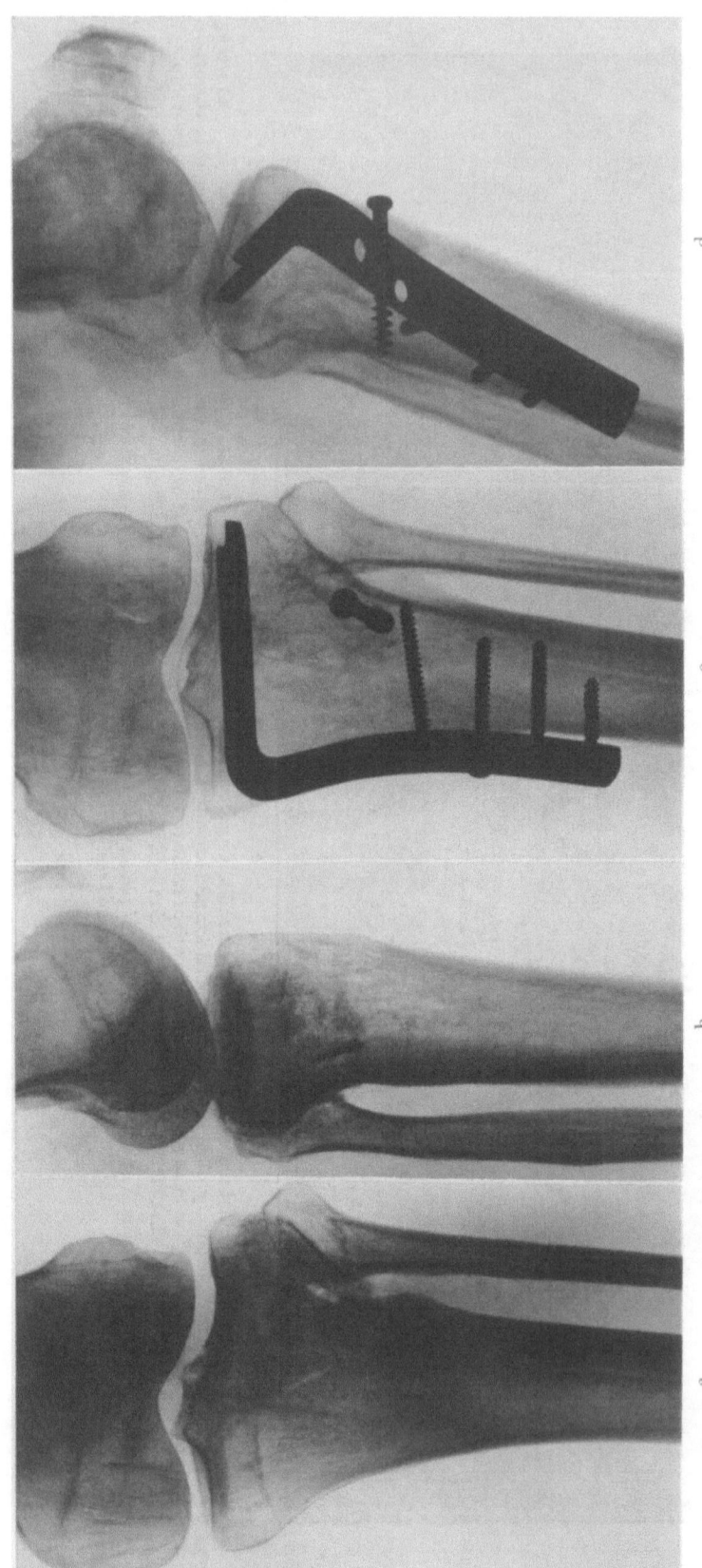

a   b   c   d

Fig. 107a—d. a and b. Comminution of the lateral tibial plateau by outward bending of the body while the position of lower leg was fixed. Depression of the plateau does not show well in the x-ray. c and d. Appearance 18 weeks after reconstruction of the lateral plateau with the patellar tendon turned upwards (temporary resection of the tibial tuberosity). Function: extension full, flexion to 80°

= Example of the use of an angulated plate to support a depressed tibial plateau, immediate postoperative mobilization of a high tibial fracture involving the joint

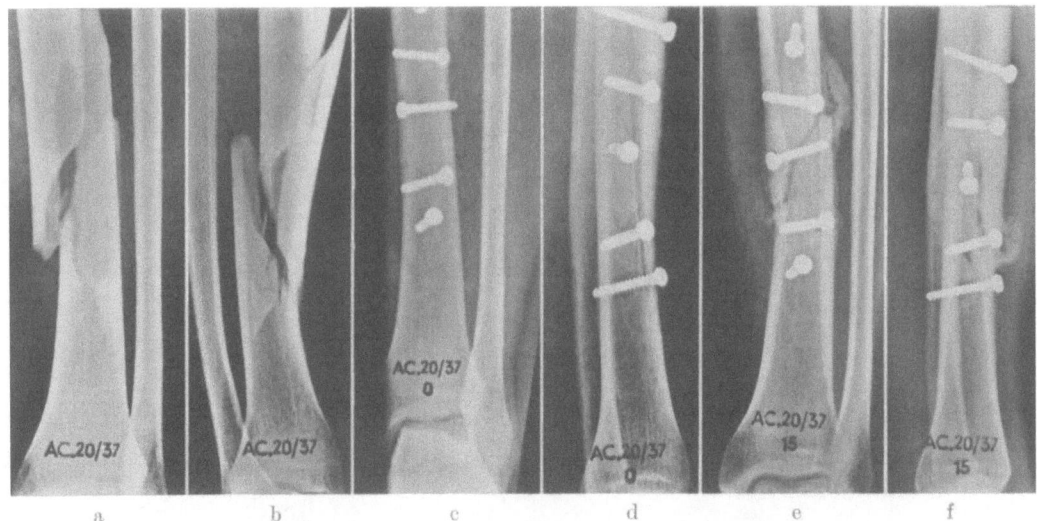

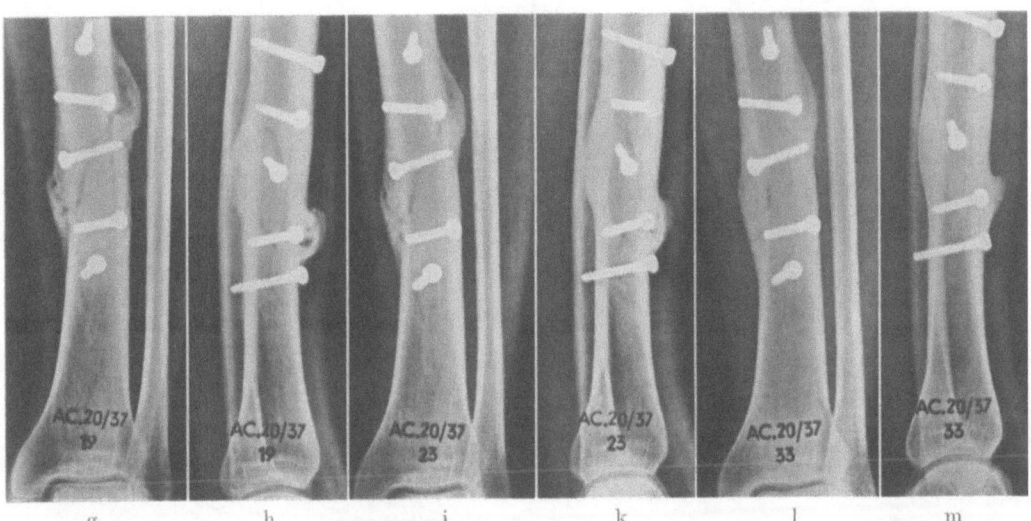

Fig. 108a—m. a and b. Butterfly fracture with additional splinters and poor contact between the two main fragments. c and d. Condition immediately after screw fixation, the screw between the main fragments has been placed very close to the fracture line. e and f. Condition 15 weeks after screwing, with early axial bending and extensive irritation callus as a sign of significant instability. Basically, indication for removal of the screws and corrective fixation with a medullary nail. g—m. Increasing transformation of irritation into fixation callus, with strictly enforced non weight bearing. Healing in a position of slight varus deformity

= *Disturbed fracture healing in a case unsuitable for screw fixation*

4. Soft Tissue Considerations in Timing Operations for Tibial Fractures

Whenever possible we operate within six to twelve hours after a fracture, before the maximal posttraumatic swelling has occurred. When for some reason surgery is impossible within this period, we delay operation until the swelling is subsiding, between the third and sixth day after the accident. When there is extensive contusion of the skin, or fracture blisters, we delay operation for a full week. By this time the condition of the skin usually will safely tolerate even major surgery. Disregard of the soft tissues will jeopardize chances of success in any internal fixation techniques and may bring them into disrepute.

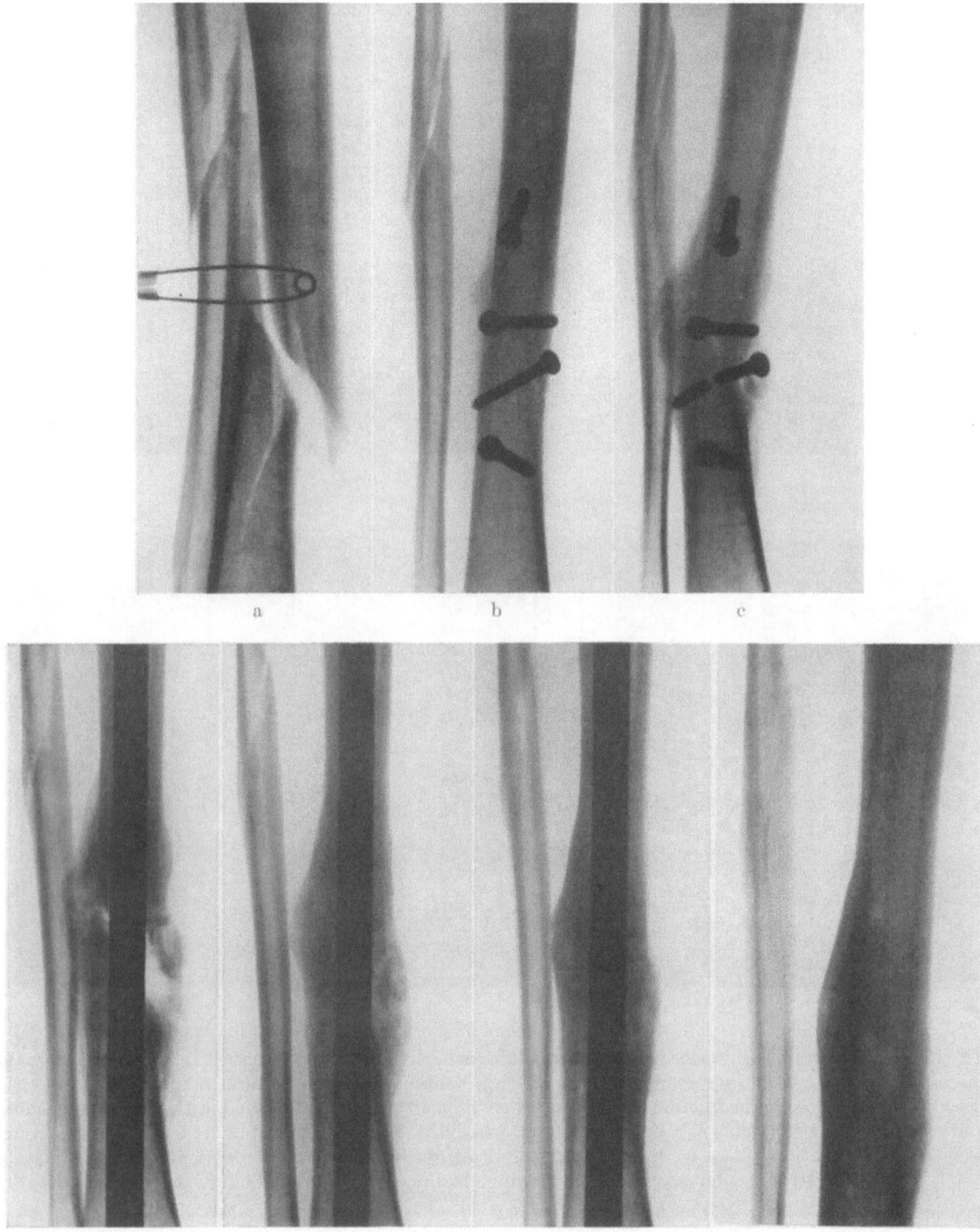

Fig. 109a—g. a Butterfly fracture with relatively short main fracture line. b Condition 11 weeks after screwing, with only 2 screws across the short fracture line. Irritation callus forming, interpreted by the doctor as a sign of union so that the patient was allowed to subject the leg to full weight bearing. c 20 weeks postop: significant formation of irritation callus. Axial bending, screw breakage, and pseudarthrosis. d—g Appearance after screw removal, reaming and internal stabilization with 12 mm. medullary nail. Rapid consolidation in the area of the pseudarthrosis. Hospitalization for 10 days, full weight bearing 8 weeks after medullary nailing

= *Appearance of irritation callus is always a sign of significant instability and, in fractures following internal fixation, is never a sign to allow weight bearing, but rather demands strict non-weight bearing. Once the development of a pseudarthrosis has begun, it should not be treated by lengthy immobilization and transplantation of bone grafts. Internal fixation with a medullary nail, or with compression plates very rapidly leads to the desired goal while allowing early postoperative mobilization*

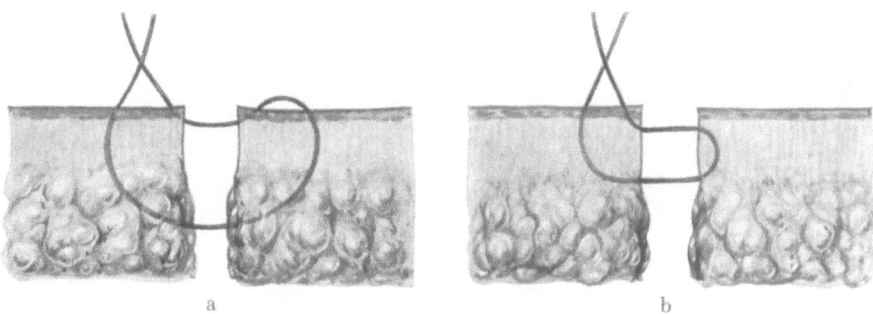

Fig. 110a and b. a DONATI's skin suture. b Subcutaneous modification of DONATI's suture: only the dermis layer is sutured

5. Technical Details in the Care of the Soft Tissues

Many surgeons are wary of internal fixation for fractures in the lower leg because of difficulties in securing good wound healing. Soft tissues of the lower leg, and especially the skin, have a relatively poor blood supply. Skin heals with less trouble and more quickly in places where the capillary net is dense. Long experience has shown that sutures on the face and neck may be removed between the second and fifth day without danger of wound dehiscence. After the same period a wound on the lower leg would open even under the slightest stress, so that tissue care is nowhere more important than in the lower leg.The need for traumatizing retraction which causes necrosis is avoided if long incisions are made here.

The technique of wound closure is also most important for smooth healing. The problem begins with the periosteum. On a growing bone, a well vascularized layer of periosteum may by seen detached from the bone and this can easily be sutured back, but a similar condition in an adult is exceptional, and it makes little sense to try to cover the bone in the middle third of the tibia with severly traumatized avascular periosteum. The growth potential of this adult periosteum is extremely low as previous attempts at growing it in tissue culture have shown (ALLGÖWER and ROSIN, 1953). It seems probable that under these circumstances bone establishes contact with surrounding blood vessels more quickly when immediately covered by well vascularized subcutaneous tissue, than when devitalised periosteum consisting almost entirely of collagen is interposed. In the middle third of the lower leg we use only a few subcutaneous sutures and close the skin itself with DONATI's delicate skin stitches (Fig. 110). Frequently we use cutaneous sutures by themselves. In the rare possibility of a tension free periosteal suture in an adult, the Redon drain must be introduced to prevent any hematoma forming in the subperiosteal or subcutaneous layers. The peroneal muscle sheath is preserved as carefully as possible during the whole operation, but if it has to be incised, or the fracture has already caused a muscle hernia, reconstruction of this compartment should be attempted. To this end the periosteum is left attached when ever possible to the anterior crest of the bone, and the peroneal muscular compartment is entered 2 to 3 mm. lateral from this crest.

In the lower third of the leg the medial surface of the tibia is covered by a thicker layer of connective tissue formed partly by the periosteum and partly by a forward extension of the fascia covering the peronei. This is strong enough to allow reconstruction of the sheath of the extensor muscles which may have been opened; it is important to close this sheath, and if the periosteum has been properly incised, closure will provide no difficulty.

Very fine material should be used for skin suture and forceps should not be used because of their traumatic effect on the skin edge. A suture of DONATI is usually indicated, but for better cosmesis we prefer an intracutaneous suture (Fig. 110b). Where there is much skin tension very fine sutures are required, inserted only 1 to 2 mm. from the edge of the wound and including epidermis and dermis only.

7*

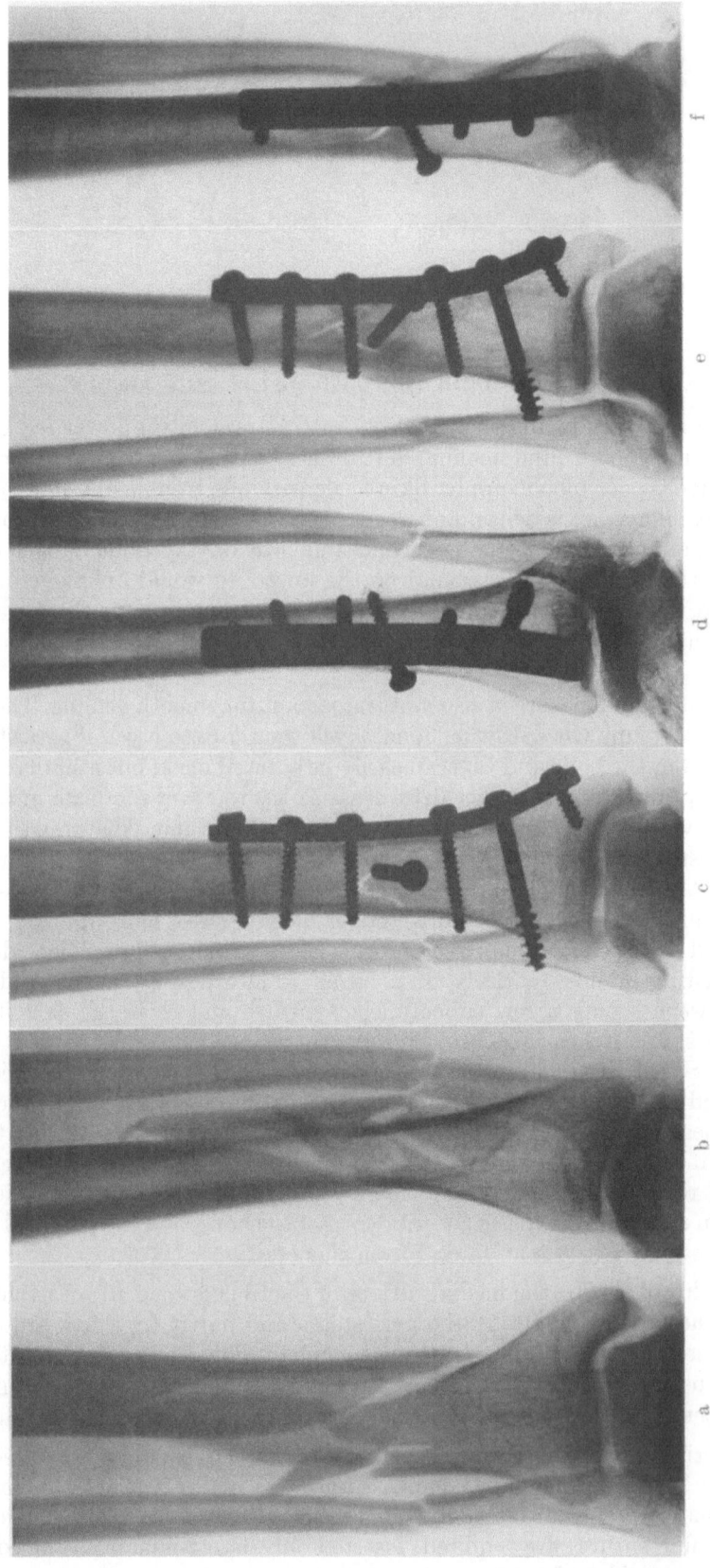

Fig. 111a—f. a and b. Comminuted fracture of the lower end of the tibia. c and d. Internal fixation with bent 6-hole plate and perpendicular screw. e and f. Condition 17 weeks after fixation: sharply defined, prognostically favourable fixation callus in the middle of the fracture region. Full restoration of function

= *The appearance of well-defined callus is evidence that nature has successfully overcome a minor instability*

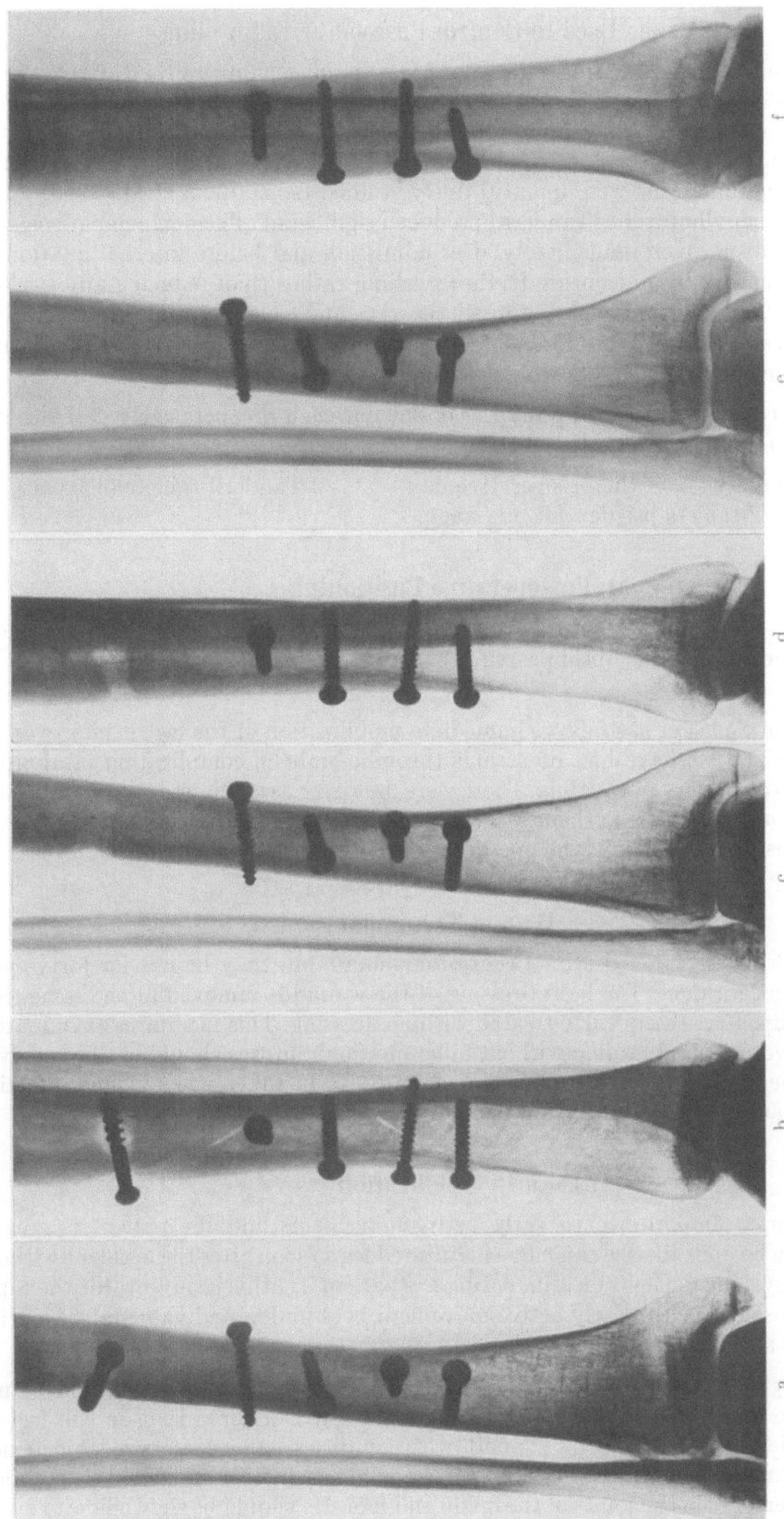

Fig. 112a—f. a and b. Condition after screw fixation of a fracture of the lower leg; infection in the area of the uppermost screw with resorption zones around the screw; screw removal. c and d. Condition 13 weeks after screw removal, filling of the bone defect. e and f. 53 weeks postop.: Resorption zone entirely bridged; elsewhere consolidation without visible callus formation

= Osteolytic zones are generally the manifestation of a latent infection in the area of the foreign object

6. Postoperative Treatment of Lower Leg Fractures

a) Drugs Used to Control Postoperative Swelling

Postoperative swelling interferes with wound healing and hampers the early return to normal of muscles and joints. The swelling that immediately follows trauma is almost exclusively due to a fracture haematoma (CLARKE, 1957, GANZONI, 1959). For about two days this swelling increases as a result of increased capillary permeability in the injured tissues. Various detumescens were quantitatively studied (ALLGÖWER et al., 1963) and it was found that Phenylbutazone (Tanderil) produced significant effects in comparison with placebos, especially if given immediately after admission and before internal fixation. It seemed to work chiefly by preventing further swelling rather than reducing any swelling already present. We have therefore adopted the pre- and postoperative use of Phenyl-butazone in all cases submitted to limb surgery, except for those that have received anti-coagulants before surgery. The following dosage is used:

a) emergencies — 2 Tanderil suppositories of 250 mg. each preoperatively, 2×2 coated tablets (400 mg.) for six days postoperatively;

b) elective surgery — on the preoperative day — 3×2 Tanderil tablets (600 mg.) and after surgery 2×2 tablets per day for one week.

b) Postoperative Positioning

To combat swelling and accelerate wound healing, the patient should rest in bed until the postoperative swelling has disappeared, i.e. for about four days with the injured leg elevated 60 cm.

The absence of a plaster cast allows immediate mobilization of the leg; it improves the patient's morale and we have had no serious thrombo-embolic complication in approximately 700 cases of surgery of the tibia. There were, however, two minor cases of embolism. When such a complication is anticipated we administer dicoumarin-derivative preparations intravenously on the day of the operation.

c) Wound Treatment

The Redon drain is removed after twenty-four hours, but may be left for forty-eight hours if drainage continues. The light dressing of the wound is removed at the same time and the wound itself is subsequently treated with no dressing. This facilitates examination and seems to favour wound healing without inflammation. Sutures should not be removed from the lower leg until the twelfth day. The measures to be taken when wound infection actually occurs are discussed in the Supplement (Chapters 2 and 3).

d) Early Mobilization

We attach great importance to **early active movements** and the patient is greatly encouraged when he finds that he can move his injured leg so soon after the accident without discomfort. Everything depends on stimulating the patient's enthusiasm towards the rapid recovery of full use of his leg. Early active movement is of undoubted value in preventing permanent joint stiffness.

Physiotherapy is begun between twelve and twenty-four hours after operation. First of all, before the first movement is attempted, the patient is assured that he will feel no pain, then the leg is lifted from its support with gentle assistance, followed by flexion exercises at the knee. The patient soon gains some confidence in his leg and will then undertake active movements in the joints of the ankle and foot. He should be shown how to dorsiflex and plantarflex his foot as well as inverting, everting and rotating it. These foot exercises should be carried out with the knee flexed to 60° to relax the calf muscles. It is important that no pain is caused and any false heroism should be discouraged. Between the fourth and the sixth day the patient may get out of bed. At this point a slight reactionary swelling is often noticed which should be used to remind the patient that during the next few weeks, he must elevate his legs often. After eight to ten days the ankle and subtalar joints are usually fully mobile.

e) Cast Support, Walking Caliper or no External Fixation

During the first week after surgery no outside support is provided except in those cases where it is found impossible to provide rigid internal fixation for badly comminuted fractures involving joints. These patients are fitted with a double U-splint in which they can practice dorsiflexion of the foot. All other patients are encouraged to exercise the foot and knee freely in their Braun's frame during the first week. After the eighth day a choice may be made between three forms of management.

External support. In cases without good fixation between two main fragments (e.g. in those where only a butterfly fragment is joining the main fragments together, or in difficult comminuted fractures), a cast is provided up to the knee in fractures of the lower third and mid-shaft, and up to the mid-thigh in upper third fractures. For the lower leg we use "Plexidon", which is a bandage of synthetic material. It provides a light, but very firm waterproof cast which is permeable to x-rays. This is left in place for ten to twelve weeks unless it becomes loose and has to be changed. After its removal the joints which were exercised energetically immediately after surgery, regain their normal function within a few days. It is quite clear, however, that joints and soft tissues do less well in comparison with cases where no cast is used.

Walking caliper. A walking device in which the weight is taken by the upper end of the tibia allows active movements to be carried out until consolidation has occurred, preventing any weight from being transmitted through the fracture. It also provides a certain amount of protection if the patient should slip because the stirrup, and not his foot touches the ground. Many of our patients quickly learn to walk in this caliper without using crutches, and housewives particularly appreciate the help it gives them by leaving their hands free. Several of our nurses who had tibial fractures found that they could resume partial duty after five weeks with the use of this caliper.

Description and Directions for Use of Röck's Below-knee Walking Caliper

1. This device is intended for use during the postoperative management of fractures of the lower leg and ankle treated by internal fixation. As it is both stabilizing and weight relieving, it obviates the need for any plaster cast (Fig. 113).

This caliper may also be used in conservative management to replace a walking cast after traction has been discontinued. Its advantages over a simple walking cast are as follows:

--- It is removable at night;
— It is washable;
— Adjustments are easily made.
— It can be worn with normal outdoor shoes.

From the surgeons point of view it is helpful in allowing constant observation of the wound and increased movement of the joints. It is available with a detachable thigh piece for use in higher fractures (Fig. 113 b).

2. **Construction.** Röck's *caliper* consists of the following parts:

a) A half shell fitting the calf made of thermoplastic material; in the "*export model*" this has a washable leatherette lining, in the *standard model* a felt lining. On the outside are four clips adjustable to five different tensions, additional adjustment being possible on the opposite side where straps are fitted with round-headed screws.

b) In front are a knee cap and a lower shin cap, both padded, fixed with adjustable straps.

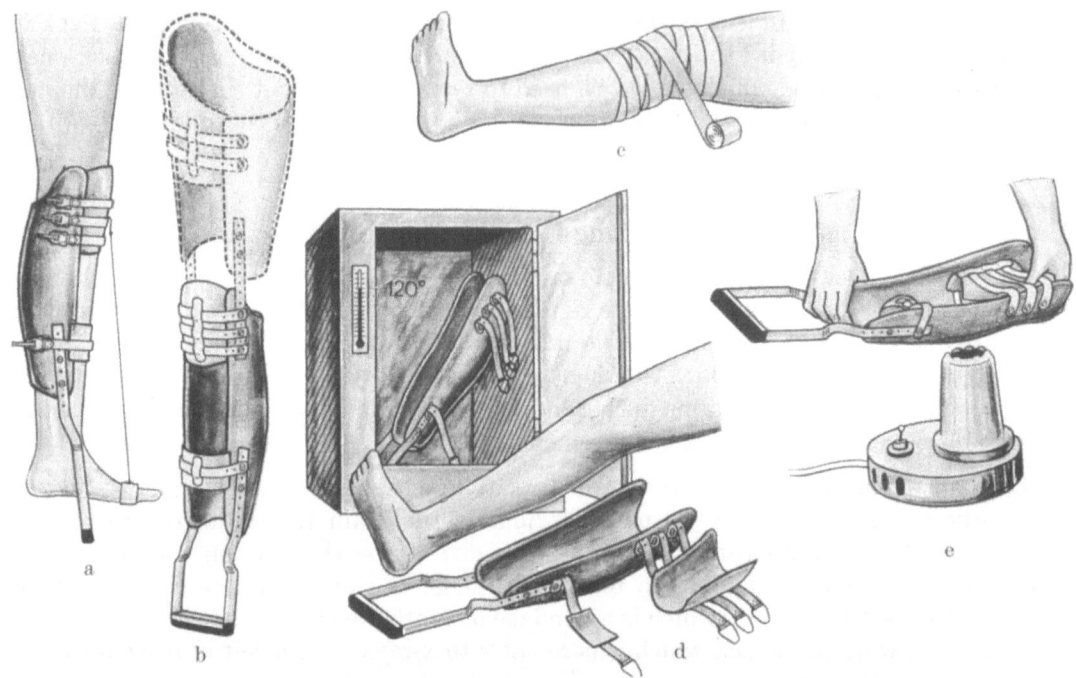

Fig. 113 a—e. Walking caliper

c) A walking iron which can be fixed at five different heights with an exchangeable block of hard rubber at the bottom. The side bars are so arranged as to allow a relatively normal gait. The adjustments extend from 5 to 15 mm. and are made on both sides with screws having hexagonal socket heads.

3. Directions for use. a) The first fitting should be done by a member of the hospital staff experienced in the procedure. Afterwards the patient can take his caliper off and replace it himself.

b) Röck's calipers come in four different sizes. Size 1 for a calf circumference of 30 to 34 cm., size 2 for a calf circumference of 34 to 38 cm., size 3 for a calf circumference of 38 to 42 cm., size 4 for a calf circumference of 42 to 45 cm.

c) Before fitting, the knee is bandaged with an elastic bandage as shown in Fig. 113 c. The right-sized shell is then fitted on the calf.

d) If any alteration in shape or size is needed, the shell can be placed in an incubator or sterilizer and heated to 120° centigrade. This softens the plastic so that it can be adapted to the form of the calf and allowed to harden (Fig. 113 d).

e) These standard sizes, however, have been selected so that little if any correction is needed. Local alteration in shape can be obtained by warming with the Röck-Horo-Electric heater which can be plugged into any 220 volt outlet (see Fig. e).

f) When the whole shell has to be heated to make it fit, it must be handled with gloves. To fit it with the right rotation an oblique box or block of wood may be placed distal to the patient's foot (Fig. f).

g) After fitting the calf shell, the walking iron is adjusted to the right length. To do this the four screws are loosened with the hexagonal key, the walking iron placed in the right position and then screwed up tight (see Fig. g).

h) When the fitting is complete, the patient tests it by walking. The clips may be re-adjusted until an optimal fit has been obtained and the patient can then put on a slipper or outdoor shoe.

Any equinus position can be corrected with a toe spring or a Plexidur scoop splint (Figs. h and i).

i) The patient may wear normal street clothing while using his caliper and carry out his normal occupation. *When walking he must be careful to put his foot down with the leg straight and to roll his weight forward.* This requires a little practice, but he soon gets used to it (Fig. k).

k) When the rubber thread on the bottom of the walking iron gets worn down it can be replaced. To do this the split pin is removed, the rubber block slid out sideways and a new one inserted. The split pin can then be re-inserted (see Fig. l).

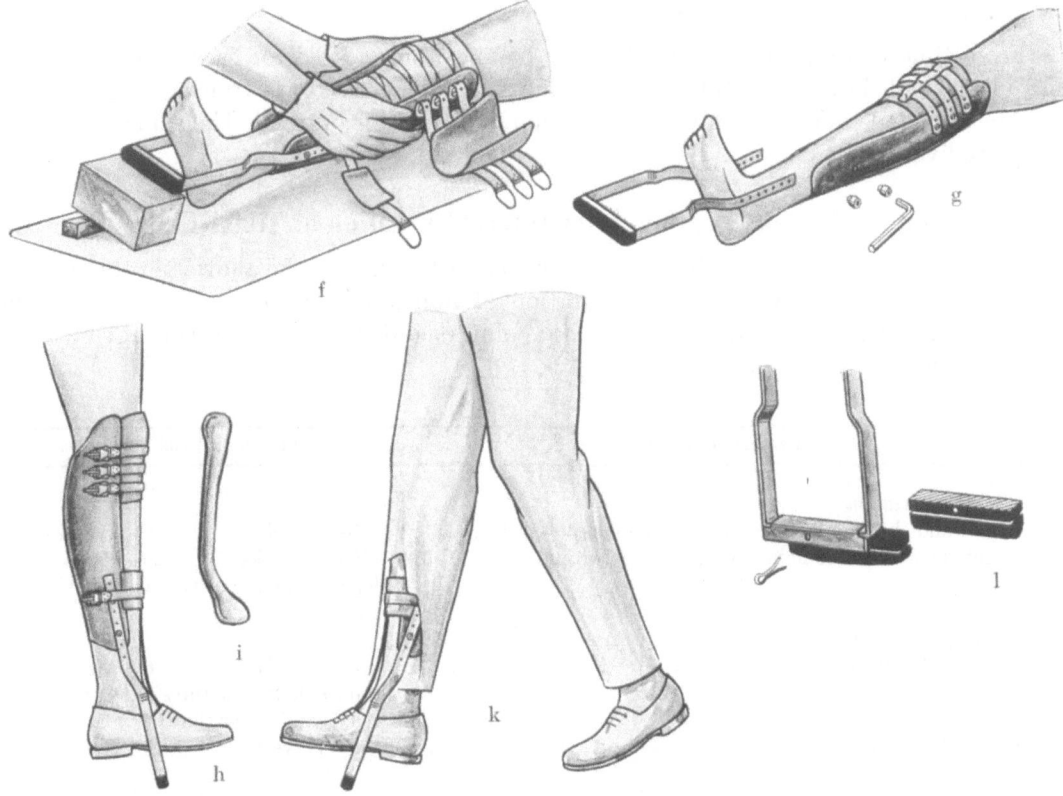

Fig. 113f—l. Walking caliper

Where an efficient orthopaedic appliance service is available, the plastic shells for the calf may be made individually. The caliper described here satisfies most people and many patients can devise small improvisations to give them comfort at pressure points. Even elderly patients and especially housewives have learned to use this caliper, and it can be said that quite two-thirds of the patients expressed their preference for this form of support over a cast. One third could not cope with it because of pain caused by pressure, e.g. in fractures of the neck of the fibula, or because of difficulty with balance. One third of the patients felt so good at using the caliper that their gait became almost normal. We treated a frontier guard, for example, who carried out his duties walking about in the mountains with his caliper for hours without any complaints. Careful fitting and correct instructions about walking are important, and patients must be shown how to extend their knee fully before putting weight on it. If the caliper is worn for too long, swelling may occur and this must also be pointed out to the patient. He should also be told to spend at least part of the day out of the caliper with the leg elevated.

Postoperative management without plaster cast and without caliper. Where it has been possible to obtain very rigid fixation, using a plate firmly secured to both main fragments by screws, or where the medullary nail traverses a transverse fracture line, it may be possible to do without either a walking plaster or a caliper if the patient cannot master the use of the latter. The surgeon also prefers to forego the use of a plaster cast where the soft tissues have doubtful vitality.

Patients in whom the tibia has been treated with screws or plates producing rigid fixation, very soon regain the feeling of having a normal leg. This may tempt them to try premature weight bearing without their caliper. If there is any doubt as to the patient's willingness or ability to co-operate, a more cautious method such as the use of a cast, should be advocated for the first eight to twelve weeks.

From time to time early weight bearing has been advocated for cases treated with a medullary nail, but this should only be allowed if the fracture is transverse or a short oblique one, and even then only if the position of the nail is optimal. The same holds true for plate fixation.

f) Time to Weight Bearing After Internal Fixation of Tibial Fractures

It is difficult to generalize about how soon weight bearing can be allowed in these cases. The following general rules for the duration of non-weight bearing are given on the understanding that they are only prognostic pointers and should be critically reviewed on each occasion.

Fracture and Treatment	Partial Weight Bearing at	Full Weight Bearing at
Medullary nail fixation		
Transverse and short oblique fractures in the middle third . . .	3—4 weeks	6—8 weeks
Comminuted fractures (combined with cerclage wiring)	10—20 weeks	20—30 weeks
	(depending state of vascularity of the fragments)	
Internal fixation with a plate		
Transverse and short oblique fractures	3—6 weeks	6—8 weeks
	(applicable for fractures in the mid-shaft and lower third)	
Comminuted fractures	8—12 weeks	10—20 weeks
Internal fixation using screws only or screws in combination with short plates		
Torsions fractures	6—8 weeks	10—12 weeks
Butterfly fractures	10—14 weeks	14—20 weeks

The surgeon who controls postoperative management, however, should rely chiefly on clinical indications and as soon as weight bearing is begun the following symptoms and signs are looked for:

Pain. Pain during the first six months after operation is seldom caused by metal corrosion, but mostly by resorption processes in the fracture area. Consequently, removing the metal is almost never indicated — what is required is weight relief. Pain localized at a fracture site is a definite danger signal; if it is only in the instep or the forefoot, some weight bearing may be allowed, but an arch support is often advisable. Sometimes a screw may be mechanically irritating a tendon or other soft tissue structure.

Localized warmth. Warmth over the fracture should always be regarded as indicating a deeper inflammatory process and sometimes a latent infection. Warmth and reddening are an absolute indication for taking the patient off his feet altogether and giving full bed rest until the symptoms have subsided. Putting the joints through an active range of movement, however, is still continued.

Swelling. This occurs particularly when the patient resumes his normal activities and instead of lying down frequently, he takes to sitting with his leg elevated, which flexes the hip joint. Swelling may also be the result of standing for too long and sometimes from using the walking caliper too much. Some swelling is often unavoidable, but the patients must be urged to try to prevent it by elevating their leg whenever possible. They must also be reminded about the correct bandaging of the leg.

When any of the above signs appear, x-rays should be taken to study the bone healing.

g) The Use of X-Rays in Assessing the Progress of Bone Healing[1]

The x-ray findings during the healing period of fractures treated by internal fixation differ in several ways from those in fractures treated conservatively. Ideally, bone healing proceeds in internally fixed fractures with little or no callus formation that can be seen on x-ray. This "primary bone healing" occurs when rigidly fixed fragments are maintained in apposition to each other with exact precision, as long as the blood supply of both fragments remains intact or is soon restored via the Haversian canals. When we began to treat fractures of the shaft of the tibia by rigid fixation, primary union occurred in 30% of 112 fractures (CORRODI, 1962). A later series of 188 fractures of the tibia however, gave a primary bone union rate of over 60%. This shows that if the correct biomechanical procedure is used, primary bone healing is the rule rather than the exception. Any deviation from the usual pattern of primary bone union must be regarded as a possibly serious danger signal.

Radiography is recommended after six, twelve and sixteen weeks. Films taken at sixteen weeks are of special importance as a majority of cases are by this time radiologically healed and do not need to be examined further until the time comes for removing the metal implants. When union has not occurred or has broken down, x-rays taken at twelve or sixteen weeks usually show this clearly, so that appropriate steps can be taken without any further delay.

Ideally, the fracture lines are almost invisible on the x-ray taken immediately after internal fixation. From this point on, the x-ray signs of fracture lines may follow one of two courses. They may disappear completely within eight to twelve weeks (as occurs in two thirds of tibial fractures), an indication that the fracture may be considered fully capable of normal weight bearing. In others, however, the fracture lines become more easily seen, which is the beginning of a process regarded by BÖHLER as practically inevitable in all fractures, being the sign of demarcation and subsequent osteolytic re-absorption of 5 to 6 mm. of the ends of fractured bones. When the fracture lines become more obvious the warning should be accepted that the fracture must be protected from any mechanical strain. This does not mean, however, that active movement apart from weight bearing should be discontinued. Bone resorption at the fracture site is usually most pronounced between eight and ten weeks after surgery, and after this the fracture lines may disappear again without any radiological evidence of periosteal or endosteal callus, as long as the fracture has not been submitted to weight bearing up to this time. Usually, however, some callus formation becomes visible in the vicinity the of fracture lines that have become more clear over the weeks, especially when strict avoidance of weight bearing has not been enforced. This callus formation in our experience is always a sign of imperfect fixation of the fracture.

We differentiate between two types of callus formation. The first we call "irritation callus" and the second "fixation callus". *"Irritation callus"* shows up as a cloudy ill-defined mass which is the bony reaction to instability at the fracture site, and this urgently needs complete relief from weight bearing (Figs. 108a to f). If a case with this appearance is firmly relieved of weight bearing, in three to four weeks the callus changes into *"fixation callus"* with clearly defined boundaries and a homogeneous structure (Figs. 108g to m). When this has occurred, weight bearing may be resumed.

If the formation of "irritation callus" is not recognized, and treated appropriately (Figs. 109a to c) the bone may bend at the fracture site and this may result in a pseudarthrosis. Even when this occurs the principle of active mobilization must not be abandoned as a nonunion following simple screwing may be treated by internal fixation with a medullary nail or by a compression plate without much detriment to the patient (Figs. 109d to g).

Well demarcated callus formation may be called actual *"fixation callus"*. The development of this shows that the callus itself has overcome any further tendency to movement.

---

[1] Together with C. WIESER, M. D., Head of the Dept. of Radiology, Kantonsspital Chur.

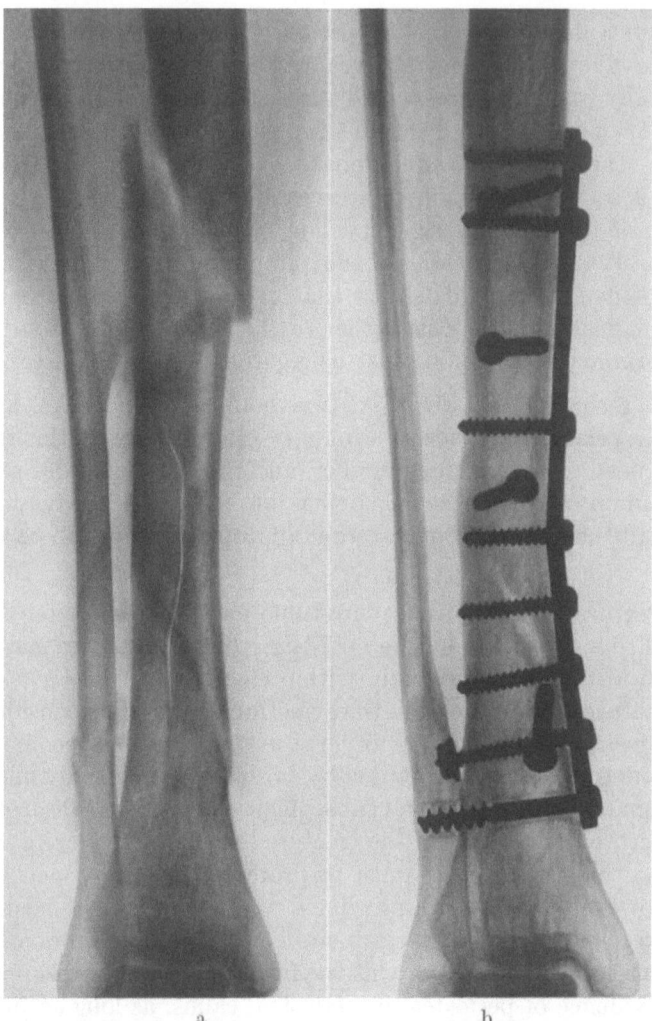

a   b

Fig. 114a and b. a Comminuted fracture of the right tibia. b Condition 26 weeks after internal fixation with long plate and additional screws applied at right angles to the plate. Note the nut on the last screw but one (it was used because this screw thread stripped), also the screw extending into the fibula: osteolysis around the screw because of movement. Full restoration of function

This is often found after medullary nailing but may also appear when screws and plates have been used (Fig. 111). If there are no clinical signs of irritation, such as pain, redness or warmth progressive weight bearing is allowed.

Osteolytic areas occurring in the vicinity of metal implants are interesting and when inferior metals were used, these areas may have been due to permeation of the tissues by metallic products (metallosis). With the development of improved metals, this should not now occur, but it may still have to be considered. The major causes of localized osteolytic processes, however, are infection (Fig. 112) and passive movement of the metal implant. The latter can occur when a screw unites two bones which normally move relative to each other such as in the inferior tibiofibular joint (Fig. 114).

7. Removal of Metal Implants Following Internal Fixation in the Leg

It is usually advisable to remove foreign metal objects that have been introduced during treatment, especially when these are plates or nails. Removal, however, should be delayed until the bone has regained a completely homogeneous structure. In tibial fractures in adults this is usually about a year after the fracture. In adolescents, the metal should be removed between eight and ten months after the operation, since the screws may otherwise become covered by periosteal callus. Before removing any of these implants a new x-ray should be taken.

Technique of removal of implants. The cosmetic result in internal fixation is usually very good if the techniques we advocate in the care of soft tissues are observed, and if straight incisions are made, the scars are barely visible (particularly appreciated by women). It is important not to spoil the result when removing plates and screws. Screws can usually be withdrawn through small puncture incisions. It is important to locate the screw exactly and to clean out any ingrown tissue from the socket of the screw head before inserting the screw driver. Removing a plate does not necessitate re-opening the entire original incision. If the screws are removed through small puncture wounds, the plate may then be withdrawn with the appropriate instruments, through an additional small incision about 2 cm. long at one end of the plate. Medullary nails can usually be withdrawn without much difficulty through the primary incision bisecting the patellar tendon. Considerable force may be needed to remove medullary nails and this carries with it the risk of some soft tissue damage during the operation. When a nail has been impacted rather flush with the surface it may be necessary to open the tibial tubercle with an osteotome.

It is better not to try to remove the nail with a few powerful blows, but to use more gentle blows in rapid succession. There have been cases in which a nail could only be removed by opening a slot in the tibia at its narrowest point where a nail would be obstructed most easily during removal. We have never needed to resort to this measure to date, but we felt it had better be mentioned for use in special cases.

Simple removal of screws requires at most a stay in hospital of twenty-four to forty-eight hours. Removing nails or plates is occasionally more traumatizing to the bone and may need a longer time in hospital. Weight bearing is allowed immediately after removal of metal, as long as the rule is observed that it is not removed until the bone has recovered a normal structure. For the next 2 months excessive activity should not be recommended, especially in the way of sport.

8. Complications of Medullary Nailing with Special Reference to the Tibia

General. Medullary nailing is a technically difficult method of internal fixation. The introduction of a metal support within the medullary canal not only requires a nail of the correct length and width, but it is also essential that the force used to obtain a perfect fit does not exceed the strength of the bone. The shape and size of the nail is important for various reasons; in the tibia its shape must allow its impaction and extraction since the medullary canal is not accessible in its long axis; a femur has a more or less pronounced anterior curve which makes it impossible to impact a rigid straight nail that is too thick.

Even in an apparently straight medullary canal the nail is subjected to a bending force because the cavity is not perfectly straight after reaming. Generally speaking, it can be said that difficulties with medullary nailing must be anticipated, where a thick nail is needed to obtain rigid fixation but where the shape of the bone varies much from that of the nail. Medullary nailing is also of doubtful value when that part of the bone that has to withstand the pressure exerted by the nail is weakened by injury, drilling or osteoporosis. For these reasons, it may be concluded that a tubular closed nail is less suitable than a slotted tube which allows a certain amount of elasticity.

For medullary nailing of the tibia experience has shown that a nail made of V 4 A steel (AISI 316) with a diameter of 11 mm. and a wall thickness of 0.9 mm. is sufficiently strong as well as flexible. Over a length of 175 mm. of such a nail a force of 46 kilograms is required to bend the nail 1 mm. In order to produce a nail of equal flexibility with a larger overall diameter, the thickness of the wall has to be reduced, so that a 13 mm. nail must have a wall no more than 0.6 mm. thick. On the other hand the thickness of the nail wall must not be diminished any further or reduced elasticity will result, producing a nail that would be permanently deformed by a lesser force. A thin walled nail demands an even better technique in insertion and extraction (see p. 58).

The dangers of wound infection with this method must be stressed since medullary nailing produces less favourable conditions than other methods of internal fixation. Filled with blood and possibly bone fragments from the drillings, the space within the nail provides a medium where the body's defence mechanisms can have little effect. We have found, therefore, that contrary to expectations, where the skin is in good condition, open nailing combined with flushing out of any bone cuttings and the application of local suction drainage is followed by a smooth postoperative course.

Complications due to the wrong position of the patient. An incorrect position makes access to the medullary canal impossible. Closed nailing can easily miss rotational deformity in transverse and short oblique fractures with small displaced fragments. If an extension apparatus is used to hold the hip and knee at right angles, the vertical position of the foot usually produces internal rotation, especially if the hip joint remains abducted. This can be prevented by open nailing.

Complications due to nailing at the wrong point of entry. It is especially important in the tibia to enter the medullary canal at the right point. This point is reached through the patellar tendon permitting the nail to be introduced in line with the axis of the tibia. If the nail is driven in at too great an angle, the posterior surface of the tibia is endangered. The thin guide rod may be bent while reaming with disastrous results. Also, even when the position of the guide rod in the medullary canal has been checked under x-ray control, there is no guarantee that the nail will necessarily follow the same path. The flexible guide rod may be correctly located in the medullary canal if introduced wrongly, but a thick nail introduced along it may split the entire bone in its long axis. If introduced at the correct point, the nail should easily be driven into the upper part of the medullary canal by hand.

Complications during reaming. Reaming has simplified and improved this method of fixation, but it is not without danger to the bone. KÜNTSCHER first reamed out the medullary canal with hand drills — a procedure which is possible up to a diameter of 9 mm. Damage to the bone produced by overheating is thus avoided, but a bone with an undetected crack can be easily split, and for this reason hand drilling over 9 mm. is not advisable. Mechanical reamers are therefore more often used today. These should have a blunt conical bit to make them self-centring in the canal, as a sharp, rapidly rotating bit might cut away the cortex on one side. The arrangement of the grooves at the cutting end should allow the bone that has been cut away to pass backwards up the canal since any bone debris in the threads would produce too much heat and damage the bone. Bone necrosis produced by heat will make the nail loose and fixation will be lost, besides increasing the likelihood of infection. Reaming should therefore be done gently with a light pressure on the drill and the reamers kept sharp and clean. The medullary canal, especially if the bone is very hard, must not be widened too much and it is best to increase the internal diameter by half millimetre increments. When the drill is removed, the bone debris lying in the grooves of the reamer should have the appearance of very small red chips. Dark yellow compressed bone in the threads is a sign that too much heat has been generated. Too energetic drilling can easily produce damage to the metal of the shaft and cutting end of the reamer, and a jammed or broken reamer may even require the bone to be trephined to extract the fragments.

Conversely, the reaming of soft bone has dangers also. If the guide rod does not remain well centred in the canal, especially if its tip is firmly anchored at the lower end, the whole thickness of the anterior or posterior cortex may be drilled away altogether. This would result in a very inefficient fixation. The posterior cortex is especially at risk from damage in this way. Medullary nailing of the tibia is only possible if the posterior cortex is intact as it will need to withstand the pressure of the nail during impaction in order to guide it down in the long axis of the bone.

Complications occurring during insertion of the nail. It has been emphasized before, that the nail must be inserted by gentle hammer blows. During the final impaction with a hammer of about 600 grams weight, it should be seen that the nail is definitely advancing with every blow. If it meets with any significant resistance the nail should be withdrawn, after which the medullary canal should be reamed out 0.5 mm. more. In the tibia we aim to ream a canal 0.5 mm. wider than the nail (in the femur 1.0 mm.), but obstruction still may occur for several reasons. A nail might be incorrectly labelled for size by the manufacturers, so it is important to measure the nail before using it with a suitable gauge. Even if the diameter of the drill and nail are equal, the nail may still become impacted since a straight nail introduced down a slightly curved medullary canal will be subjected to a bending strain. The flexible shaft of the drill with its short bit can traverse a curved path, but a straight nail cannot. Another reason is that with blind nailing, the end of the nail may strike the cortex of the distal fragment. In such a case, continued hammering will split the distal fragment. It is to prevent this that the AOI nail has been provided with a conical end. In one case we found that a small fragment had broken away and became jammed in the medullary canal of the distal fragment. This produces distraction of the fragments and if left alone may result in the later extrusion of the upper end of the nail.

Complications of re-nailing. In exceptional cases the nail may need to be replaced some weeks later by a shorter nail if a joint is in danger, or by one that is thicker if fixation proves to be non rigid. This procedure would seem to be simple, but surprises may occur and displacement of the fracture is sometimes produced during extraction of the nail, making it dangerous to insert a new nail blindly. An intact fibula may also prevent a closed reduction of the tibia. When replacing a nail the original one should be removed over the thick guide rod to prevent any displacement at the fracture site.

Complications during extraction. Removal of a medullary nail, especially when it has been in the bone for several years, can be very difficult. An extracting tool that gains a purchase on the whole of the upper end of the tube at the top of the nail is mechanically better than a hook which only gets a purchase on a small area. Thick walled nails can be more conveniently extracted with a hook inserted into a slot, though such nails of a given diameter are somewhat too rigid. During extraction, nails are subjected to a great bending force and an inferior tibial fragment can be split off while extracting a very rigid nail.

Complications resulting from improper postoperative care. Medullary nailing seldom provides as good immobilization of a fracture as can be obtained by other methods of internal fixation. It allows earlier weight bearing, however, since it supports the bone internally and a variable amount of callus may therefore be formed after operation, depending on the relationship between rigidity and the forces applied by weight bearing. When there is no complaint of discomfort, even a large amount of callus need not be regarded as disadvantageous.

Careful consideration must be given before weight bearing is allowed. A transverse fracture in the middle third may be allowed to bear weight in the third week without any ill effect. In fractures of other parts of the bone, medullary nailing provides less good fixation and weight bearing should not be allowed for six weeks. Oblique fractures, or fractures with more than two fragments, should be treated even more cautiously, as too early weight bearing may result in shortening of the bone so that the nail becomes relatively too long. This results in extrusion at the upper end with pain at the patella, or even damage to the knee joint. Re-nailing may save the situation, but proper postoperative care should prevent this from being necessary.

Precautions to be Taken to Avoid Complications.

1. Accurate estimation of the shape and width of the medullary canal and of the hardness of the cortex.

2. Selection of a nail of the right length. X-rays should be used to show where the upper end of the nail should be on the skin and the angle it should be introduced at, with reference to the anterior edge of the tibia. The length of the guide rod and the flexible shaft should be known.

3. In medullary nailing of the tibia, the condition of the posterior cortex of the shaft must be studied. It should be intact and sufficiently strong to stand up to pressure from the nail. Where the medullary canal is wide and the bone porotic, beware of an over-rigid or thick medullary nail.

4. The use of an image intensifier can prevent many complications. Open nailing may also do so and it is the only method that permits a genuinely exact reduction, ensuring that the drill can be centered equally in both fragments.

5. The degree of rigidity obtained and the possibility of shortening of the bone must be taken into account in assessing the time that must elapse before weight bearing is allowed.

II. Malleolar Fractures

1. Functional Anatomy

In ankle fractures it is tempting to concentrate too much on the bone as it appears on the x-ray while ignoring the injury to soft parts, which always accompanies such fractures. LAUGE-HANSEN in 1952 emphasized the close relationship between ligament injuries and the bony lesions in this area. Thus, equal importance must be given to both types of lesions.

Especially important is the inferior tibiofibular joint (Fig. 115) which is held together by the following components:

a) the posterior tibiofibular ligament,

b) the anterior tibiofibular ligament and

c) the interosseus membrane extending proximally.

The mortise of the ankle joint is held together more by the ligaments than by the interosseus membrane itself. As these two ligaments are elastic and the fibula capable of some flexibility and torsion, the mortise has a dynamic function while supporting the complex actions of the ankle joint.

Behaviour of ankle joint on passing from stance phase to walking: During the stance phase the ankle joint axis inclines by inversion by about 5° from the horizontal with, depending on the positive torsion of the leg, a displacement of about 25° to the frontal plane through outward rotation. During the dynamic take-on phase the malleolus fibularis and the dorsal tibial lip, both connected by the posterior syndesmosis, absorb the backward thrust of deceleration, i.e. the lateral malleolus has a weight bearing function. The pressure forces, exerted on the lateral malleolus by the talus, are transferred to the lower tibia by the syndesmotic ligaments and the interosseous membrane. There are no similar laterally-directed forces of clinical importance in the supporting or take-off positions of the stance phase.

Such considerations support the opinion expressed in French literature since the late 18th century that the lateral malleolus has priority in the mortise. The deltoid ligament

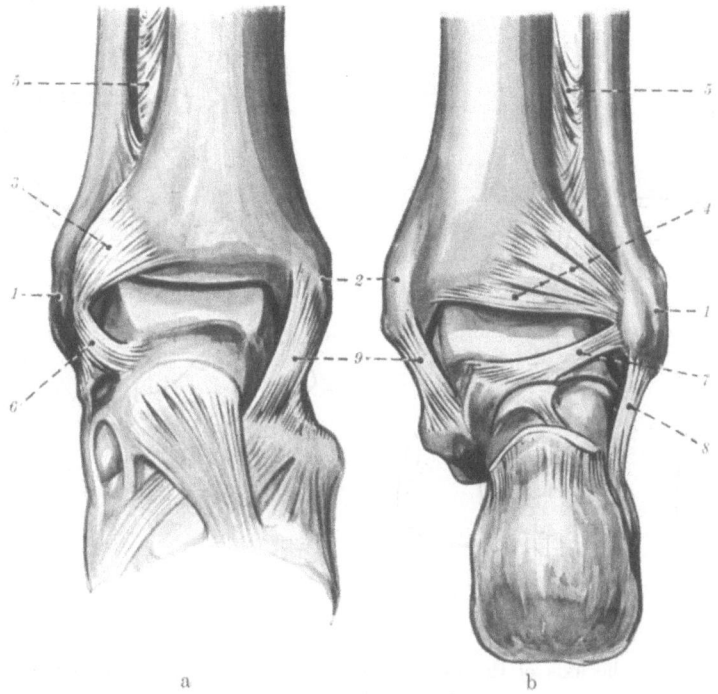

Fig. 115a and b. Anatomy of the ankle

1 Lateral malleolus	4 Posterior tibiofibular ligament	7 Posterior talofibular ligament
2 Medial malleolus	5 Interosseus membrane	8 Calcaneofibular ligament
3 Anterior tibio-fibular ligament	6 Anterior talofibular ligament	9 Deltoid ligament

offers no efficient resistance to the lateral mortise-opening forces, as NAVARRE (1962) showed experimentally: if the syndesmosis is dissected, the talus can easily be displaced laterally by two to three millimetres although the deltoid ligament is intact. The literature does not record the effect of the opposite experiment, namely the transverse resection of the medial malleolus. Our clinical studies, however, showed that the loss of the medial malleolus allows the talus to be pushed manually about 2 mm. towards the medial side, but that this displacement does not occur while walking. This is in agreement with BOLIN's assumption (1961), based on x-ray evidence, that the lateral malleolus must carry up to one-sixth of the moving body's weight. This weight bearing function must not be under-estimated. The lateral malleolus together with the inferior tibiofibular joint has a greater functional importance in supporting the talus statically and dynamically than does the medial malleolus. The rigid medial malleolus on the other hand has a purely static function and, together with the deltoid ligament, prevents eversion at the ankle joint. BARNET and NAPIER's (1952) observations have helped to clarify the mechanics of the ankle joint. During plantar- and dorsiflexion the position of the transverse axis of the talus changes (Fig. 116) so that the medial axial point during plantarflexion is displaced distally. The medial radius of rotation becomes longer (Fig. 116b) and the axis of rotation lies at right angles to the lateral articular surface of the talus. This shows, when movement occurs, the function of the lateral malleolus as a weight bearing and supporting pillar. During dorsi-flexion the axis of rotation comes to lie at right angles to the articular surface with the medial malleolus, which then takes the pressure (Fig. 116a). If it is also remembered that the articular surface of the talus is wider at the front than at the back, it is clear that the movement at the ankle joint is one of considerable complexity.

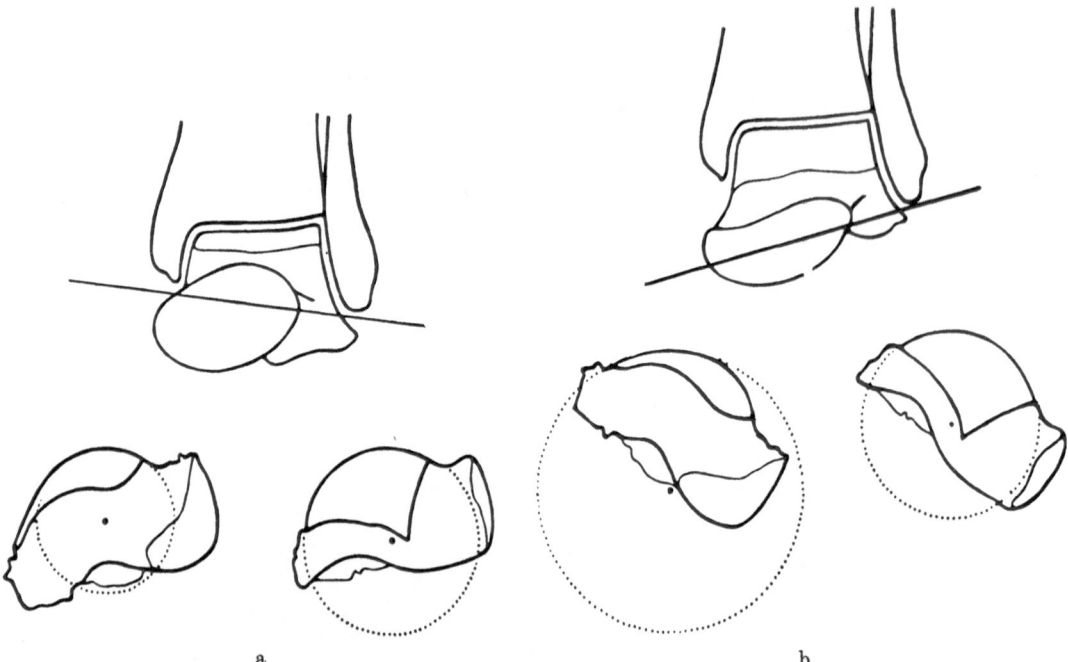

Fig. 116a and b. Shift in the axis of the talus during dorsiflexion (a) and plantarflexion (b). (After C. H. BARNETT and J. R. NAPIER)

2. Pathological and Physiological Considerations

The more a joint is used, the more significant become malalignments as a cause of later trouble. Even a small incongruity of joint surfaces can cause a load to fall at certain points on the articular cartilage beyond their physiological capacity. This produces degenerative changes in the articular cartilage and eventually in the bone, leading to osteoarthritis. PAUWELS calculates that a small reduction in the weight bearing surface at the hip joint considerably increases the pressure falling per square centimetre.

To investigate what happens at the ankle joint, we examined the behavior of the articular surface in different displacements of the talus which have practical importance.

We tilted the vertical axis by 2° and 4° in a lateral direction and displaced the talus 2 mm. towards the lateral malleolus. The small posterolateral displacement thus produced resulted in an impressive reduction of the area of the weight bearing surfaces in contact (Fig. 117). BREITENFELDER (1957) showed on the cadaver that a 2 to 3 mm. backward displacement of the lateral malleolus moves the vertical axis of the talus by 10°. Of equal significance is the shortening of the fibula so that, in fractures at the level of the inferior tibiofibular joint, a valgus displacement of the talus results (Fig. 118). When the fibula is fractured above the inferior tibiofibular joint, the shortening produces, beside the valgus deformity of the talus, an additional spreading of the ankle mortise with a lateral displacement of the talus (Fig. 119).

These findings show that even a slight displacement of the lateral malleolus can be of serious consequence to the mechanics of the joint. The fibula is the mainstay in the support of the talus and it is not surprising that even when slight displacement remains, secondary osteoarthritis is likely (Fig. 120).

It is not certain, however, whether the slight displacements we studied experimentally have the same significance in vivo. It is possible that the ligaments may provide enough compensation to prevent the talus from subluxating as much as the fracture displacement

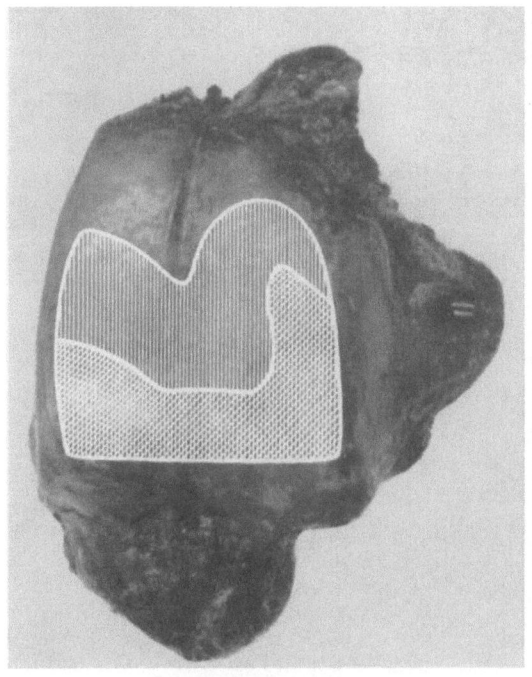

a

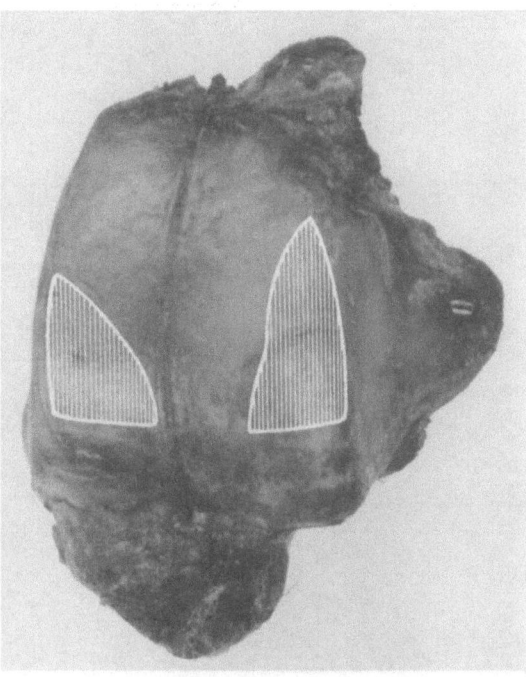

b

▦ Contact area between the upper surface of the talus and the mortise during a normal hinge movement of 10°.

▨ Reduction of this contact area during external rotation of the axis of the talus by 2°

Reduction of the contact area during external rotation of the axis of the talus by 4°

Reduction of the contact area after linear shift of the upper end of the talus towards the lateral malleolus by 2 mm.

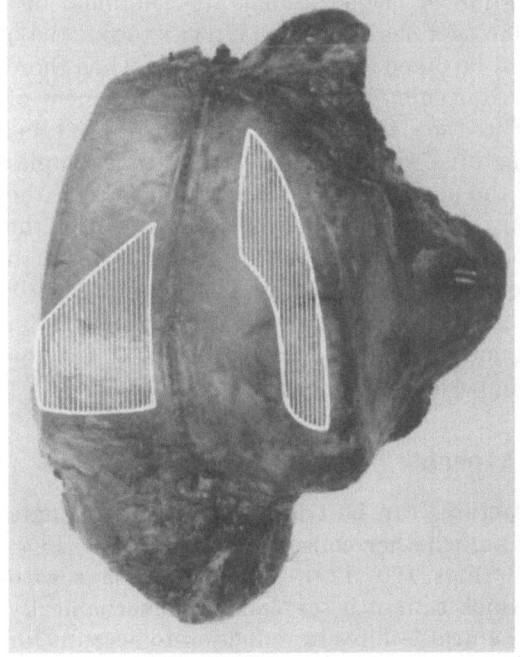

c

Fig. 117a—c. Showing the contact surfaces in the ankle joint during a hinge movement of 10⁰ (5⁰ plantar and 5⁰ dorsiflexion). a Normal contact area and its reduction when the vertical axis of the talus is rotated externally by 2⁰. b When external rotation is 4⁰. c With a lateral displacement of 2 mm. of the top of the talus

8*

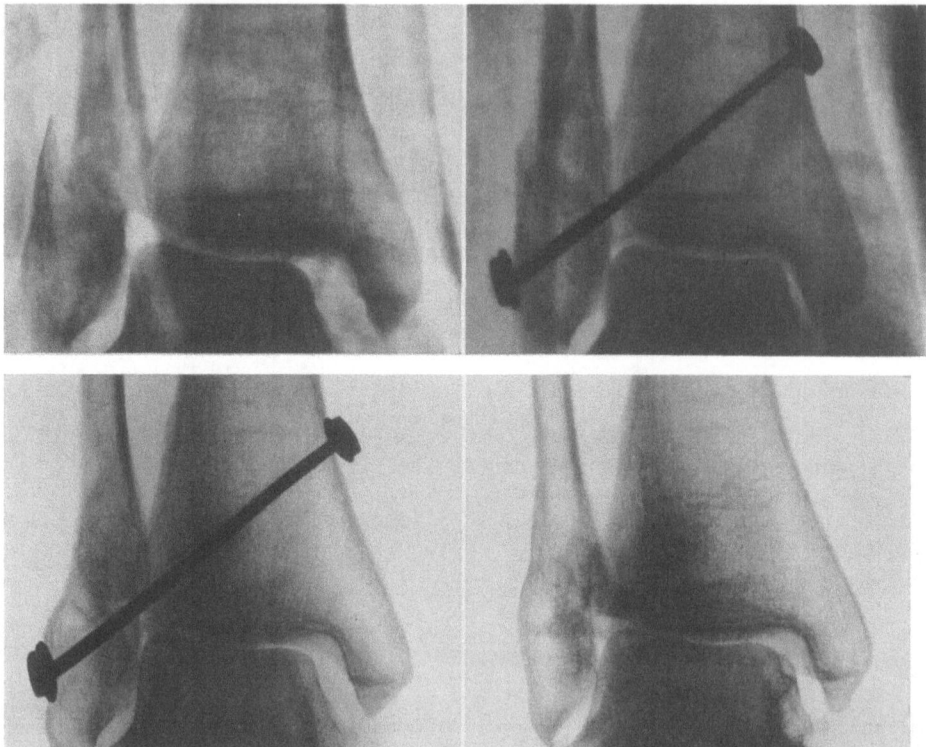

Fig. 118. Secondary osteoarthritis after surgical treatment. The primary reduction was already inadequate. Further displacement occurred with a bolt in place

would allow, but we have no certain knowledge whether this takes place. Further experiments and accurate postoperative observation of healed lesions after minimal displacement of malleolar fractures are needed. Our own observations (WILLENEGGER 1961) suggest that even the slightest displacement must be taken seriously, especially when there are several components as in the simultaneous shortening and backward displacement of the fibula. The only insignificant displacements are those in which the position of the talus is maintained and where the fractures do not involve weight bearing surfaces. Examples of these are: 1) the rather comminuted zone of the medial inferior articular surface of the tibia in an inversion fracture (Fig. 121) and 2) fractures of the posterior margin of the tibia when the amount of the articular surface borne by the separated fragment is less than one quarter to one fifth of the antero-posterior diameter of the joint. If the fragments bearing articular cartilage are larger than this, imperfect reduction always results in secondary osteoarthritis (Fig. 122). Finally it must be emphasized that metal fixation has especially bad results when fragments are imperfectly reduced (Fig. 123).

3. Clinical Aspects

Almost all late disability after malleolar fractures can be traced back to inadequate reduction and resultant secondary osteoarthritis, whether conservative measures (Figs. 118, 123) or operative fixation has been used (Figs. 120, 122). Apart from cases with infection inside the joint, secondary arthritis which cannot be explained biomechanically is very rare and it is important to look for mechanical failures in reduction to account for late arthritis in malleolar fractures.

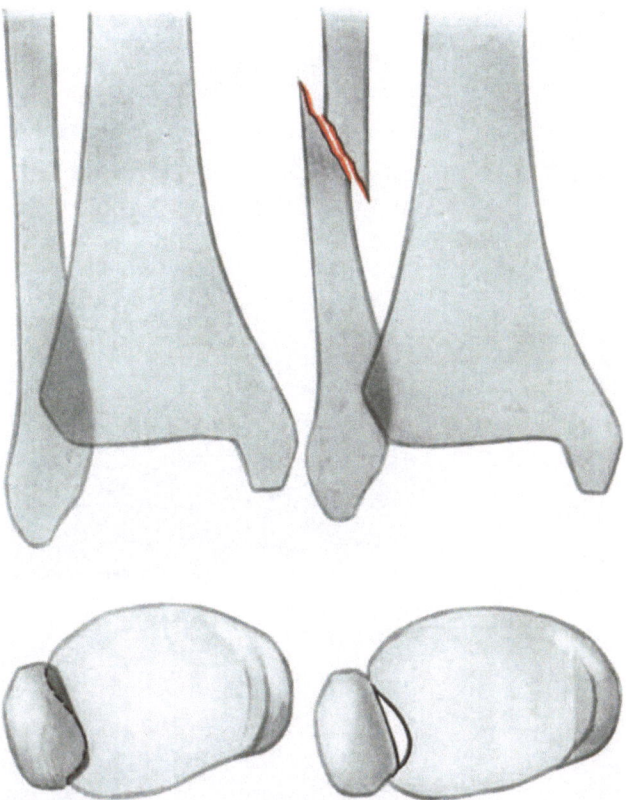

Fig. 119. Displacement of the fibula in the incisura fibularis of the tibia due to shortening

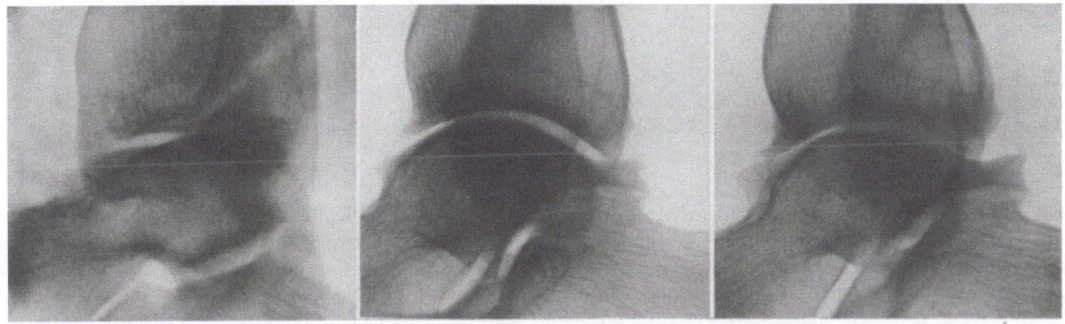

Fig. 120. Although reduction was good otherwise, an upward displacement by 3 mm. of the lateral malleolus remained. The slight rotation of the upper surface of the talus thus produced resulted in osteoarthritis accompanied by chronic synovitis and discomfort (reviewed at 3 and 6 years)

The ankle joint's weight bearing function makes it very liable to osteoarthritis, a condition which is usually progressive and presents itself as a painful chronic synovitis with a reduced range of movement. Sometimes, a relatively good early result with little discomfort and a good range of movement may conceal early osteoarthritis which is visible on x-ray. The first signs of a developing arthritis are areas of sclerosis, which can be seen quite early at points under increased pressure. In follow-up examinations, all cases of inadequate reduction showed signs of osteoarthritis within eighteen months of the injury (WILLENEGGER 1961).

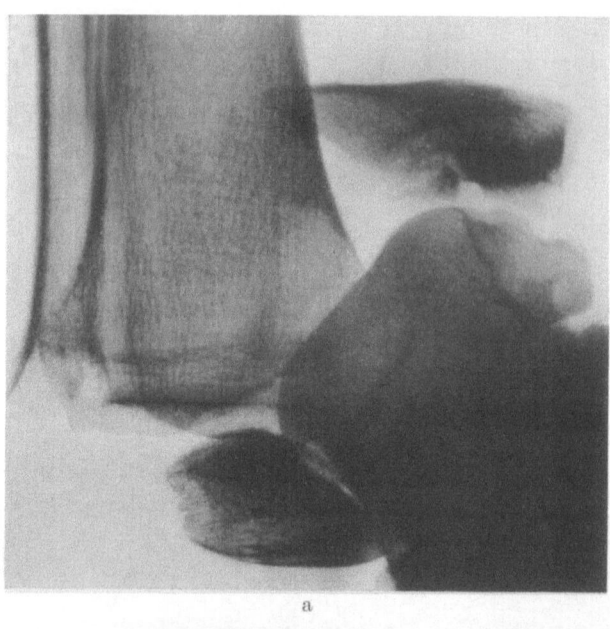

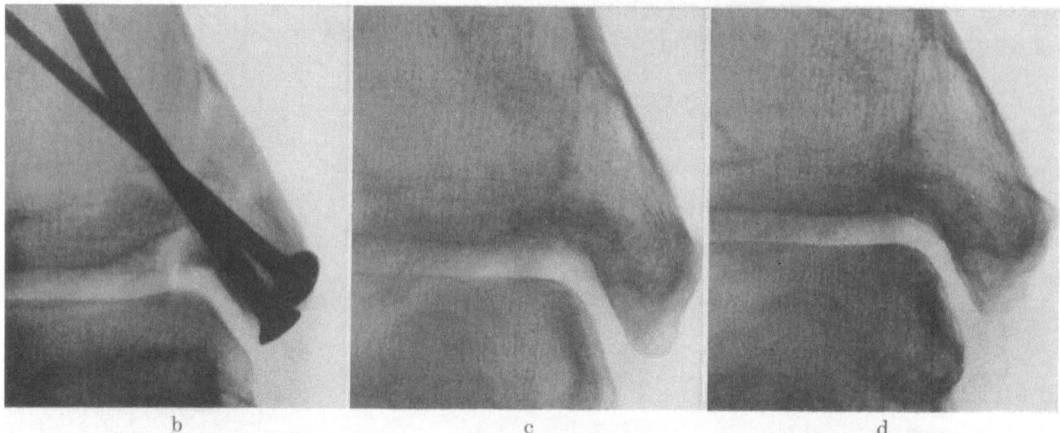

Fig. 121 a—d. The comminuted nature of the fracture of the medial malleolus including its articular surface did not cause secondary osteoarthritis because no lack of congruity between the upper surface of the talus and the mortise remained. On review at 6 and again at 9 years, full function had been regained at the joints of foot and tarsus and there was only slight capsular thickening. No compensation was payable

Osteoarthritis is one of the most important criteria in assessing the results in malleolar fractures, and when it occurs it means that reduction was imperfect. When there is no osteoarthritis it can be concluded that the reduction was biomechanically adequate and that no areas were left in which articular cartilage had to bear abnormal pressure. The end result should also be judged by exact measurements of joint function, observation on capsular thickening, persistent synovitis and the amount of discomfort. It is only by using such criteria that it is possible to compare critically the end results of different theories and methods of treatment. Results judged on criteria such as "good", "moderate", "poor" are of little value since these terms are interpreted differently by each surgeon. For example, KIRSCHNER (1949) compiling the results of reduction after LAUGE-HANSEN speaks of "good clinical results" when the joint movement was only half of normal range.

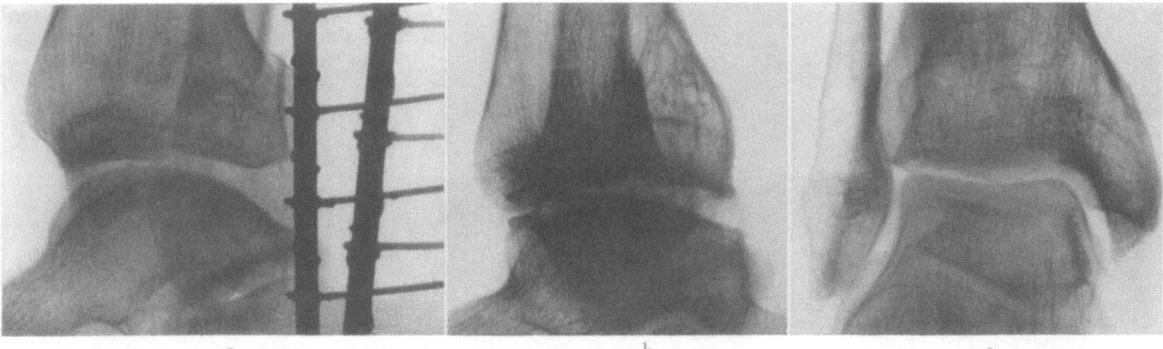

Fig. 122 a—c. Osteoarthritis following inadequate reduction of a large posterior marginal fragment of the tibia

4. Pros and Cons of Operative Treatment

The most important thing in the ankle joint is to close the mortise. Ligaments and bones must both be considered. The lateral malleolus is especially important because it has both a weight bearing function and it also controls the position of the talus.

Good conservative methods are capable of producing a good reduction in many malleolar fractures allowing a diastasis of the mortise to be closed. Frequently, however, slight displacement persists, which may be mechanically significant. Furthermore, an initial good position may deteriorate when the swelling subsides, necessitating a second reduction. The possibility of interposition of soft tissues, preventing accurate reduction, has also to be taken into consideration. To this must be added the disadvantages of prolonged immobilization in a plaster cast. In general, the end results of conservatively treated ankle fractures are unsatisfactory in about 30% of cases according to a survey by REIMERS (1953). In consequence, the number of surgeons who advocate operation on malleolar fractures has increased greatly during the past ten to twenty years.

As a result, the medical literature contains such a mass of different techniques that it would be impossible to deal with all of the suggested methods individually, and we are confining ourselves to those that have proved effective in our hands (see page 126).

There are two main advantages to primary internal fixation for malleolar fractures:

1) anatomical reduction of the mechanically important elements can be carried out with the greatest degree of certainty,

2) any ligamentous injury, especially of the anterior inferior tibiofibular joint, can be exposed and repaired. No compromise should be accepted when restoring the anatomical mortise if a permanent good result is to be obtained; and if the operation has not produced an anatomically exact result, a second intervention should be undertaken.

A really rigid internal fixation will allow early mobilization of the joints after operation. Such mobilization has an especially beneficial effect on the articular cartilage since it can only be kept anatomically normal if it is subjected to continual movement and variations in pressure ("cartilage massage", as put forward by PAUWELS). This is especially important as injuries to the articular cartilage always complicate malleolar fractures. In one center 200 ankle fractures treated by primary fixation were followed-up postoperatively. According to LAUGE-HANSEN's classification 75% of these were in either stage 3 or 4. Secondary

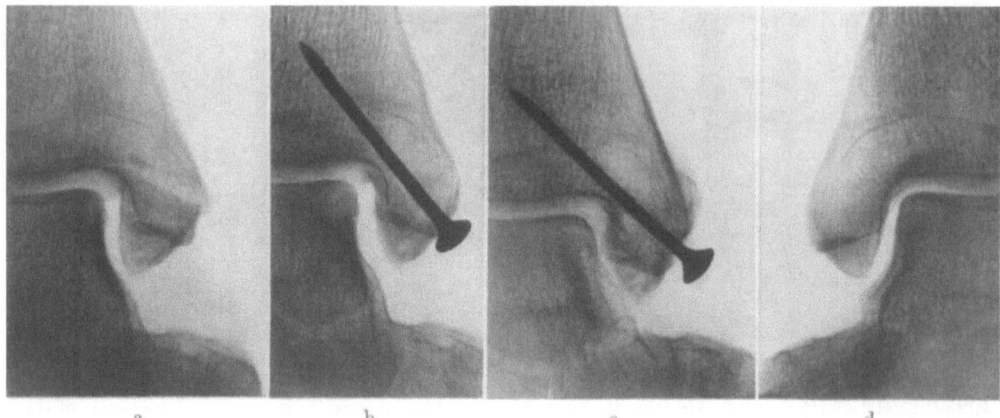

a   b   c   d

Fig. 123a—d. Osteoarthritis following imperfect fixation of an avulsed medial malleolus. The method itself was not at fault, but the reduction was inadequate. X-rays taken a immediately after the accident, b after operation, c at two years, d the normal opposite side

arthritis was found in 6%, full restoration of function in 92%, while there was a permanent disability in 7.5%.

It is easier to reconstruct both bone and ligaments during the first few hours after the injury as the reactive process after injury rapidly weakens both the cancellous bone and the connective tissue. All dislocation fractures of the ankle joint should therefore be submitted to emergency operation, especially when the skin of the fracture site is stretched tautly over it. A rapidly progressive soft tissue swelling, fracture blisters, or injury from the bone to the subcutaneous tissues represent a contra-indication to surgery after a few hours (Fig. 127). When a case comes up late, and especially where there is severe injury to the soft tissues or doubt about the blood supply, it is absolutely essential to postpone surgery for even as long as ten days. A temporary reduction and immobilization of the displaced fracture must be undertaken, however, and the soft tissues protected by elevation of the limb during the waiting period.

5. Classification of Malleolar Fractures

In these fractures there is a close correlation between the type of accident and the nature of the resulting injury. They were first classified by ASHURST and BROMER (1922) and their work was developed in further detail by LAUGE-HANSEN (1952). We have found, however, together with others, that using such a scheme is somewhat cumbersome, and as modern accidents often occur at high velocity, the original classification does not always apply. As internal fixation is directed towards accurate reconstruction of the injured bone and ligament, it is more important to assess in detail the components of the actual injured structure rather than the causative factors.

It is more useful therefore to use a simpler method of classification as advocated in recent papers. DANIS (1956), who was one of the first to adopt the routine treatment by surgery of malleolar fractures, drew attention to the great importance of the lateral malleolus. From the situation and type of fibular fracture, it is possible to deduce the nature of ligament injury. This may need more careful x-ray studies (on the everted and inverted foot) and sometimes the extent of the ligament injury is not realized until actual operation, especially in cases of rupture of the deltoid ligament and the ligaments of the

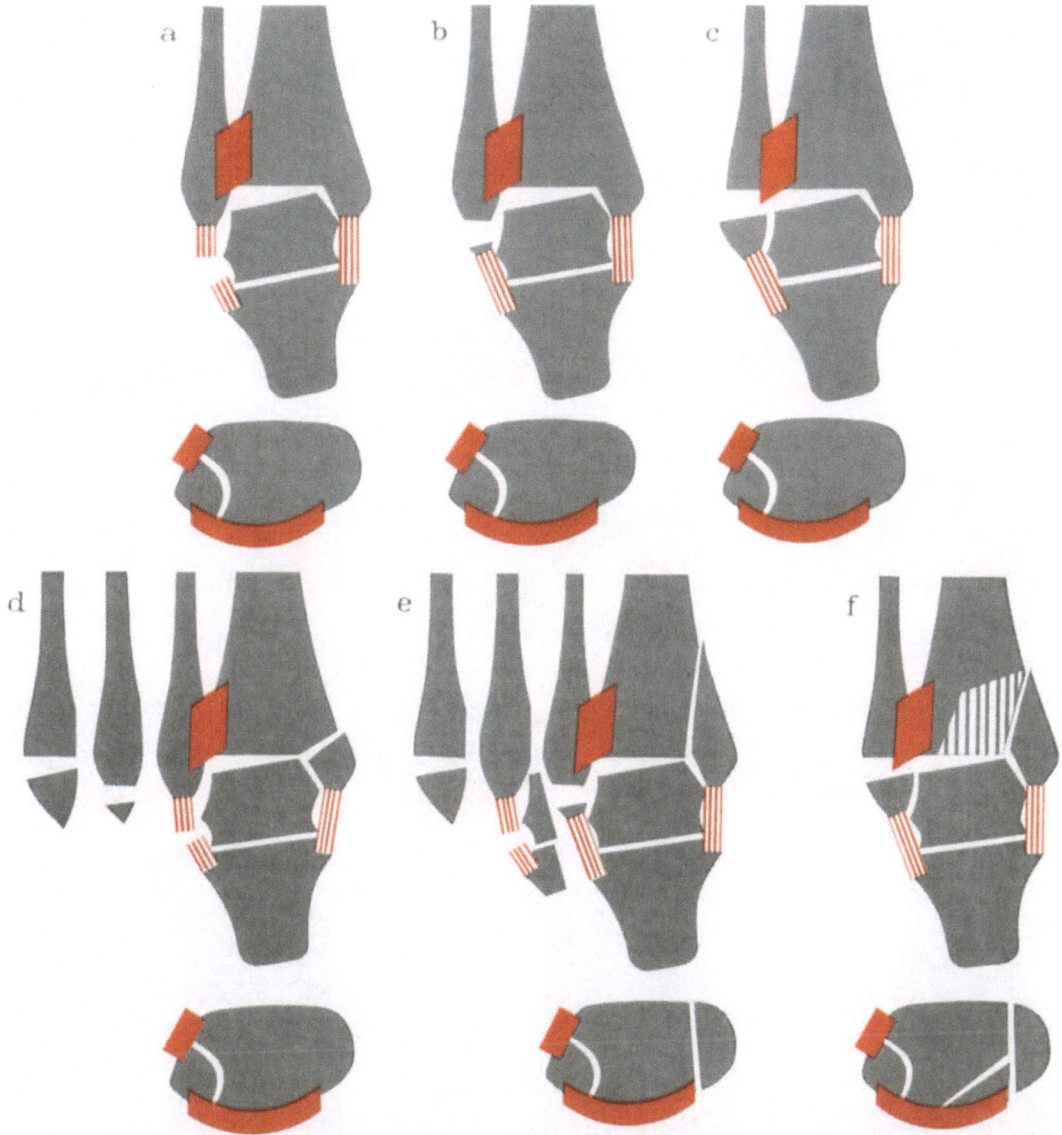

Fig. 124a—f. Malleolar fractures with injury to the fibula distal to the syndesmosis. a Rupture of the lateral fibular ligament. b Avulsion fracture of the tip of the fibula. c Transverse fracture at the level of the joint line. d Additional oblique fracture of the medial malleolus. e Additional vertical fracture of the medial malleolus. f Additional fracture of the posterior margin of the tibia

inferior tibiofibular joint. Our experience is that any classification should concentrate chiefly on the condition of the fibula. The injuries then fall into two main groups:

a) Injuries below the tibiofibular joint, b) Injuries level with it or above.

Group a) includes the inversion fractures in which there may be a medial malleolar fracture also. The tibiofibular joint, however, usually remains intact.

Group b) includes the external rotation, eversion and abduction fractures which, with the exception of pure external rotation fractures, usually involve injury to the mortise. On this basis the following classification has evolved:

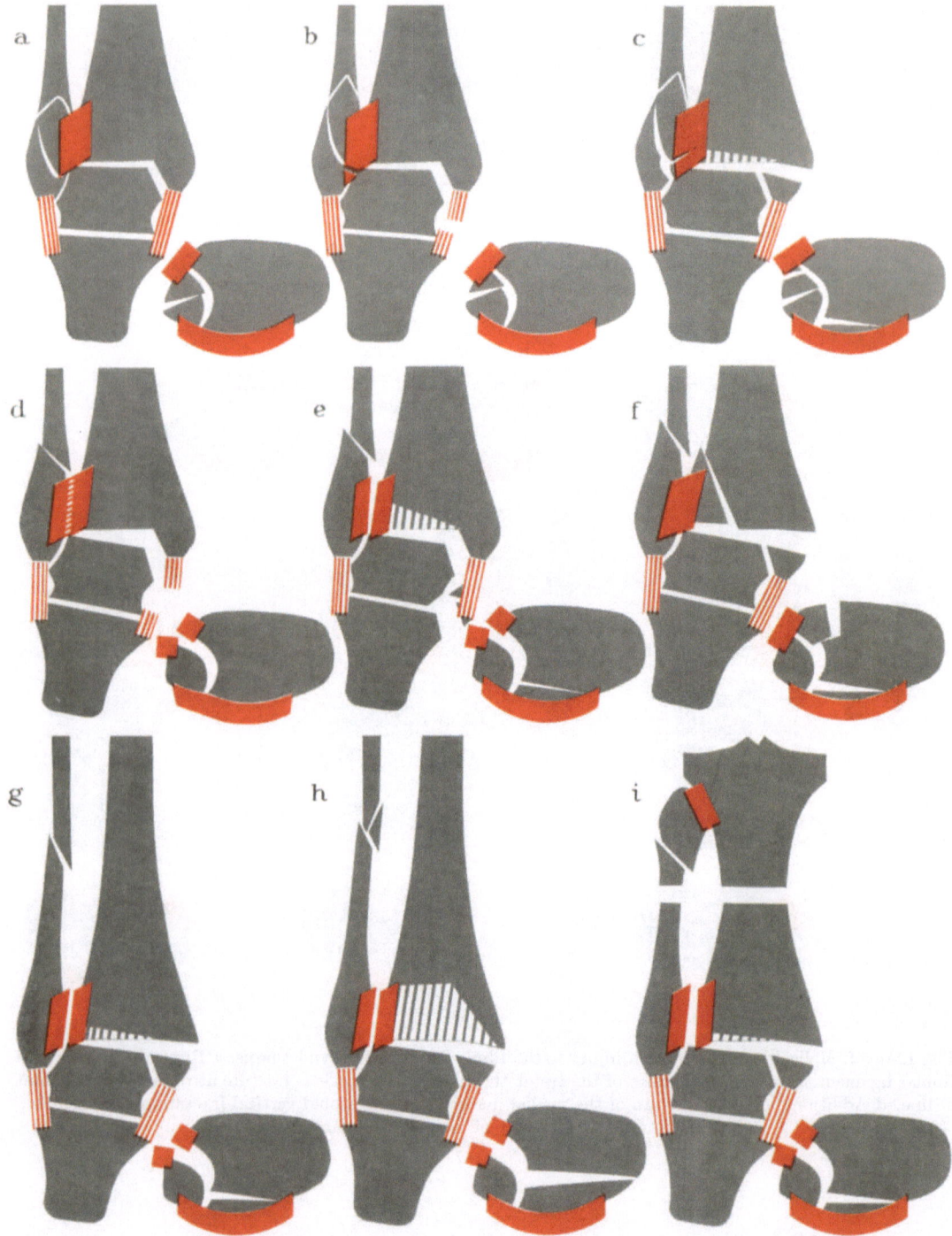

Fig. 125a—i. Malleolar fractures with injury to the fibula at or above the level of the syndesmosis. a Isolated oblique fracture of the lateral malleolus. b Additional rupture of the deltoid ligament. c Additional avulsion fracture of the medial malleolus and of the posterior margin of the tibia. d Oblique fracture of the fibula just above the syndesmosis with rupture of the A.I.T.F. ligament and the deltoid ligament. e Additional avulsion fracture of the posterior margin of the tibia. f As in e but with a large avulsion fracture of the tibial attachment of the A.I.T.F. joint and the medial malleolus. g Fracture of the shaft of the fibula with complete disruption of the syndesmosis and avulsion fracture of the medial malleolus. h As in g but with a significant fracture of the posterior margin of the tibia. i As in g, fracture of the neck of the fibula

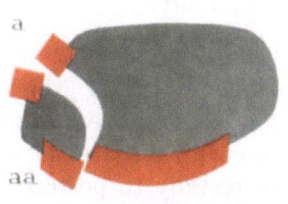

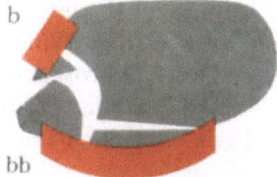

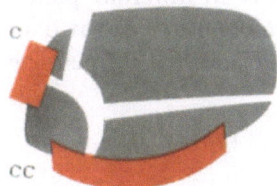

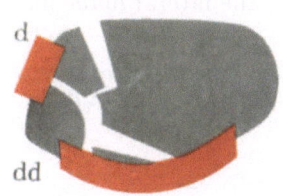

Fig. 126. Types of injury to the A.I.T.F. joint. a Isolated rupture of the ligament (*Clairmont* type). b Avulsion fracture of the anterior edge of the lateral malleolus (*LeFort-Wagstafe* type). c Avulsion fracture of the tibia with formation of an antero-lateral fragment, "Tubercule de Tillaux Chaput". d As in c with a larger fragment involving cartilage

Types of injury to the P.I.T.F. joint. aa Isolated rupture of the ligament. bb Segmental avulsion at the posterior margin of the tibia. cc Formation of a large triangular fragment at the posterior margin of the tibia (*Earle-Volkmann* type). dd Small avulsion fracture

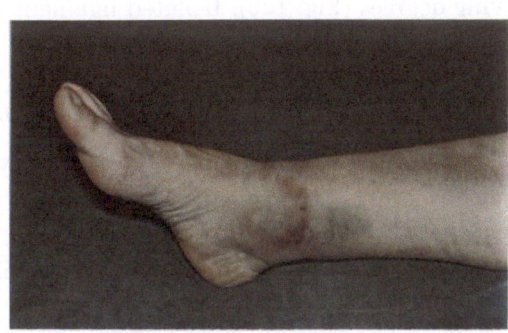

Fig. 127. Significant skin damage above the medial malleolus with an eversion fracture dislocation

a) Malleolar Fractures with Lesions of the Fibula Distal to the Inferior Tibiofibular Joint

Below the level of the ankle joint, the fibula breaks by way of traction on the ligaments when the afterfoot is bent over into inversion. According to the degree and direction of additional forces (internal rotation, adduction) the following types of injury are produced (Fig. 124).

α) Isolated Injury to the Lateral Malleolus

aa) Rupture of the fibular ligament (Fig. 124a)

bb) Avulsion fracture of the tip of the fibula (Fig. 124b)

cc) Transverse fracture at the level of the ankle joint line (Fig. 124c).

β) Combination with Fracture of the Medial Malleolus

aa) or bb) or cc) combined with a fracture of the medial malleolus which has a more or less vertical line (Fig. 124d or e).

γ) Combined with a Fracture of the Posterior Margin of the Tibia

This posterior fragment lies medially and does not involve the posterior inferior tibiofibular joint (Fig. 124f). In all of these fractures the tibiofibular joint is intact and as a result there is no liability of diastasis. Should the mortise become instable, however, it is because the fracture has weakened the support given by the malleoli, and this determines the amount of dislocation of the talus.

b) Malleolar Fractures with Injury to the Fibula at or above the Level of the Tibiofibular Joint

Here the fibula breaks from the combined effect of torsion, shearing and flexion, which are due to forcible external rotation, eversion and abduction of the foot. In a pure external rotation of the foot, or internal rotation of the leg if the foot position is fixed to the floor, the fracture of the fibula is typically oblique running from anterior distally to posterior proximally.

In the commonest and simplest type — isolated external rotation fracture of the lateral malleolus — the medial malleolus and the tibiofibular joint remain intact (Fig. 125a). The higher the site of the oblique fracture, the greater was the additional external rotation causing the injury. The higher the fracture also, the greater the amount of damage to the tibiofibular ligaments, the interosseus membrane and to the deltoid ligament which may be completely ruptured (Figs. 125b—i).

The anterior and posterior tibiofibular ligaments can tear at several different points and to varying degrees (Fig. 126). Isolated ligament injury is seldom complete but it does occur, though rarely. More often there are avulsion fractures at the points to which the ligaments are attached.

The following lesions of the anterior inferior tibiofibular ligament are typical

1. A simple rupture of the ligament (*Clairmont* type).

2. Avulsion fracture of varying dimensions at the anterior edge of the lateral malleolus (*Lefort-Wagstafe* type).

3. Avulsion fracture of the anterior lateral tubercle of the tibia of various size, sometimes involving part of the articular surface of the distal tibia ("Tubercule de *Tillaux-Chaput*").

Types of injury to the posterior inferior tibiofibular ligament are:

1. A simple ligament rupture,

2. The most common injury involving an avulsion fracture of the posterior surface of the tibia, ranging from a radiologically scarcely visible flake to a large triangular fragment, of the so-called "third malleolus" (EARLE-VOLKMANN). Characteristic of this posterior fragment is its lateral position (Figs. 125, 126).

An isolated diastasis of the mortise is rare. MAGNUSSON (1945) could only find fifteen cases in medical literature, plus one case which he observed himself. We have seen one such case ourselves (MÜLLER — personal communication). If a pure separation of the mortise is relatively often diagnosed it is because the average x-rays have not shown the accompanying fracture high up on the fibular shaft, and that instead of a medial malleolar fracture there is a rupture of the deltoid ligament which has gone unrecognized.

This shows that the inversion type of injury described under a) is due to a fairly simple mechanism, whereas the influences causing the external rotation, abduction and eversion types are more complex.

Despite the complexity of forces causing the latter types of fractures we have tried to classify them generally, as shown below (Fig. 125):

α) Fractures with Mainly External Rotation

Characteristics. Oblique fibular fracture level with the tibiofibular joint. Little if any damage to the distal tibiofibular ligaments.

aa) Isolated oblique fracture of the lateral malleolus (Fig. 125a).

bb) Oblique fracture of the lateral malleolus with rupture of the deltoid ligament. In this case there may be partial damage to the anterior inferior tibiofibular ligament (Fig. 125b).

cc) Oblique fracture of the lateral malleolus with a transverse fracture of the medial malleolus, anterior inferior tibiofibular ligament injured minimally, posterior ligament injured as avulsion fracture at the posterior margin of the tibia (Fig. 125c).

β) Fractures with Additional Eversion and Abduction

Characteristics. Oblique fibular fracture running up the shaft. Tibiofibular joint markedly injured in all cases.

dd) Oblique fracture of the fibula slightly above the tibiofibular joint with rupture of the deltoid ligament, or avulsion or marginal fracture at the medial malleolus (Fig. 125d). Extensive injury to the anterior inferior tibiofibular ligament in (Fig. 126a to d). Posterior ligament of the tibiofibular joint remains intact.

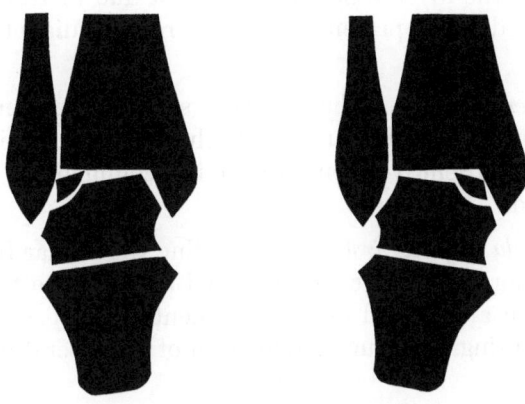

Fig. 128. Flake fracture

ee) as in dd) but the fibular fracture runs higher up the shaft (Fig. 125e). In this case the posterior tibiofibular ligament is injured in the form of a small triangle (EARLE-VOLKMANN).

ff) as in dd) but with the addition of a large triangle fractured off the anterio-lateral margin of the lower end of the tibia (Fig. 125f) (Tubercule de TILLAUX-CHAPUT).

gg) Fracture further up the fibular shaft and rupture of the deltoid ligament or avulsion fracture resp. transverse fracture of the medial malleolus: Both anterior and posterior ligaments of the inferior tibiofibular joint are ruptured as is the interosseus membrane (Fig. 125g).

hh) as in gg) but with the presence of a large fragment from the posterior margin of the tibia (Fig. 125h).

ii) as in gg) but with a fracture of the shaft or at the neck of the fibula (Fig. 125i). Everyone of these fractures has diastasis at the ankle mortise and there is often severe displacement of the talus laterally or in another direction.

It should also be pointed out that with all fractures where the talus is displaced, there may be an accompanying injury that does not show on x-ray. There may be damage to articular cartilage which can occur on the articular surface of each malleolus or on the dorsum of the talus. There may be some articular cartilage damage in any avulsion fracture. In the talus the cartilage is injured on the medial or lateral side, depending on whether it is an eversion or inversion fracture (Fig. 128). This is known as a "flake fracture".

6. Operative Technique

Objects. a) Anatomical reconstruction of the bony parts and restoration of congruity to the ankle joint.

b) Repair of ligaments.

c) Achievement of a sufficiently rigid fixation to allow early mobilization, thus preventing damage resulting from immobility.

Timing of operation: Emergency operation whenever possible.

Contra-indication: Poor skin condition or arterial circulatory disturbance.

a) General Technique

1. *A pneumatic tourniquet* is essential to give a bloodless field. Only when the skin condition is doubtful or the arterial supply disturbed due to trauma, or in cases where there are other vascular diseases present (arteriosclerosis or diabetes) should the use of a tourniquet be foregone.

2. *Position on the operating table.* When only one side is to be operated upon the leg may be placed with this part uppermost; but when both malleoli are going to be approached a normal position with the patient lying on his back is recommended, tilting the table to one or other side as required.

3. As a rule, the *fibula is fixed first.* By controlling the fibular fracture, alignment and stability of the ankle mortise may be well restored at the same time. This rule must be modified, however, when an avulsed deltoid ligament is trapped between the talus and medial malleolus, preventing an accurate reduction of the lateral malleolus.

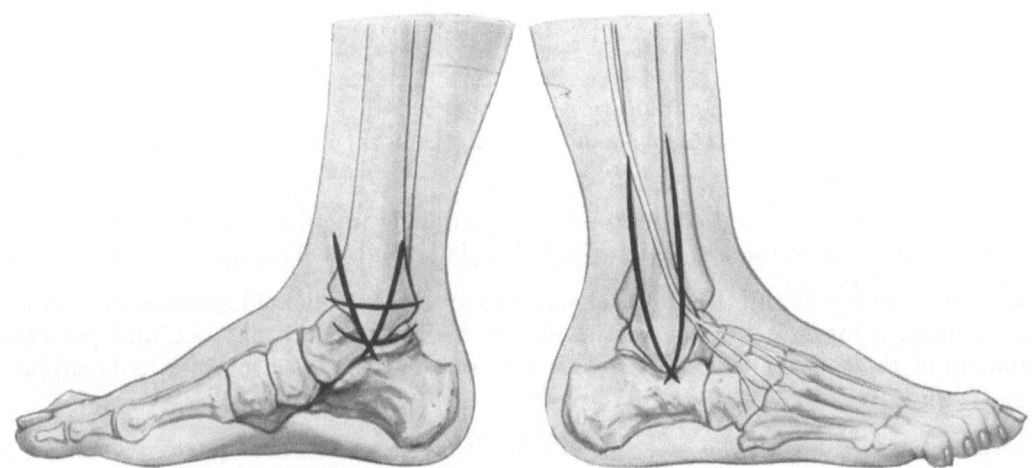

Fig. 129a and b. Skin incisions for approach to the (a) medial and (b) lateral aspects of the ankle

4. *Skin incisions:*

Lateral side. A slightly curved incision, convex anteriorly or posteriorly, is equally useful (Fig. 129a and b). The cutaneous branch of the lateral popliteal nerve should be preserved as its division results in an unpleasant loss of sensation in the lateral aspect of the foot.

Medial side. A slightly curved incision, convex anteriorly or posteriorly is used. If no extensive inspection is anticipated, a transverse incision or one slightly curved down towards the heel may be made level with the ankle joint.

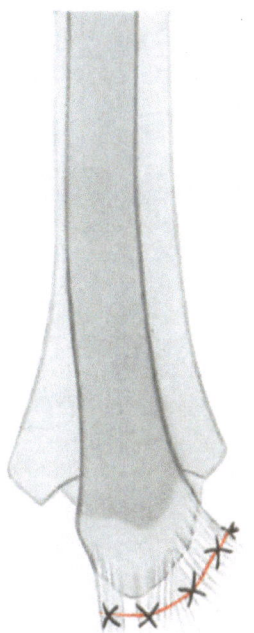 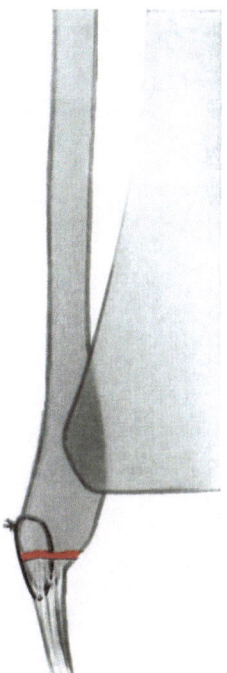

Fig. 130. Running suture of the lateral ligament   Fig. 131. Wire suture for avulsion fracture of the tip of
the fibula

5. A *perfect reduction* of the fracture line is the object and though it may appear to have been achieved, there can always be hidden inaccuracies. The operation should therefore not be concluded before a final x-ray examination has been made. In difficult cases, especially when repair has been delayed, it may be useful to make comparable x-ray studies on the uninjured side. An accurate reading of the condition of the mortise is only possible if the x-rays are taken in an a.p. view with the tibia internally rotated about 30°. To allow for individual variation in the amount of torsion of the tibia this can best be achieved by placing the axis through both malleoli parallel with the x-ray plate.

6. At the end of the operation a *suction drain* (Redon) should be inserted on each side.

7. We consider that *elevation of the leg* after operation is especially important with malleolar fracture-dislocations.

b) Special Operative Technique

There is already extensive literature on the repair of individual fractures and ligament injuries around the ankle joint (see WILLENEGGER 1961). Methods should be used that meet the following requirements:

1. Rigid fixation with accurate anatomical reduction.

2. Methods which produce some compression between bony fragments, and therefore increased accuracy of reduction and rigidity of fixation.

3. Preservation of the elasticity of the ankle mortise.

4. Procedures should be simple.

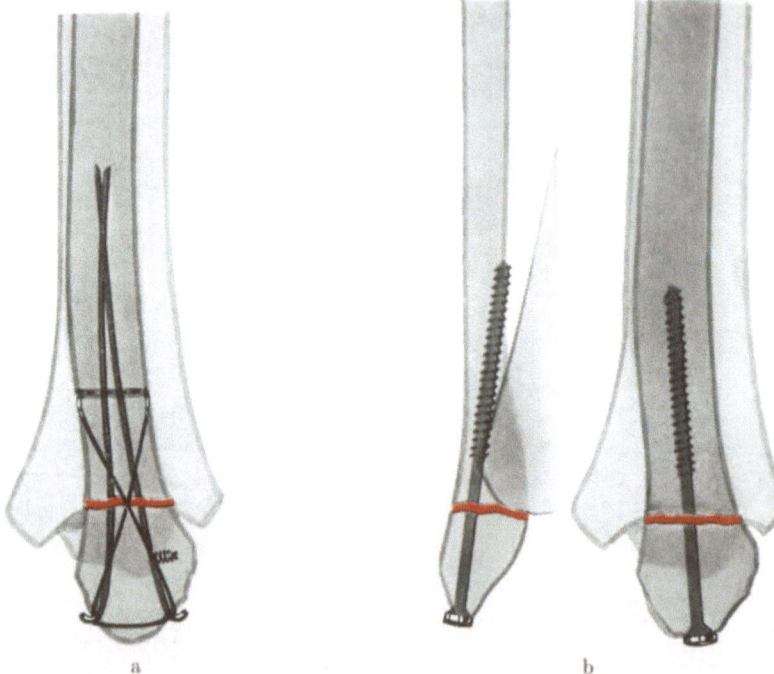

Fig. 132a and b. Treatment of transverse fracture of the fibula at the level of the joint line. a Figure of eight traction absorbing wiring. b Lag screw

The treatment of the inferior tibiofibular joint is an involved one and a final perfect solution has not yet been obtained. We will now describe the methods which, with their variants based on current literature and our own experience, have been found to meet best the basic requirements.

α) Management of the Fibula

1. Rupture of the Lateral Fibulotalar Ligament

Findings. There is often a wide transverse rupture of the ligament and the capsule is usually also torn at the distal and anterior aspect of the lateral malleolus. The articular surface of the talus may be displaced forward and is then visible.

Procedure. Reduction is obtained by externally rotating and everting the foot. When the joint surfaces have been brought into line, the ruptured ligament and capsule are usually found to be lying in good apposition. A double-running suture beginning at the front, using some material such as braided nylon No. 0, is recommended. The individual stitches should be made with the finest needle possible (Fig. 130).

2. Avulsion Fracture of the Tip of the Fibula

Findings. In this injury the lateral ligament is intact though a few fibres may have been ruptured anteriorly. The joint is opened and subluxed as in (1).

Procedure Reduction as in (1), the bony fragment being held back with a fine hook. Fixation is achieved by a hemi-cerclage wire introduced through an a.p. drill hole in the malleolus itself, then running round the tip of the detached fragment through the ligament at its insertion.

3. Transverse Fracture Level with the Joint Line

Findings. There is usually a simple transverse fracture.

Procedure. Reduction is by external rotation and eversion. Exact replacement of the fracture is held with the help of a fine hook. The following procedures have been found to give the best fixation:

traction absorbing wiring (Fig. 132a);

oblique screwing using a lag screw such as for the medial malleolus (Fig. 132b);

and crossed pins as in Figs. 133b and 152b.

4. Oblique Fracture of the Fibula Level with the Joint Line of the Tibiofibular Joint, Usually External Rotation Fracture

This fracture runs from the front below to the back above, and all types of fractures occur from short oblique to long spiral types. There may be butterfly fragments and irregular comminution. The joint is not usually visible unless the fracture interval is very wide or there is much comminution.

Treatment of the oblique fracture of the fibula (Fig. 133). Exact reduction and temporary fixation with bone forceps present no problem with fresh fractures in bone of normal density. If the proximal fragment is firmly attached, at least with the anterior tibiofibular ligament, it is sufficient to hold the distal fragment up to it. The anatomical position of the lateral malleolus can then be assured. More complicated are the problems of final fixation, since in addition to stability there is also the importance of the anatomically normal valgus position of the fibular malleolus to be stressed. It is important to hold the reduction firmly during the whole process of internal fixation.

Internal fixation by medullary nailing does not always give sufficient rigidity and on removing the temporary support it is sometimes possible to see the fracture opening up with loss of the above mentioned valgus position of the malleolus. There are, however, some cases where a medullary nail is undoubtedly adequate, but in our experience we have had better results when internal fixation directly holds the correctly reduced fragments together. To this end the following procedures have proved useful and reliable.

A *lag screw* is used as for the medial malleolus. It must be introduced from the posterior part of the distal fragment, aiming at a right angle to the fracture line, if possible. A 3.2 mm. drill is used. As these malleolar type screws are self-tapping it is not necessary to tap a thread. If the fracture is a longer one a second screw introduced more proximally may be needed; for a very narrow shaft of the fibula a scaphoid screw may be preferable (Fig. 133a).

Pinning with KIRSCHNER *wires* has been found to be useful, with one wire introduced towards the front and the other towards the back of the distal fragment. Both wires are placed so that they cross over at an acute angle and the wire driven from the back above the tibiofibular joint is anchored in the lateral cortex (Fig. 133b) of the tibia.

In some cases *medullary splinting* may be combined with cerclage or traction absorbing wiring (Fig. 133c). In our hands a KIRSCHNER wire of 2 mm. diameter, an equally thin RUSH pin or a triangular OBERHOLZER nail, have proved effective in medullary nailing. All of these are driven in, not drilled; and in all cases without exception, the last 4 cm. must be bent to allow for normal valgus position of the distal fibula.

Comminuted fractures present greater problems since the anatomical reduction itself, to say nothing of rigid fixation, approaches the limits that are possible in surgery. If the comminution is irregular and unsupported by any main fragments, anatomical reconstruction may be altogether impossible.

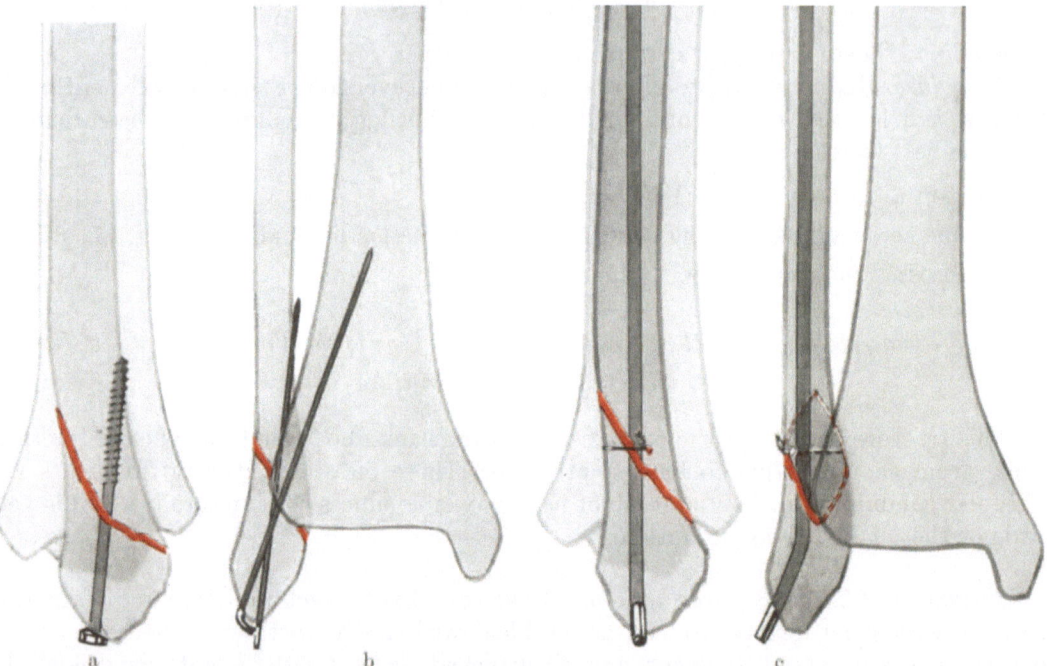

Fig. 133a—c. Treatment of oblique fractures of the fibula at the level of the tibiofibular joint. a Lag screw.
b KIRSCHNER wire fixation of the lateral malleolus with one of the wires penetrating the tibia. c Medullary nail
combined with hemi-cerclage wiring to prevent rotation

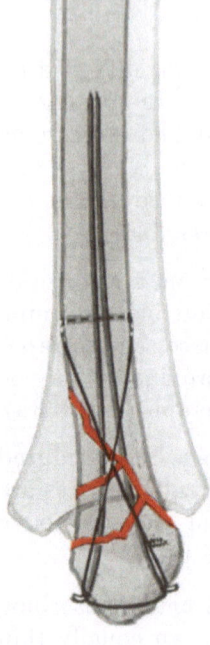

Fig. 134. A lag screw
is used for fractures
with one large frag-
ment of the lateral
malleolus and figure
of eight traction ab-
sorbing wiring for
comminuted
fractures

The primary requirement in open fixation is to preserve the remains
of the periosteal sheath at al lcosts. Its anterior edge and the connection with the anterior inferior tibiofibular ligament are most commonly
intact. With the thumb, fragments can sometimes quite easily be
pressed medially and anteriorly against the remaining supporting
layer of periosteum. Once the general shape of the fibula has been
restored in this manner, two or more thin wires of not more than
1.2 mm. diameter can be driven from the front and back of the lower
end of the malleolus longitudinally up into the shaft. The distal ends
of the wires are then bent at a right angle and clipped off short. Round
these projecting ends a traction absorbing wire is passed over the
surface of the bone and through a transverse hole drilled above the
fracture in the shaft of the fibula as shown in Fig. 134 to complete
the final fixation. In addition, any individual splinters can be fastened
to one another by fine periosteal or interosseous catgut stitches, especially in a transverse direction.

If restoration of the shape of the bone is more difficult due to bad
comminution it is wise to adjust the length of the fibula with the help
of x-rays taken in the operating room, using the opposite leg for comparison. Fixation in these cases can never be really rigid and is best
performed by oblique wiring with relatively thin KIRSCHNER wires
passed more or less parallel to the axis of the bone, possibly supplemented by a medullary nail.

5. Fractures of the Fibula Above the Tibiofibular Joint

Unlike the previous injuries this group is accompanied by damage to the tibiofibular joint (Fig. 125). The operative treatment here requires different procedures for internal fixation and for the closure of the joint. The object of internal fixation of the shaft of the fibula is the accurate replacement of the lateral malleolus which has been displaced in a backwards and upwards direction and externally rotated.

Treatment of fractures of the fibula slightly above the tibiofibular joint:

The *short oblique fracture*: Hemi-cerclage wire combined with a scaphoid screw traversing the fracture line as nearly as possible perpendicular to its mid point (Fig. 135a).

With a *longer oblique fracture* two or three scaphoid screws may be used (Fig. 135b). Effective use has also been made of two or more cerclage or, better, hemi-cerclage wires using thin stainless steel wire.

Treatment of fractures of the shaft of the fibula:

In our experience treatment of the shaft of the fibula is *important up to the mid-shaft*, in order to restore the congruity of the inferior tibiofibular joint, not only to restore length to the fibula, but to control rotational and valgus deformity. Procedures that are suitable are as follows:

In the *short oblique fracture* and when the *medullary canal is narrow*, transfixion with a scaphoid screw is combined with a hemi-cerclage wire (Fig. 136a). With *short oblique fractures of the fibula* and *wide medullary canal*, medullary nailing is advocated using the trifin nail developed by OBERHOLZER (2.5 and 3.5 mm. diameter). This nail should only be driven across fractures that have been exposed, accurately reduced and temporarily held with forceps, so that no displacement, especially in a rotational or a longitudinal direction is possible while the nail is being driven in (Fig. 136b).

In *higher fractures, transverse or butterfly-type*, causing shortening of the fibula, or involving changes of the valgus position of the lateral malleolus, a screwed-on plate using compression has proved to be a very reliable method, especially when a late repair has to be performed (Fig. 136c).

β) Surgical Treatment of the Inferior Tibiofibular Joint

With all injuries of this joint, even if only the anterior or the posterior ligaments are involved in isolation, there is some loosening of the joint itself which can easily be verified during the operation. The details of the injury (diastasis, fracture of the posterior margin of the tibia and any avulsion fractures in the area) can be shown by x-rays and by direct inspection of the ligaments of the mortise at the time of operation.

When only a small fragment is avulsed from the tibia by the posterior inferior tibiofibular ligament, enough connective fibres are usually left to hold the back of the joint together. Fixation of the fractured lateral malleolus is therefore sufficient to restore the strength of the posterior part of the joint. With a large posterior tibial fragment, the situation is different as it must be accepted that continuity has been lost between the posterior ligament and the tibia. Such a large fragment does not always have to be reduced, but it is then necessary not only to reform the tibiofibular joint, but to suture the anterior tibiofibular ligament and to stabilize the inferior tibiofibular joint.

1. Loss of Continuity of the Anterior Part of the Inferior Tibiofibular Joint

Pure ligament sprain. If the posterior ligament is intact either originally or because of surgical intervention, it is sufficient to unite the anterior ligament by suture.

Wide separation of the mortise is more difficult.

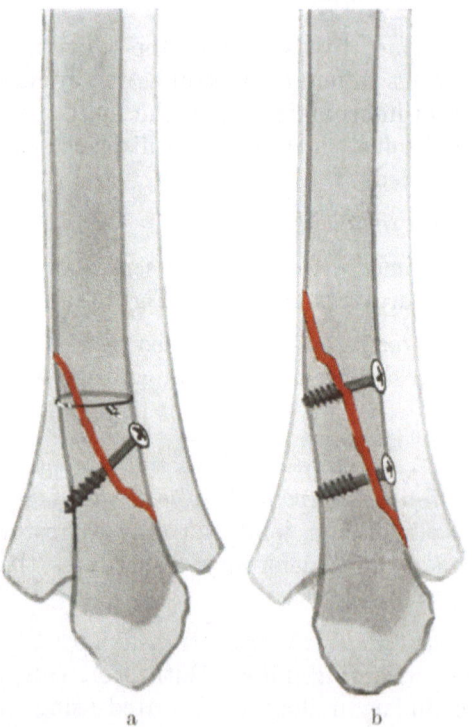

Fig. 135a and b. Treatment of oblique fractures
of the fibula above the syndesmosis. a Screwing
and hemi-cerclage wire for short oblique fractures.
b Screwing for long oblique fractures

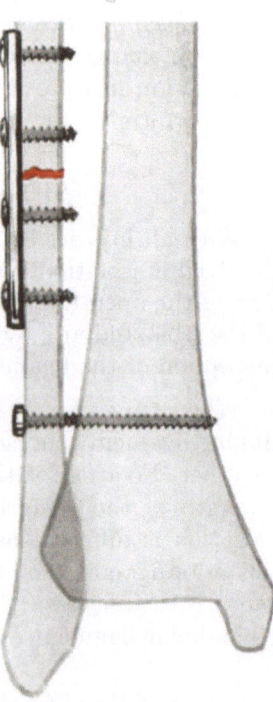

Fig. 136b

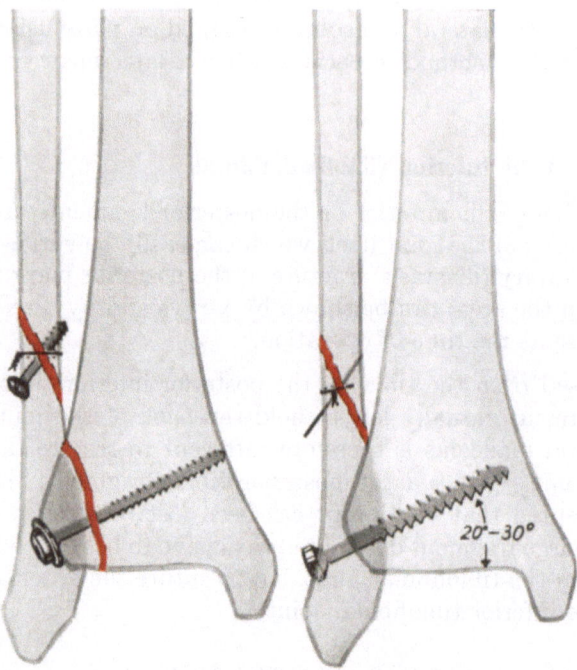

Fig. 136a—c. Treatment of fractures of the shaft of the fibula. a Transfixion with a scaphoid screw or wire
pin combined with hemi-cerclage wiring if the medullary canal is narrow. b Medullary nailing if there is a
wide canal. c Plate and screws for a transverse fracture or an oblique fracture high on the bone with a butterfly
fragment

One of the oldest procedures, originated by LAMBOTTE and adopted later by SCHÜRCH and MERLE D'AUBIGNÉ, was to use a threaded bolt. The danger of this technique is that excessive pressure can be exerted, making the mortise rigid. Our own case histories (WILLENEGGER) show, besides some very good results, several incidents where the inferior tibiofibular joint ossified and pressure-induced osteoarthritis occurred. We have therefore abandoned in general the use of bolts for fresh diastasis here.

Similar disadvantages apply to screwing the mortise at the level of the joint. DANIS's proposal to insert the screw at an angle of 25° or 30° to the horizontal (Fig. 136) does not diminish the disadvantages of this method, but in the absence of other suitable methods we use screwing as a short term mechanical method of fixation, especially when combined with suture of the anterior ligament. In spite of removing the screws at two months, some cases of fusion of the joint continued to occur, so that we are progressively reducing the number of cases treated with screws.

At present we feel that diastasis must be corrected by attacking the anterior ligament when, for any reason, there remains a lack of continuity in the posterior ligamentous connections. This is fairly easy when there is a large triangular fragment avulsed from the tibia (Tillaux-Chaput's tubercle). Such a fragment can be accurately reduced and fixed with a lag screw which may be of scaphoid, malleolar or cancellous type according to the size of the fragment (Fig. 136a). More difficult are the cases where the ligamentous damage is isolated, and in avulsion-fractures of the anterior edge of the fibula. In such cases we more often try to suture the anterior ligament, sometimes passing the suture through the bone, and to stabilize the mortise with a transverse screw placed *above* the tibiofibular joint. It is important to place this screw carefully, avoiding any compression force which would imperil the inferior tibiofibular joint itself (Fig. 136b). This screw should be removed at not later than eight weeks.

2. Loss of Continuity of the Posterior Inferior Tibiofibular Ligament

The posterior tibiofibular ligament does not tear off at its lateral (fibular) insertion. This ligament remains always attached to a fragment of the fibula. In the case of au intact anterior ligament this fragment will reunite easily without surgical intervention.

The avulsion fracture on the tibial side (EARLE-VOLKMANN) must, for mechanical reasons, be very exactly replaced and fixed, if the fragment comprises more than a fifth of the inferior articular surface of the tibia.

If dorsiflexion does not succeed in securing reduction, open reduction must be undertaken. Reduction of the fibular fracture in most instances reduces the EARLE-VOLKMANN fragment as to height, so that it can be fixed by a screw inserted from the medial side of the tibia. If such is not the case, approach is from the medial side, mobilizing the tendon of tibialis posterior by incising the periosteum along the posteromedial aspect of the tibia and retracting it backwards, together with the other soft tissues (blood vessels, nerve). The posterior surface of the tibia is thus exposed subperiosteally. The fragment can then be fixed with an awl and moved distally into a reduced position. It can be held temporarily with one or two transfixion wires introduced from the front of the tibia and an x-ray is then taken. Final fixation is obtained by a single lag screw inserted from the front of the tibia very close to the articulation via a small longitudinal incision (Fig. 137b); but a smaller and more medial fragment as seen in inversion type fractures (Fig. 124f) is better screwed from behind or fixed with one or more wires of not more than 1.4 mm. diameter. The wires can be bent and clipped off not quite flush with the bone.

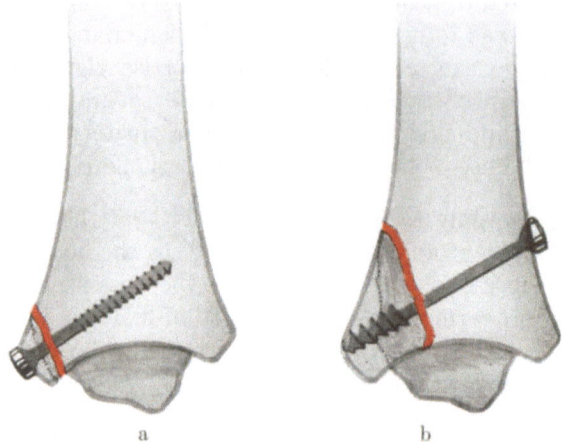

Fig. 137a and b. Screwing of a large posterior marginal
fragment of the tibia

γ) Management of the Medial Malleolus

1. Rupture of the Deltoid Ligament

Findings. As with the lateral ligament, there may also be a simple rupture of the ligament, though avulsion of its lower end at the talus may occur too. The retinaculum of the flexor tendon may be torn. Frequently, a large piece of ligament is interposed between the malleolus and the talus.

Procedure. For a wide transverse rupture, a double running suture is advisable as described for the lateral ligament (Fig. 138a).

2. Avulsion Fracture of the Tip of the Medial Malleolus

Findings. The deltoid ligament itself is intact, but there are bony fragments ranging from tiny flakes to large fragments.

Procedure. As with avulsion fractures of the lateral malleolus, hemi-cerclage wiring is indicated here (Fig. 138b). When much of the deltoid ligament is separately involved, additional sutures in the ligament may be needed, both in front of and behind the reduced fragment.

3. Marginal Fracture of a Small Malleolar Fragment

Findings. Transverse, oblique and sometimes irregular fractures with some cancellous involvement occur.

Procedure. Some of these fragments go on to necrosis, often dating from the injury itself, so that any manipulation of the fragment must be carried out with great care, reducing the fracture with fine hooks and fixing it with wires of between 0.8 and 1 mm. diameter passed across the fracture line and left with their ends projecting and bent over to allow fixation with the additional traction absorbing wires, as shown in Fig. 138c.

4. Separation of a Large Fragment from the Malleolus

Findings. Here the fracture line may vary in direction from transverse to vertical. There is often interposed periosteum which may originate from the edge of either the main

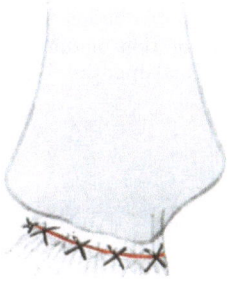 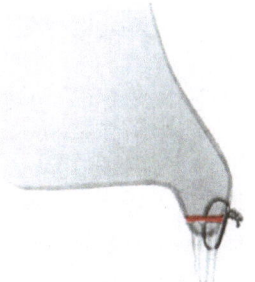

Fig. 138a. Continuous suture of the medial ligament   Fig. 138b. Wire suture for avulsion fracture of the tip
of the medial malleolus

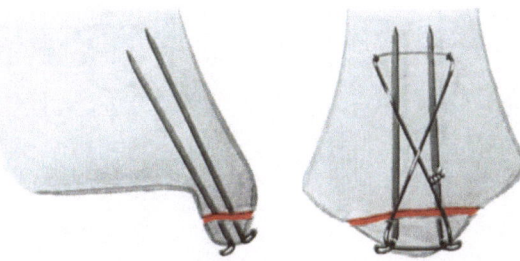

Fig. 138c. KIRSCHNER wire fixation on the left and the same on the right with additional traction absorbing
wire for an avulsion fracture of the medial malleolus

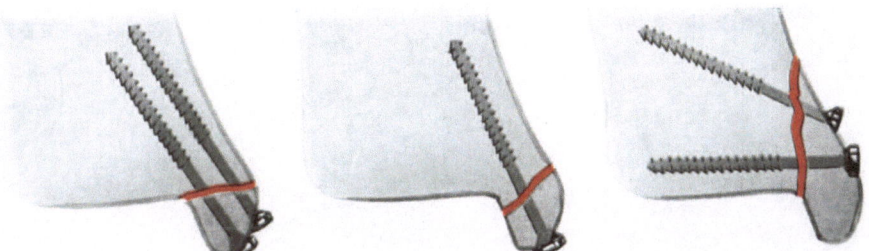

Fig. 139. Lag screw fixation for large fragment of the medial malleolus

fragment or the separated malleolus. The joint should be opened and inspected to determine how much injury has been caused to the articular cartilage of the talus. When the
fragments are large there has usually been little damage to their viability.

Procedure. Using fine hooks these fragments can almost always be reduced accurately.

The anterior tibial margin must be examined, for if reduction has not been exact, this
can easily be seen at this point. Reduction is held with two pronged hooks and a temporary
fixation obtained with one or more Kirschner wires. Application of a lag screw of malleolar type is the method of choice for final fixation, after drilling a hole with a 3.2 mm. bit.
No tapping is necessary (self tapping screw). If there is any evidence of rotation still being
possible after this, a second screw should be used. Sometimes it is necessary to use a small
scaphoid screw or a KIRSCHNER wire for the anterior spur of the fragment (Fig. 139).

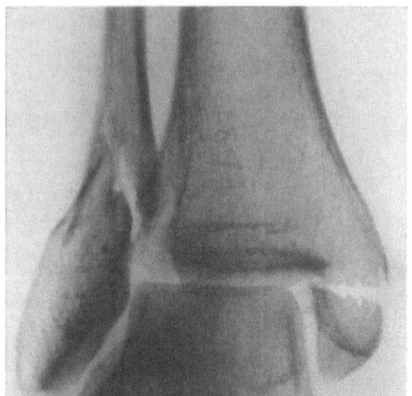

Fig. 140a—d. a Eversion abduction fracture. b Wire pin
fixation. c Complete restoration of function at 5 year review.
d The normal opposite side to c

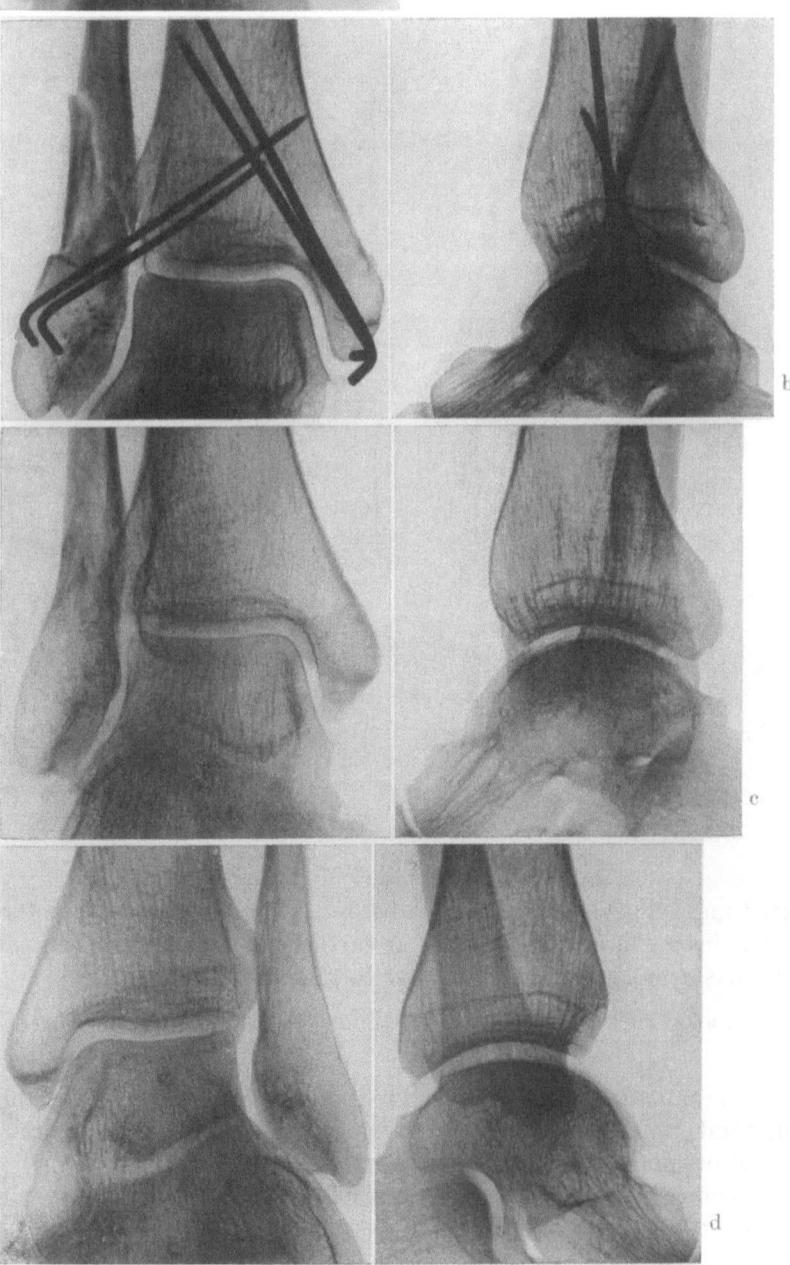

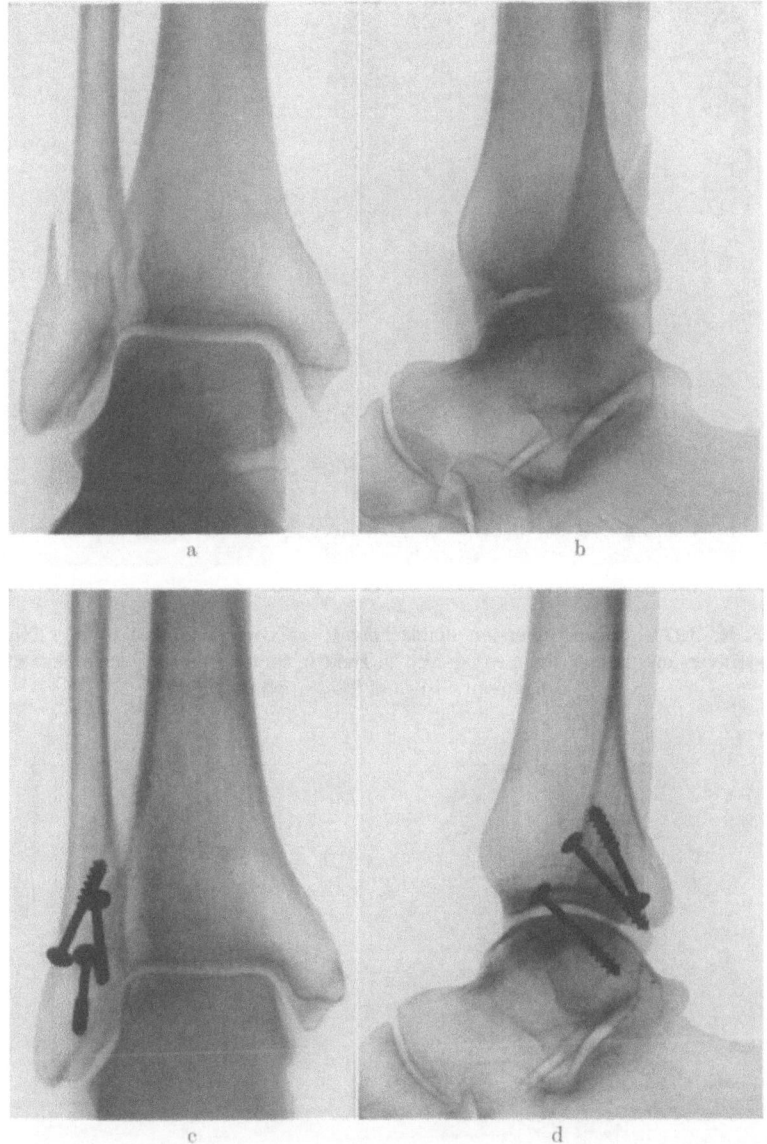

Fig. 141 a—d. Z. J., 1897. Displaced external rotation fracture. a and b. X-rays taken after the accident. c and d. 17 weeks after internal fixation, suture of the A.I.T.F. and deltoid ligaments

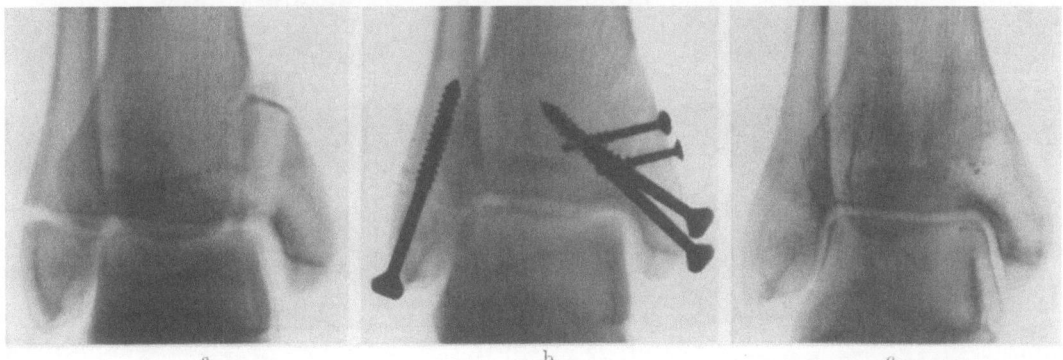

Fig. 142 a—c. S. F., 1944. Displaced inversion fracture. a X-ray at time of injury. b After internal fixation. c 20 weeks later

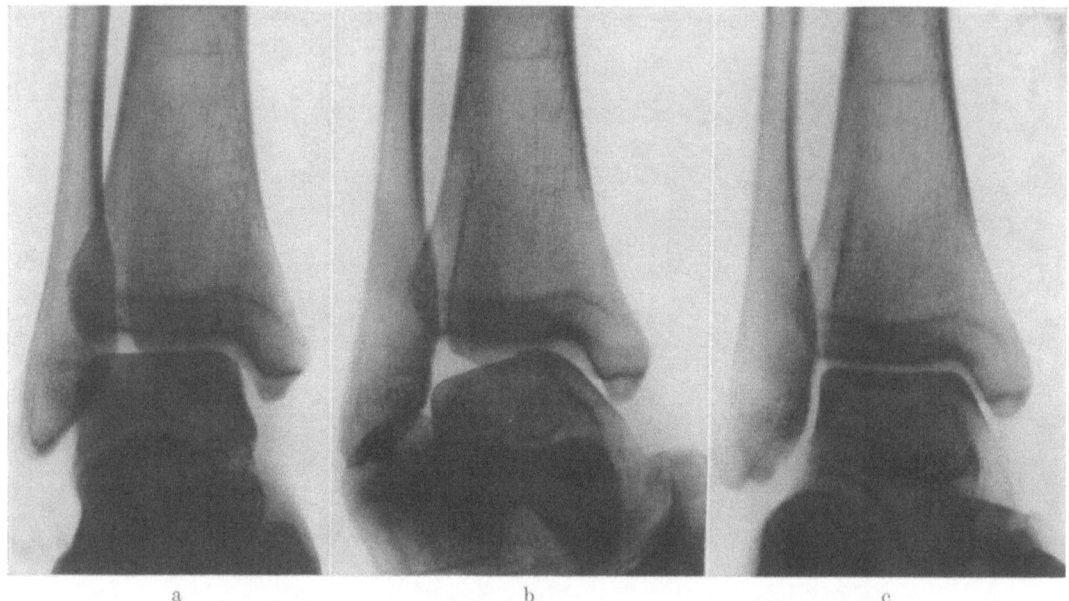

Fig. 143 a—c. S. H., 1939. Severe inversion displacement. a X-ray after the injury. No fracture visible.
b Held in forced inversion: lateral ligament defect. c Held in forced inversion six weeks after suture of the
ligament. Normal joint apposition

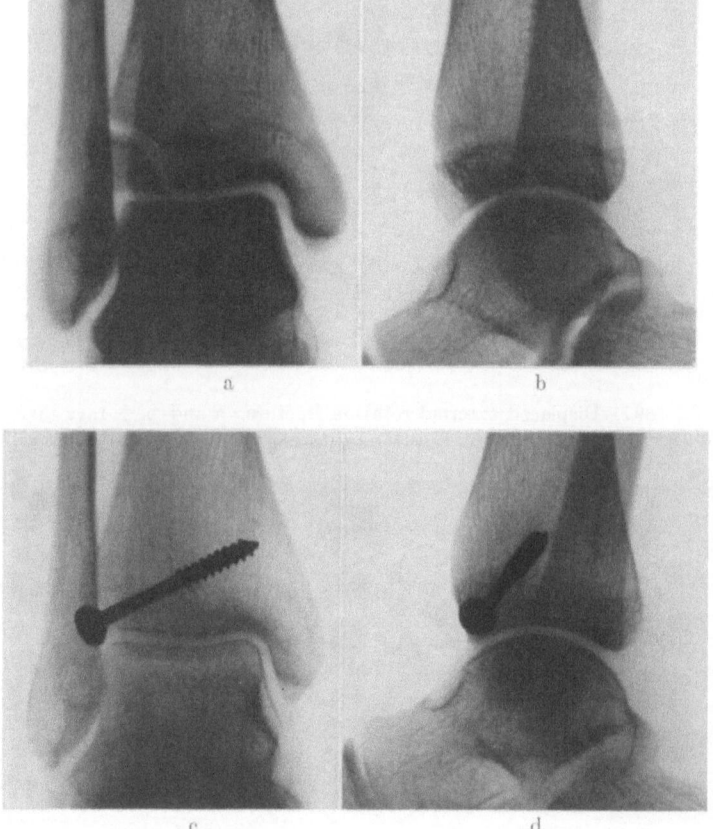

Fig. 144 a—d. B. M., 1946. Displaced external rotation fracture with an intact fibula. a and b. X-ray taken
after the accident: large Tillaux-Chaput tubercle. c and d. 6 weeks after internal fixation

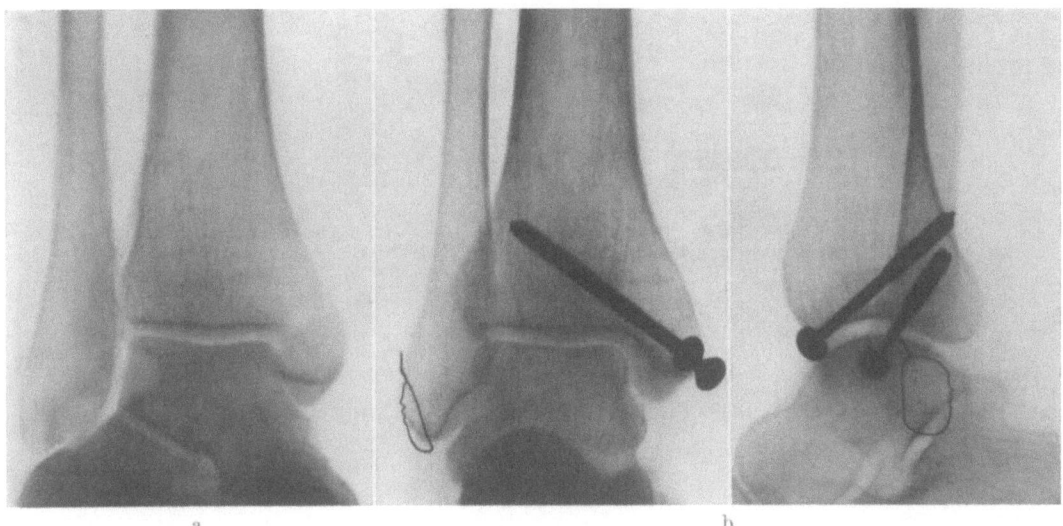

Fig. 145a and b. B. V., 1886. Displaced inversion fracture. a X-ray after injury. b 25 weeks after internal fixation

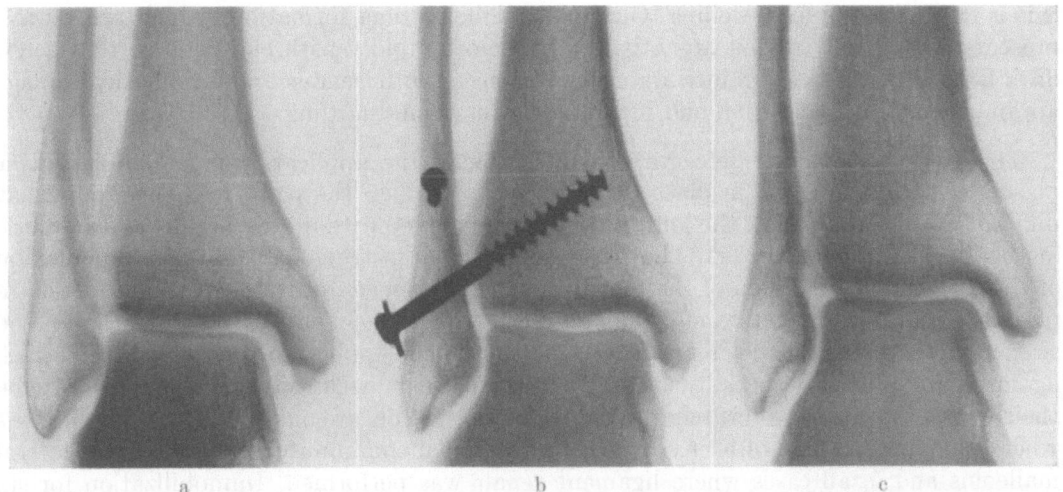

Fig. 146a—c. B. T., 1943. Ossification in the region of the tibiofibular joint following screwing by DANIS's method. a X-ray of injury. b Internal fixation and screwing of the syndesmosis. c 8 months after fixation, 6 months after removal of the screw from the tibiofibular joint: considerable bony reaction within and above the joint

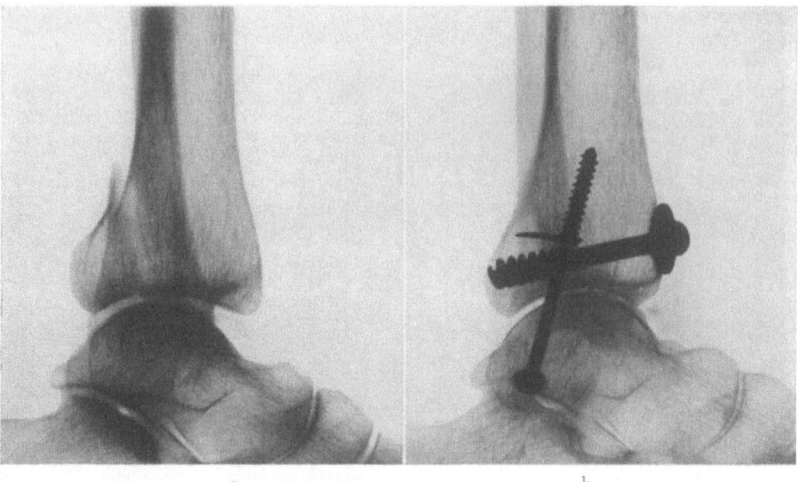

Fig. 147 a and b. S. M., 1898. Displaced eversion fracture. a X-ray of the injury. b 13 weeks after internal fixation

c) Postoperative Treatment

The importance of elevation of the leg after operation cannot be overstressed, for when this is done there is less swelling. Oedema and hematoma formation, which are always present in cases not treated urgently, subside more rapidly with elevation so that a few days later the skin has regained its normal creases. Both venous and lymphatic drainage are improved in this position and make for better wound healing.

To avoid any equinus deformity we recommend the application of a double gutter plaster cast (Fig. 22), left in place for four days. By then the pain from the wound has diminished enough to allow the joint to be actively moved without discomfort and supporting bandages can be discarded. The patient should be instructed to practice dorsiflexion of the foot and mobilization of the toes to some extent even during the four day period in plaster. From now on, active movements must be vigorously carried out, but there is no reason why a removable plaster back slab should not be applied to the leg as a protection against injury. This is especially useful when the patients need to travel or wish to resume their work with the use of crutches. Exceptions to this rule are only made in difficult cases where rigid fixation has not been secured, as in irregular comminuted fractures of the lateral malleolus and in all cases where ligament repair was performed. Immobilization for six weeks cannot then be avoided.

After malleolar fractures, weight bearing depends on the severity of the injury, but early mobilization is still advocated. In pure external rotation fractures of the lateral malleolus where there is no diastasis or other accompanying injuries, early weight bearing can be allowed when the skin wound has healed. When the ligaments are also injured, however, weight bearing should be postponed for four to six weeks. When the inferior tibiofibular joint has been held by screws they should be removed before full weight bearing, at about eight weeks. Three months after the accident, the patients are usually back to normal.

Fig. 148a—c. S. M., 1929.
Displaced eversion fracture

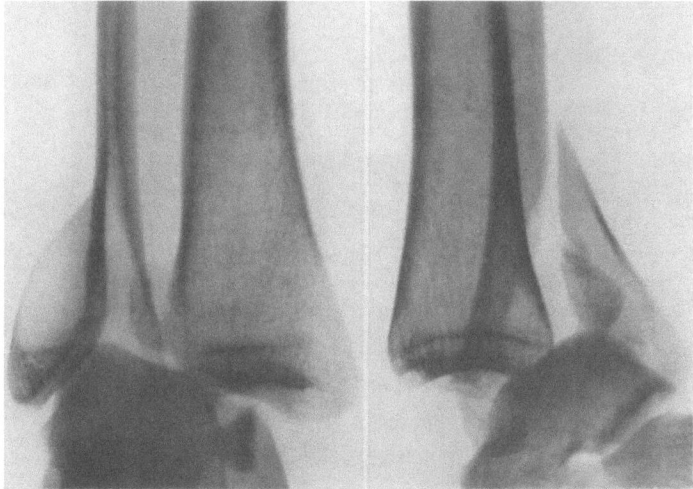

a X-ray of the injury

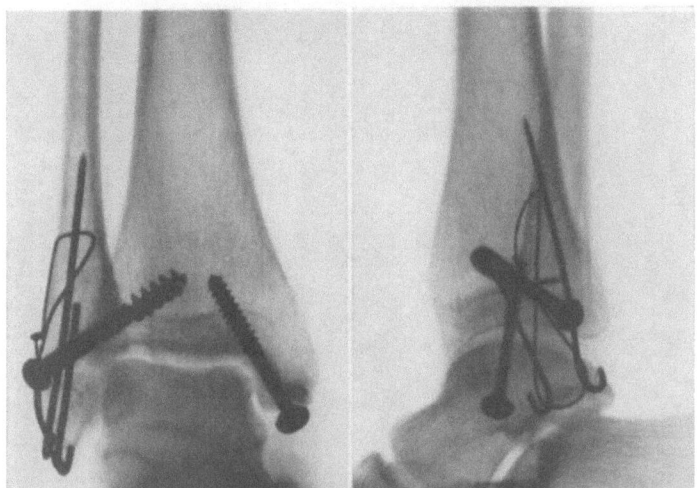

b 8 weeks after internal fixation

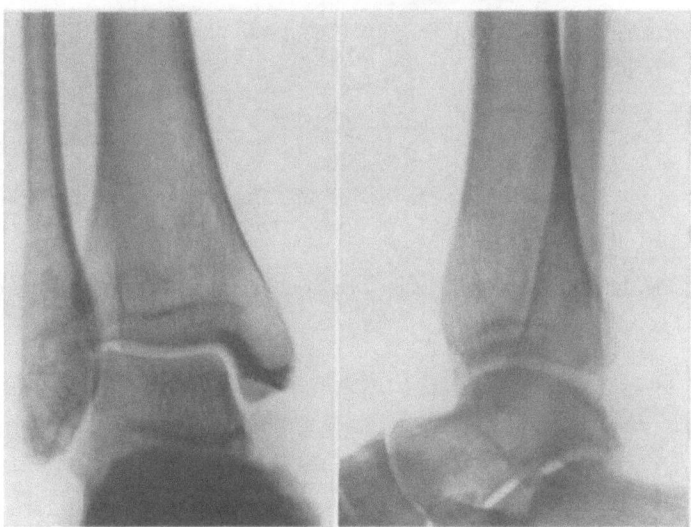

c 16 weeks after internal fixation and 8 weeks after removal of the metal

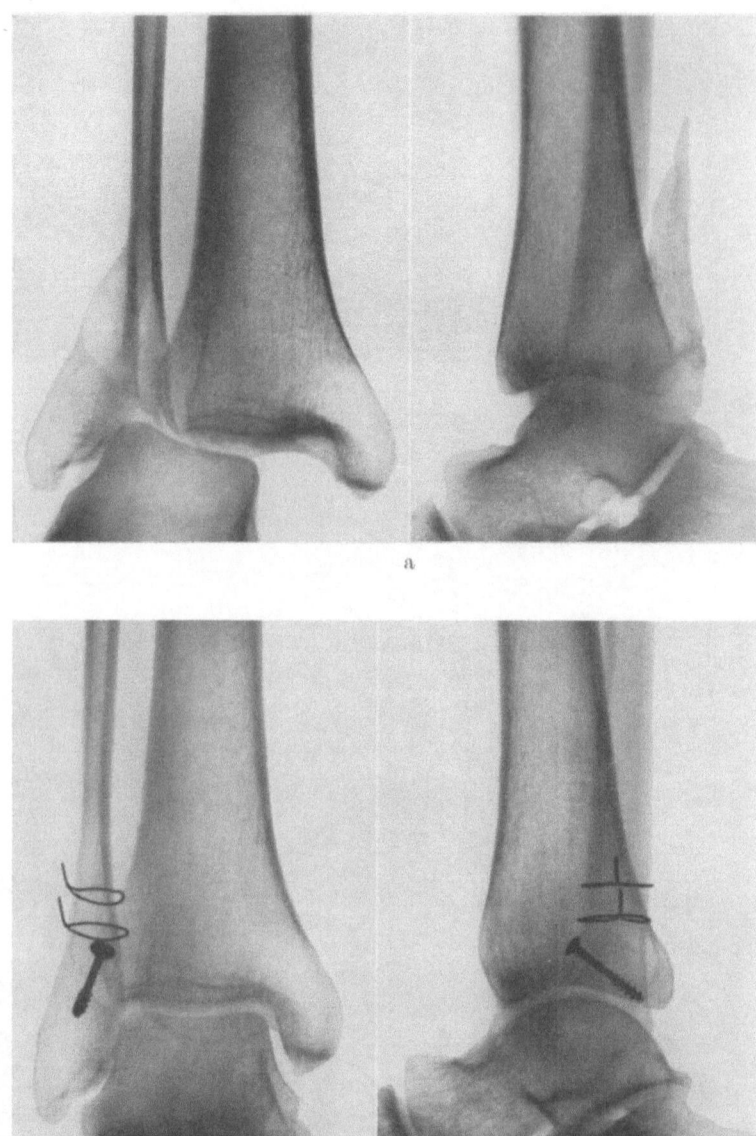

a

b

Fig. 149a and b. H. J., 1936. Displaced eversion fracture. a X-ray of the injury. b 10 weeks after internal fixation

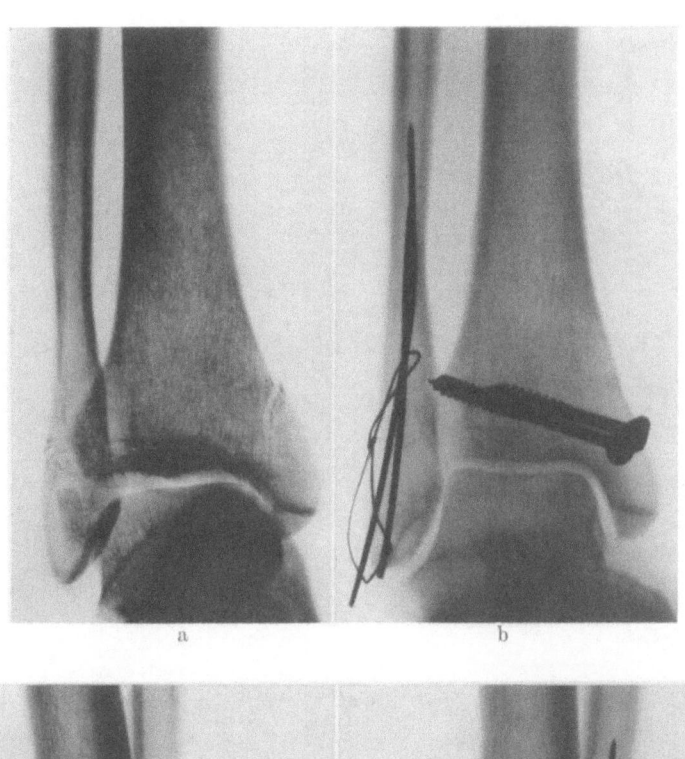

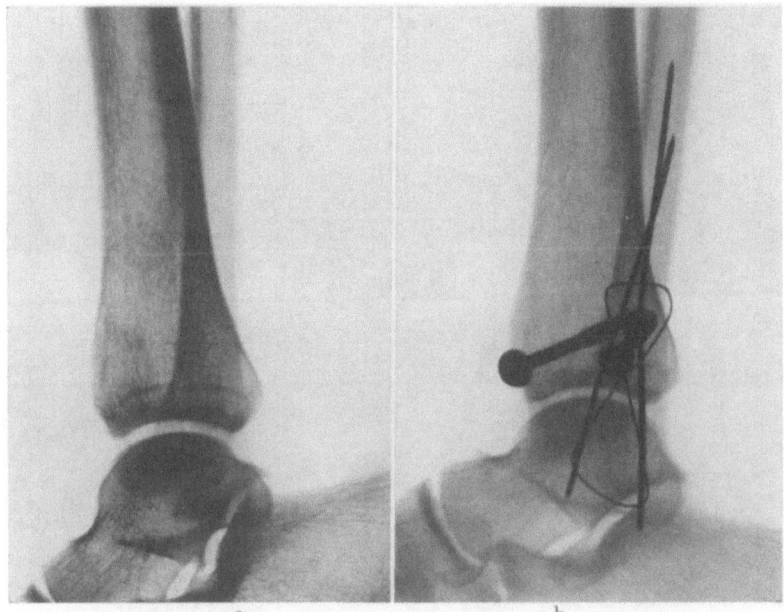

Fig. 150a and b. S. L., 1931. Displaced inversion fracture. a X-ray of the injury. b 1 year after internal
fixation

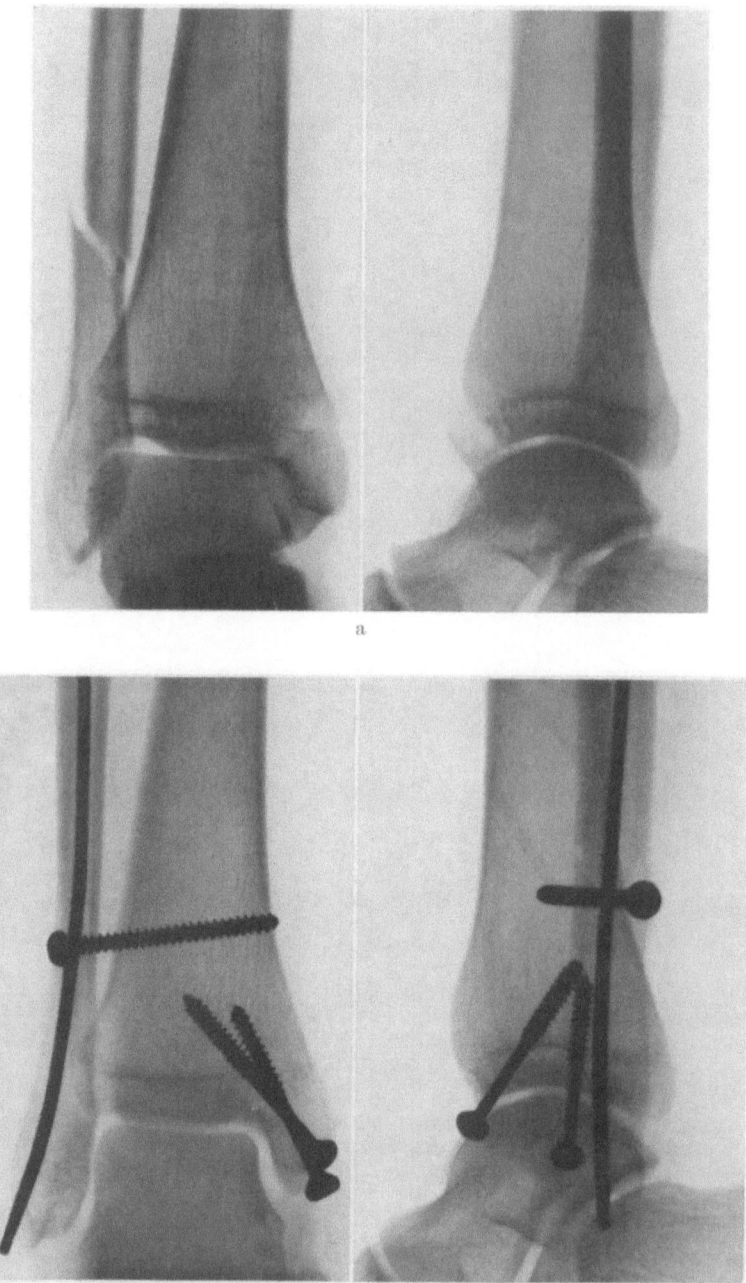

Fig. 151 a and b. U. J., 1945. Displaced eversion fracture. a X-ray of injury. b Postoperative result

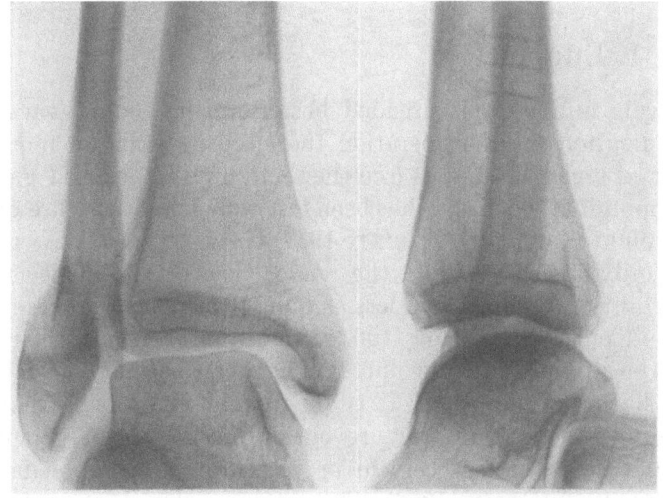
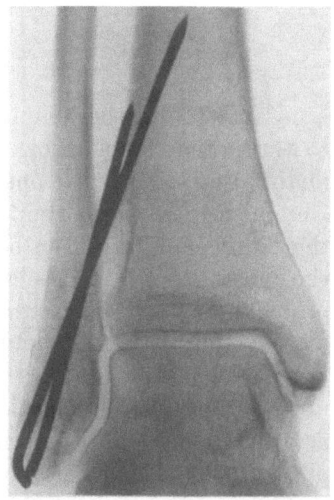

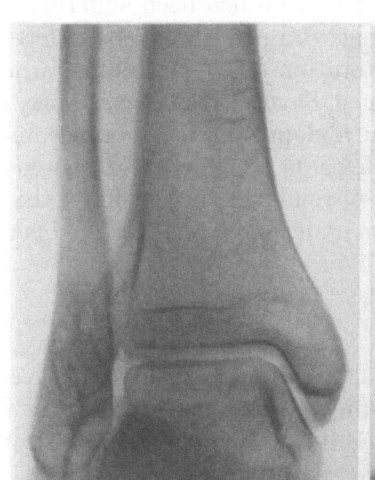
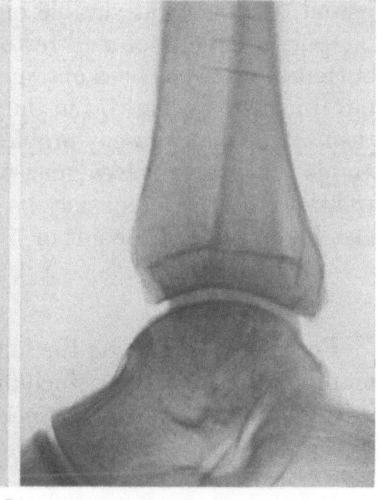

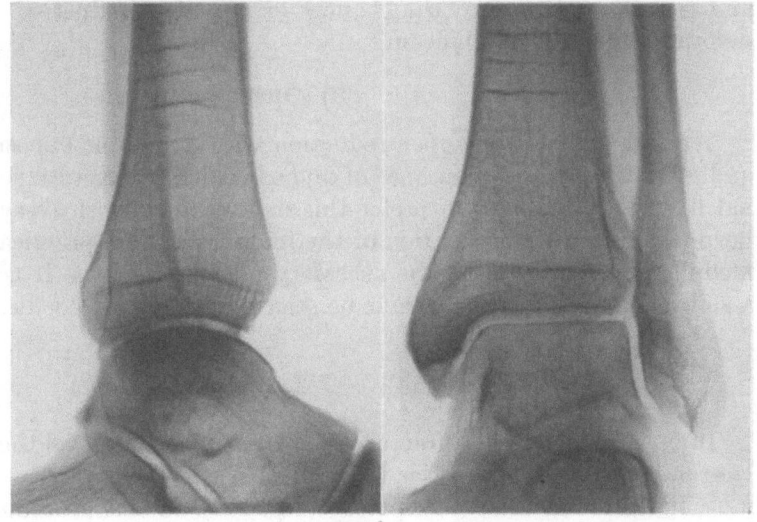

Fig. 152 a—d. Crossed wire pinning of oblique fracture of the lateral malleolus and tilting of the talus. a X-ray of the injury. b Cross pins in the lateral malleolus. c 6 years after internal fixation. d The normal opposite side

III. Fractures of the Femur

1. Introduction

A fracture of the femur is a severe injury; it is dreaded because of its consequences to the patient as a whole. The indication for the operation therefore depends on more factors than simply the operative and technical details (see the section on Shock and Fat Embolism). Very important is the amount of blood that has been lost, which in a fracture of the femur can vary from between 500 to 3000 ml. (CLARKE, 1957, GANZONI, 1959). As to the question of fat embolism, we only wish to remind the reader that this is a special problem (SEVITT, 1962). It is important to replace blood loss as quickly as possible, aiming at a systolic pressure about 100 and pulse rate below 100. In addition Rheomacrodex (low molecular weight Dextran) can be administered in volumes of between 500 and 1500 ml. until a good microcirculation has been re-established. It is our distinct impression that as a supplement to these measures in the treatment or prevention of shock, emergency operation and energetic postoperative care have a certain prophylactic effect upon fat embolism (KNISELY, 1942, THORSEN, 1950, GELIN, 1956). The reaching of a decision for surgery, especially on any patient who has been suffering from clinical shock for a long period, is thus a responsible one. Surgery should be deferred until there is an adequate peripheral circulation and restoration of blood volume, or at least until a normal hourly output of urine has been obtained. Severe brain damage may constitute a contraindication, but injuries elsewhere, as in the abdomen and thorax, need not delay surgery, though they themselves may present problems as to which area should be approached first. For example, a ruptured spleen must be removed at once, but if the condition allows, the primary treatment of the femur may be undertaken at the same operating session. This holds true also for injuries of the gut or liver.

2. Position

For any operation on the femur, the patient is best placed on his side to facilitate free manipulation of the leg including flexion of the hip to a right angle, which allows the introduction of a medullary nail into the bone with the least damage to soft tissues.

a) Closed Reduction

In specialized clinics this method may be preferred with the help of image intensifiers and television. However, the chances of imperfect reduction, especially with rotational deformity, are not insignificant.

b) Open Reduction

We feel that primary open reduction with a suitable exposure has few disadvantages and gives the greatest assurance of an anatomically exact reduction and really rigid internal fixation. We therefore prefer this method in almost every case. In a medium sized hospital, open internal fixation of the femur is a more practical procedure than is closed medullary nailing without the necessary technical means. It is important, however, that a suitable approach to the femur be selected to give as bloodless a field as possible.

3. Approach

In open reduction of a fracture of the femur at any level the best approach is posterolateral, first splitting the fascia lata and then separating the vastus lateralis from the intermuscular septum, using a raspatory (Fig. 154). In this procedure four or five perforating arteries are encountered and these require preliminary ligation. In supracondylar fractures

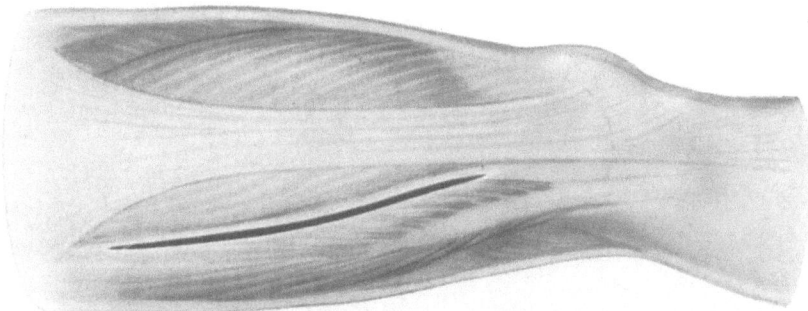

Fig. 153. Surgical approach for fractures of the middle and distal thirds of the femur

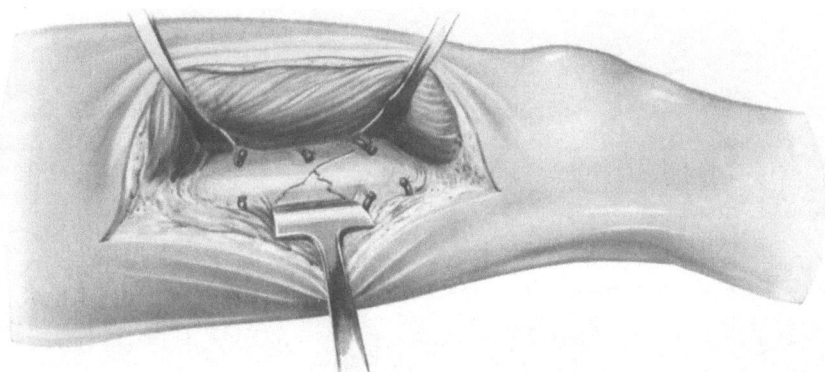

Fig. 154. The vastus lateralis is drawn back from the intermuscular septum with preliminary ligation of the perforating vessels

partial or complete division of the iliotibial tract is often unavoidable. Fractures of the distal shaft and the condyles can be operated on under tourniquet with advantage.

4. Fractures of the Middle Third of the Shaft

The approach is as described above. In all fractures of the femur the fracture zone must be bridged by either double plates or by an intramedullary nail (after reaming the medullary canal). *The use of screws alone is absolutely contra-indicated* as refracture almost always follows (in a very long oblique fracture occurring in adolescence, an exeptional case may be suitable for screwing).

a) Open Medullary Nailing

The fracture site is exposed as described above, from behind the vastus lateralis. The fracture is reduced and held as firmly as possible by forceps (or it may be bridged over temporarily with a plate which is fixed to the bone with forceps). The medullary cavity is opened up on the lateral side of the trochanter major, close to its upper end, with an awl, leaving intact the muscular insertions. The guide rod is introduced and the reaming done to a width of 12 to 14 mm. in women and 14 to 16 mm. (rarely up to 18 mm.) in men. The reaming should only continue to a level just distal to the narrowest point of the medullary canal so that the distal end of the nail may be firmly held in undamaged cancellous bone. Remaining rotational instability after nailing can be eliminated by a supplementary 4 to 6 hole compression plate using short screws that penetrate one cortex only, to avoid any conflict with the nail.

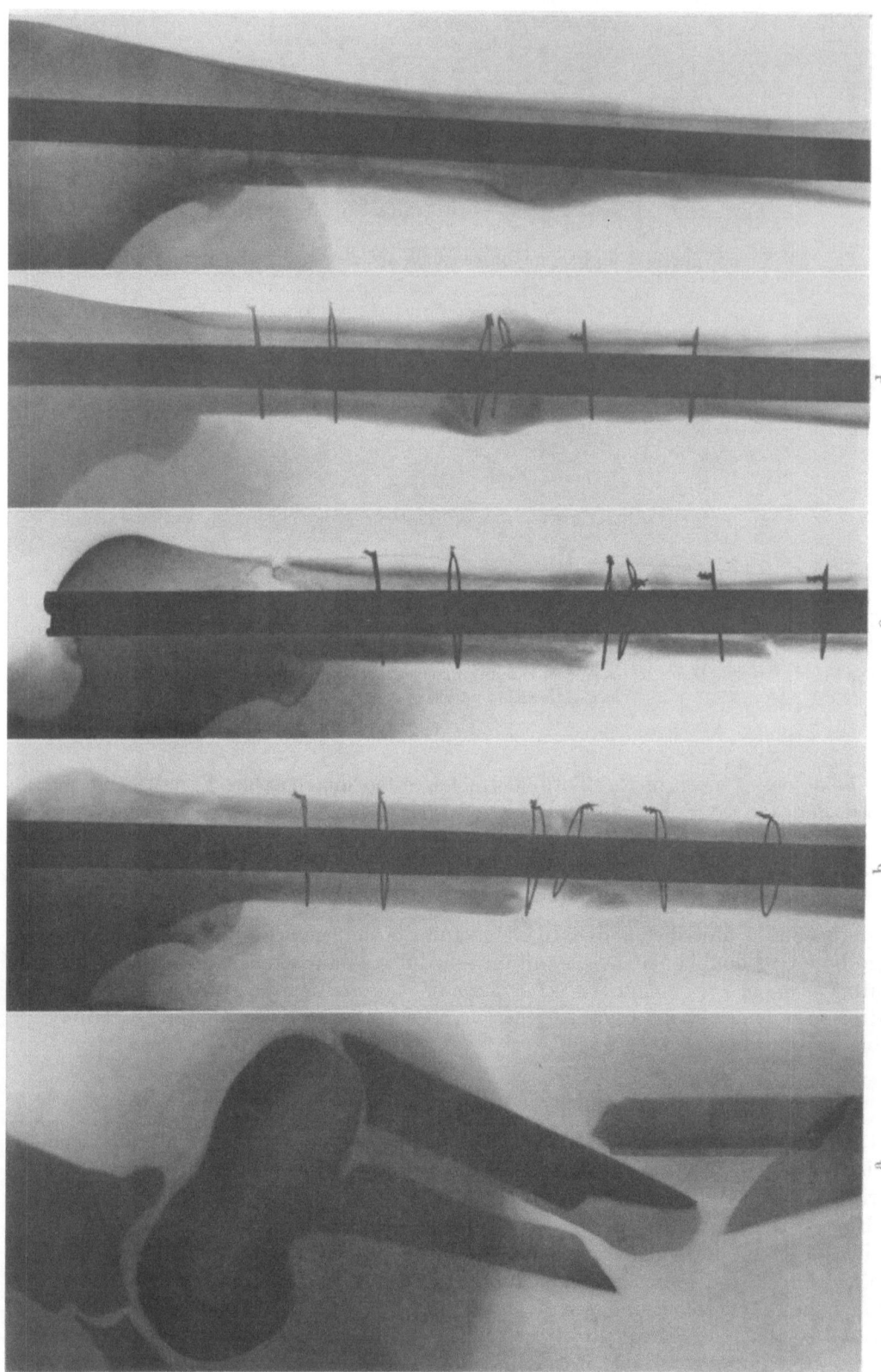

Fig. 155a—e. a Comminuted fracture of the left femur due to a road accident. In addition, the patient had the following injuries: compound comminuted fracture of the right tibia, fracture of the pelvis, contusion of the left kidney, rupture of the bladder and urethra, lacerations and contusions of the left elbow with an opened bursa and avulsion of the triceps tendon, multiple lacerations and contusion of the head. Emergency internal fixation of the left femur and the right tibia. b Postoperative x-ray after open medullary nailing and supplementary cerclage wiring of the femur. c 11 weeks after operation: No weight bearing, but active exercises. d 41 weeks after operation before removing the cerclage wires. e 58 weeks after operation

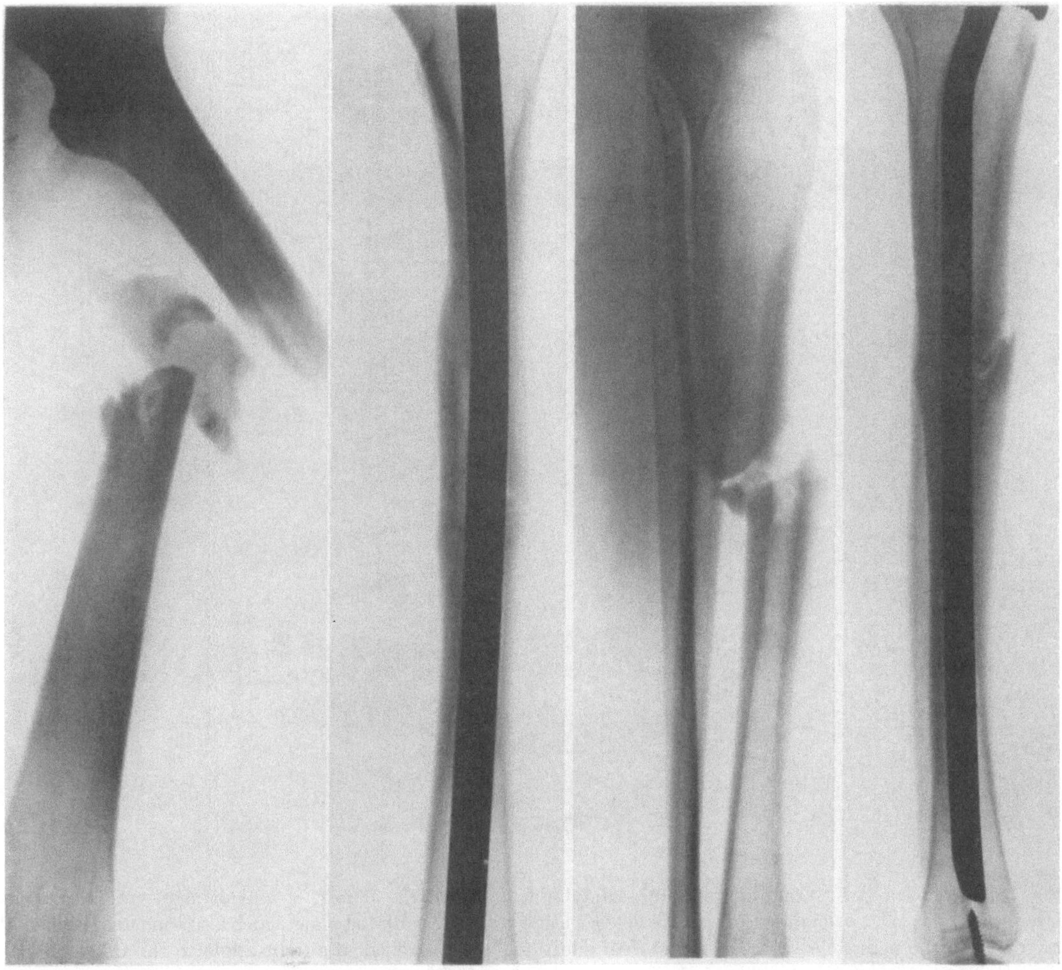

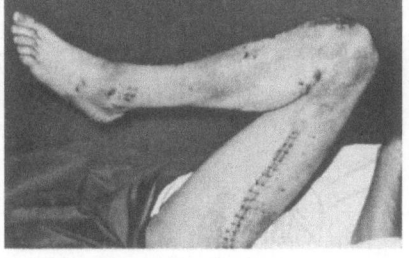

Fig. 156 a—g. a Compound comminuted fracture of the left
femur due to a road accident. b 29 weeks after medullary
nailing. Patient had the following additional injuries: compound transverse fracture of the left tibia, fracture of the left
medial malleolus, lacerations and contusions of the head.
c and d. Treatment with primary internal fixation of the
femur, of the tibia and the malleolus, hospitalization for 23
days. e Positioning after internal fixation of the femur. f and g.
Range of active movements 18 days after primary fixation of
the femur, the tibia and the medial malleolus

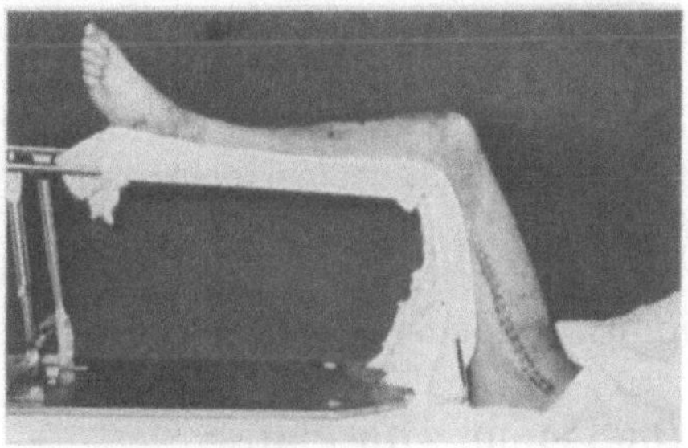

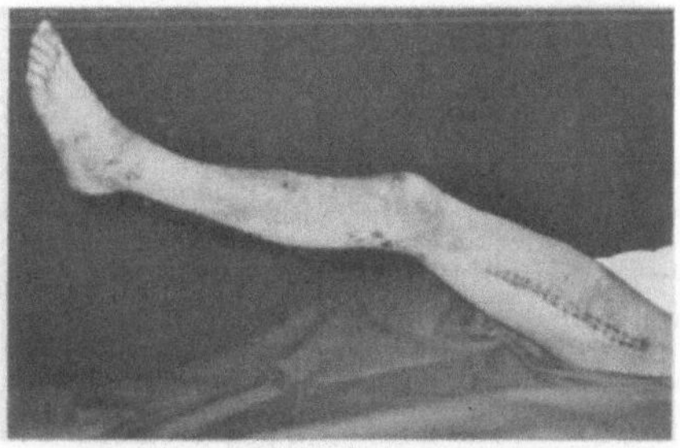

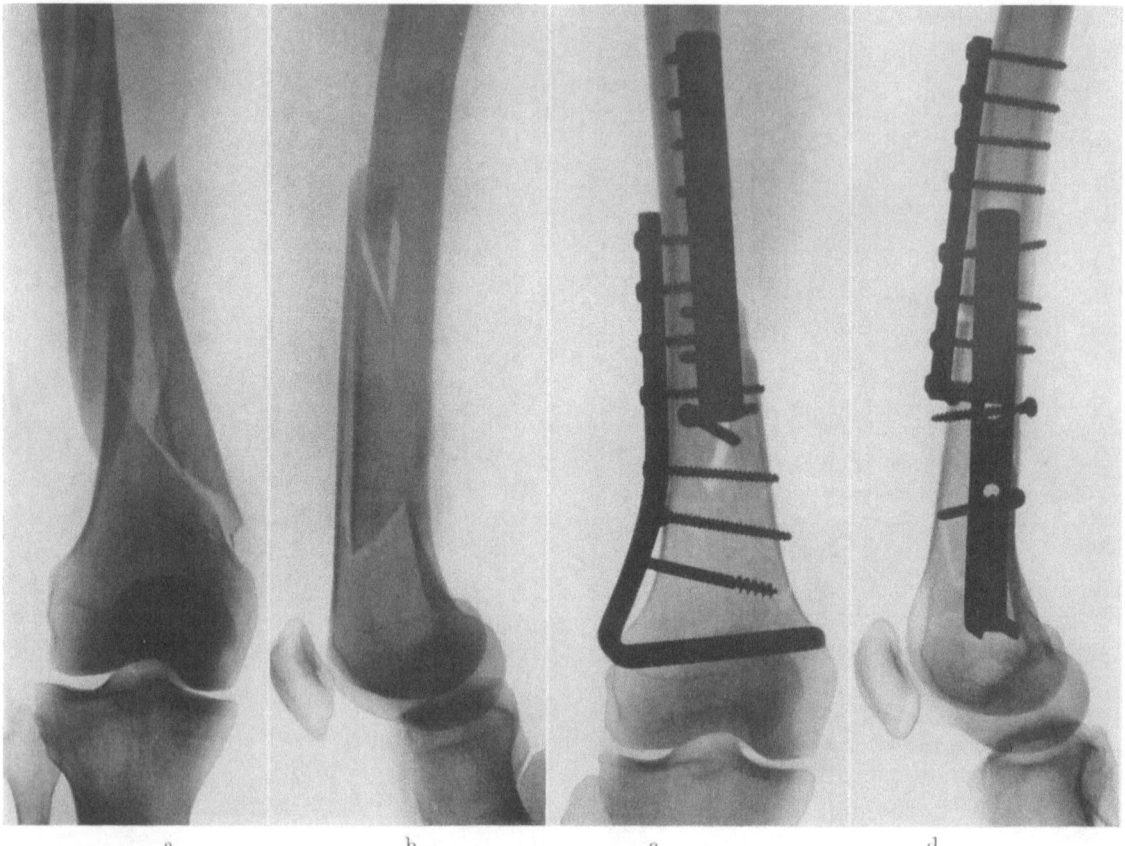

Fig. 157 a—d. a and b. Comminuted supracondylar fracture of the femur. c and d. Appearance 7 weeks after operation: the two main fragments are held together with an angulated plate which also connects the medial fragment to the main ones with lag screws. An additional plate applied at a right angle to the first one also fixes the two main fragments. The patient remained in hospital for 16 days. The fracture healed by primary bone union

As an alternative one might consider in rare cases reaming the proximal fragment before reduction from the fracture site, a procedure which seems technically easier but which carries the risk of directing the nail too much to the medial side of the femoral neck, with impairment of the capsule of the hip joint, and which may lead to a deposit of bone chips in the region of the gluteus minimus, producing calcification.

b) Internal Fixation of the Femur with Plates

The fracture is exposed as described above and the reduction held with forceps or temporary cerclage wires. Two compression plates are then applied, simultaneously if possible, so that one plate lies on the anterior and the other on the lateral surface of the femur. It is valuable to put both plates under compression simultaneously, using 2 devices. Nothing smaller than the broad eight-hole plates should be used, and longer plates may be necessary though they need not be of the same length (Fig. 157). Only part of the screws should be anchored in both cortices.

c) Wound Closure and Postoperative Positioning

The vastus lateralis which had been displaced forwards is held back in position by two or three loose catgut sutures. Redon drains are brought out from the fracture site proxi-

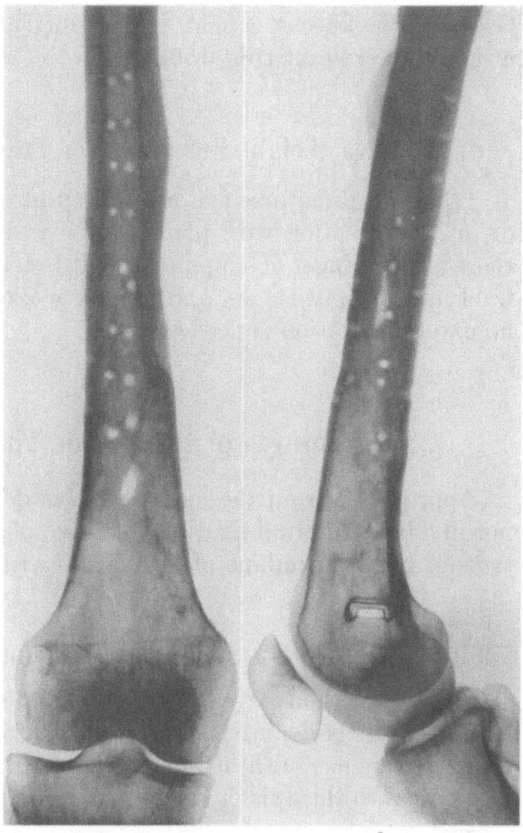

Fig. 157 e and f. Appearance 61 weeks after operation, immediately after removal of the metal

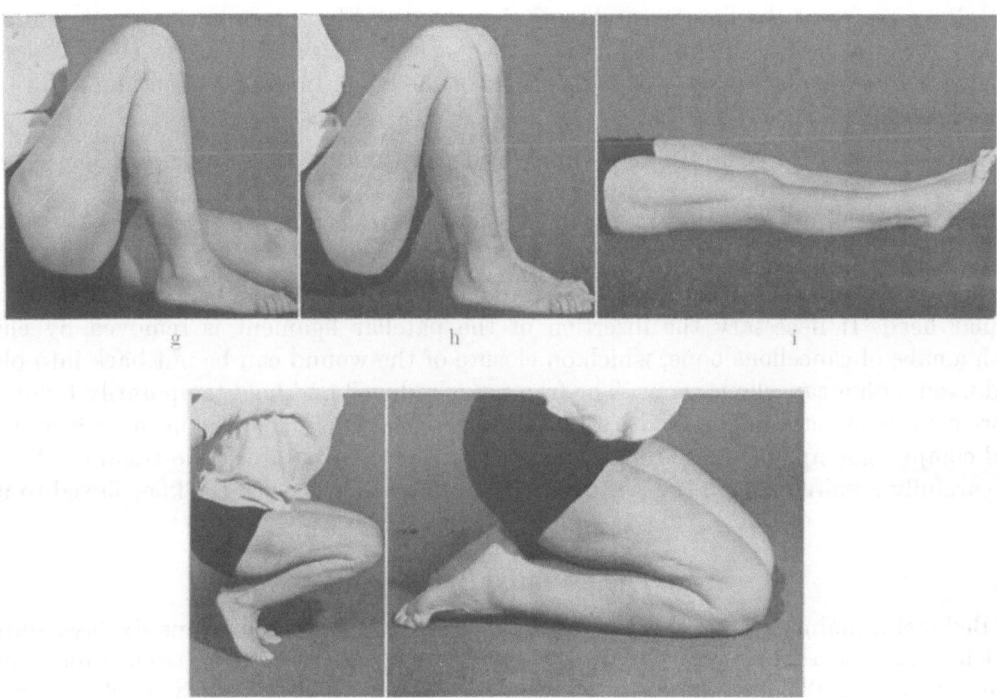

Fig. 157 g—l. Range of movement 101 weeks after first operation, 40 weeks after removal of the metal

mally through the skin and the fascia lata is carefully repaired. The leg is held after operation with the knee at a right angle, which allows full movement of the knee to be regained at about two weeks (Fig. 156).

d) Time to Weight Bearing after Fractures of the Middle Third of the Femur

Transverse fractures can be allowed to take their full weight after either a rigid nailing or internal fixation with plates, three weeks after the operation. In oblique fractures if there is any danger of slipping, weight bearing should be delayed, depending on the type of fracture, for between six and twenty weeks. If rigid internal fixation has been achieved, no external fixation is needed.

5. Fractures of the Lower Third and of the Femoral Condyles

Approach is from the lateral side as described above. If the condyles themselves are not involved, internal fixation with two plates is usually adequate (Fig. 157). It is advantageous here to combine plate fixation with a primary cancellous autograft.

a) Supracondylar Fractures

The best method of treating a supracondylar fracture is with an angulated plate (Fig. 158). The shaft of the femur must be clearly visualized, but the position of the plate is determined by the line of the articular surface. First of all, therefore, a KIRSCHNER wire is driven in paralled to the axis of the joint and its position checked radiographically.

The physiological angle between the axis of shaft and that of the articular surface is 95°. The AOI blade-plate has this angle and if the blade is driven parallel to the axis of the joint, the shaft is fixed at the correct angle. Individual variations can always be estimated by taking x-rays of the uninjured side. Fixing the distal fragment to the angulated plate makes the otherwise difficult reduction much easier. In suitable cases compression is applied before the plate is screwed to the shaft of the bone. In oblique fractures additional screws can be used.

Subtrochanteric fractures are very suitable for this kind of right angle fixation as well.

b) Transcondylar Fractures, Y-Fractures

A lateral approach is used as described above splitting the ilio-tibial tract down to the fibular head. If necessary the insertion of the patellar ligament is removed by chisel with a cube of cancellous bone, which on closure of the wound can be put back into place and fixed with a cancellous screw. The fracture is reduced and held temporarily by one or more cancellous screws. The blade of the angulated plate is introduced as described above and compression applied (Fig. 158). During closure of the wound the ilio-tibial tract must be carefully repaired. Again the postoperative position is that with the knee flexed to 90°.

c) Postoperative Management

Bed rest is maintained until the wound is securely healed, which means six days, during which anticoagulants are started. Progressive active exercises begin twenty-four hours after operation. Weight bearing is allowed between eight and twenty weeks after the injury, depending on its severity. If rigid internal fixation has been obtained, no external fixation will be needed.

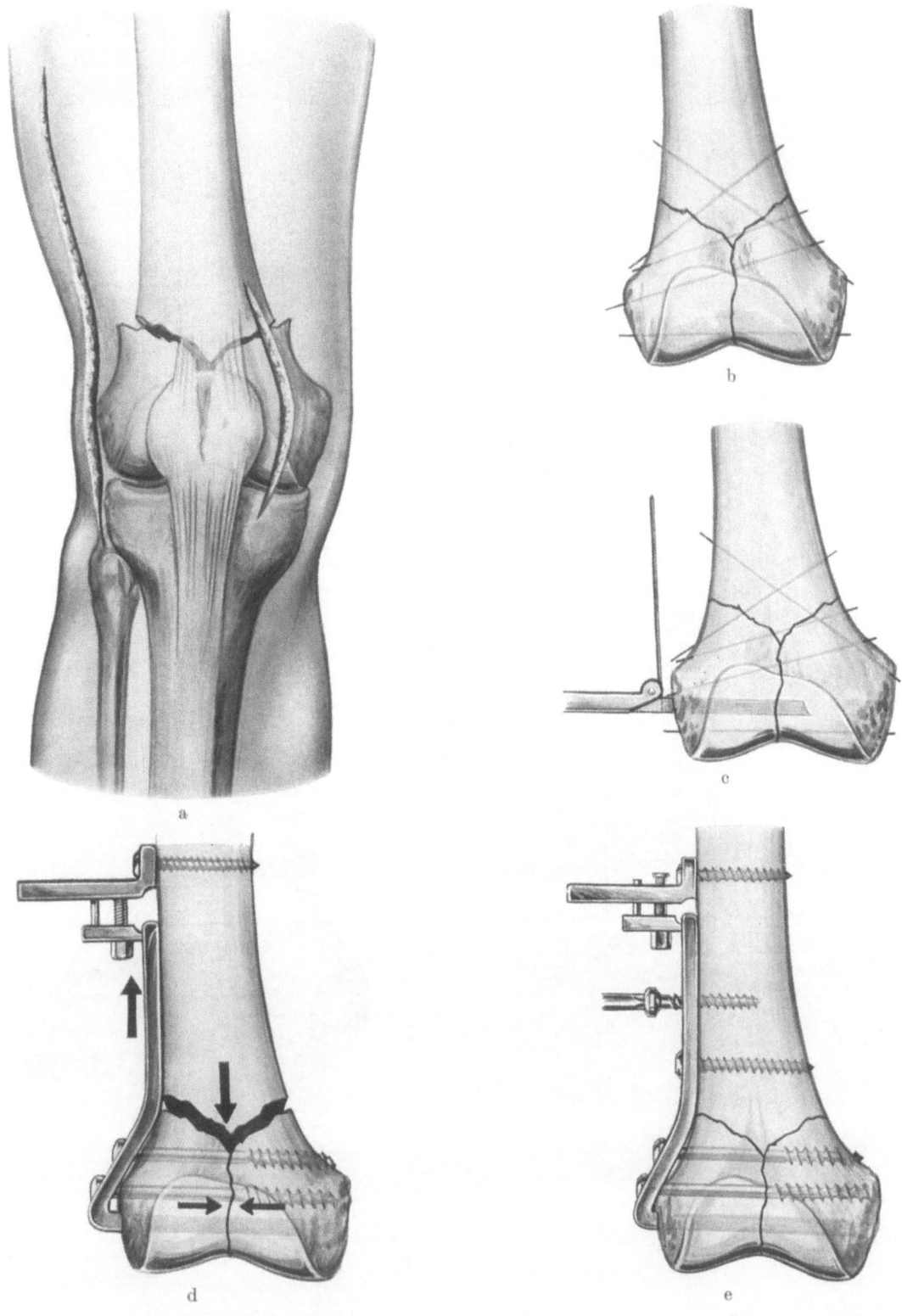

Fig. 158a—e. Surgical procedures for Y-fractures of the femoral condyles. a Approaches. b Temporary alignment with KIRSCHNER wires (1 wire parallel to the articular surface). c Introduction of the special chisel. d Internal fixation of the condyles and thereafter compression towards the shaft of the femur. e Fixation of the plate with screws to the shaft

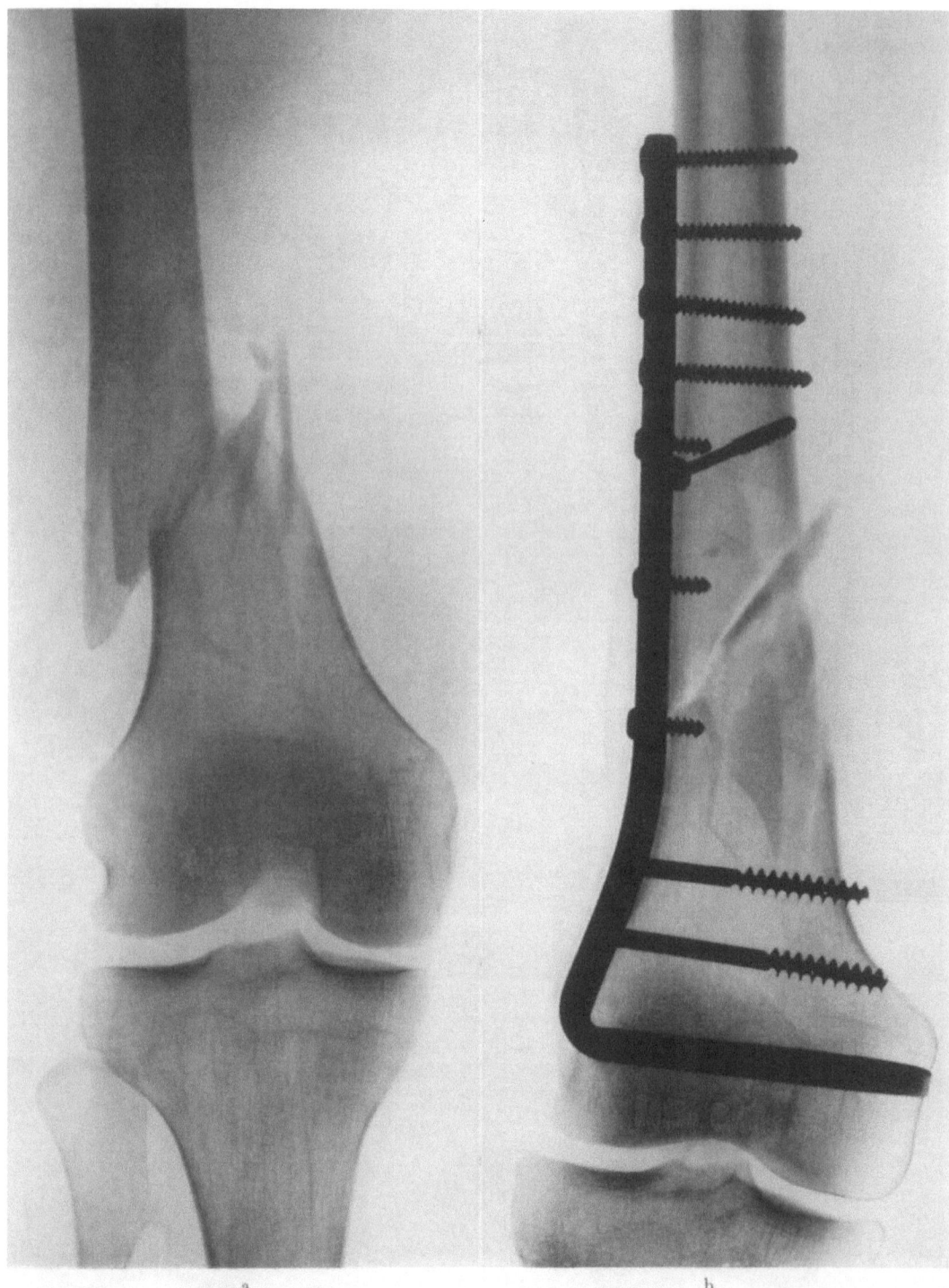

Fig. 159a and b. a Compound comminuted fracture of the lower end of the femur. b 4 weeks after operation:
The fracture is spanned by a long condylar plate and active knee flexion is possible up to 70⁰

IV. Fractures of the Patella

The appropriate treatment of a fractured patella depends on its type and the time that has elapsed since the accident, especially when there is contusion of the knee. Conservative treatment is satisfactory when the fracture is not displaced and the extensor mechanism is intact. Fixation with a simple encircling wire (as described by BERGER, KOCHER, NICOLET) though still commonly used is not very effective as the muscle pull soon opens out the fracture line towards the anterior surface of the patella (Fig. 160b). The fragments then become tilted and the stage is set for traumatic osteoarthritis.

The *double traction absorbing wiring* prevents any postoperative shift of the fragments and allows active movements to be begun in the knee within a few days. We have therefore adopted this technique, when the fracture is comminuted, eventually in combination with

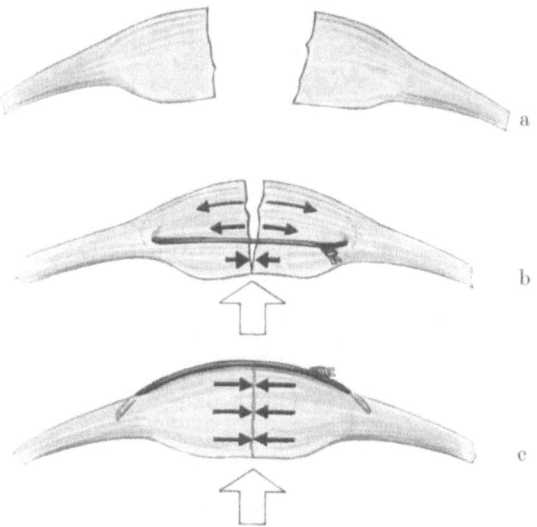

Fig. 160a—c. a Fracture of the patella. Extension strain has torn the fragments apart. b After simple cerclage or screwing, separation of the anterior part of the fracture through traction is still possible, and some tilting of the fragments is unavoidable. c If, however, the wire is placed anteriorly, it can absorb all traction forces and result in simple compression; tilting is no longer possible

KIRSCHNER wires. We only do a partial or total patellectomy when the articular surface of the patella cannot be reconstructed, or when we are treating old fractures. In the early period the functional results of patellectomy, if the muscles are in good condition may be good even with much use, but as time goes on the joint becomes weaker and degenerative arthritic changes usually develop.

The basic principles of traction absorbing wiring have been outlined, both when discussing cerclage wiring (page 38) and in fractures of the olecranon (page 169). It is important that the encircling wire lies over the anterior surface of the patella and that the wire is tightened until the fragments separate slightly at the back (Fig. 161a). When the knee is flexed, or the quadriceps tightened, the fracture surfaces are subjected to very high compression so that any slipping is impossible. One traction absorbing wire alone in which only the tendineous attachments at the extremities of the patella are fixed has usually proved ineffective since the constant pull of the muscles may produce a fatigue fracture in the wire. The second small traction absorbing wire is inserted on the patella passing through Sharpey's fibres only, as in Fig. 161b. Both wires are of V 4 A stainless steel (AISI 316) 1.5 to 2.0 mm. in diameter. Finally, the collateral ligaments are carefully repaired.

Postoperative management. After operation the leg is placed in a foam rubber splint in which the knee joint is held at 150°. After five or six days the knee is actively extended and the whole leg lifted up. Flexion is not allowed to exceed a position of 120°. The patient is discharged from the hospital after ten to twelve days when the joint swelling has sub-

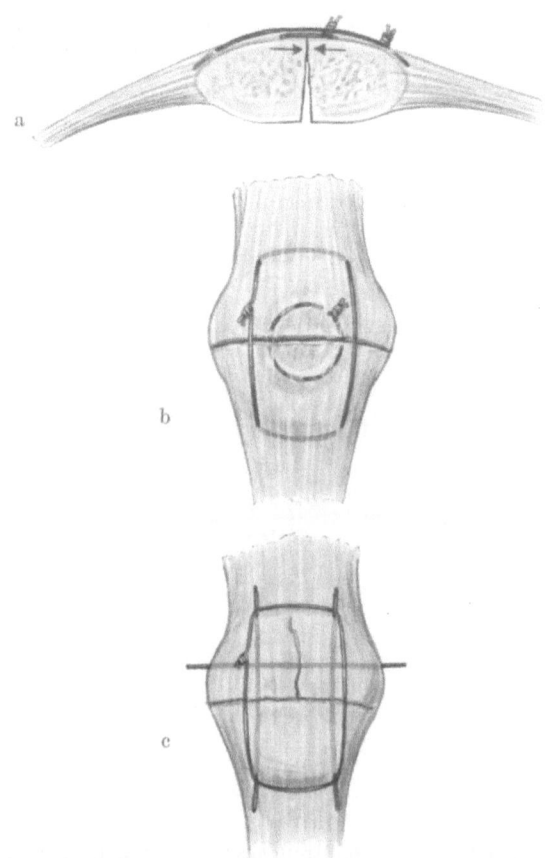

Fig. 161 a—c. Position of the traction absorbing wires at the end of the operation for internal fixation of the patella. The fragments appear to be somewhat over-corrected. a Lateral view. b Anterior view of a simple transverse fracture. c Supplementary pinning for a fracture with multiple components. The ends of the longitudinal wires are united under considerable tension by the circumferential wire

sided and the knee can be extended even against resistance. A plaster cylinder is then applied, to be worn for a month.

After removal of the plaster cylinder, check x-rays are taken and active and passive mobilization begun. At four months a further x-ray examination is carried out.

For the *treatment of patellar fractures*, the following *guide rules* have been evolved.

1. Undisplaced fractures: *Conservative or operative treatment.* The extensor apparatus is usually intact and active extension is possible.

Conservative treatment. The hemarthrosis is aspirated and a compression bandage applied. After two days, when a further aspiration may be necessary, a plaster cylinder extending to the mid-calf is applied with the knee extended but not hyper-extended. This is kept on for a month during which quadriceps exercises, straight leg raising and walking are allowed. The plaster is removed at a month, after which an elastic bandage is worn and physiotherapy is started for two to three weeks.

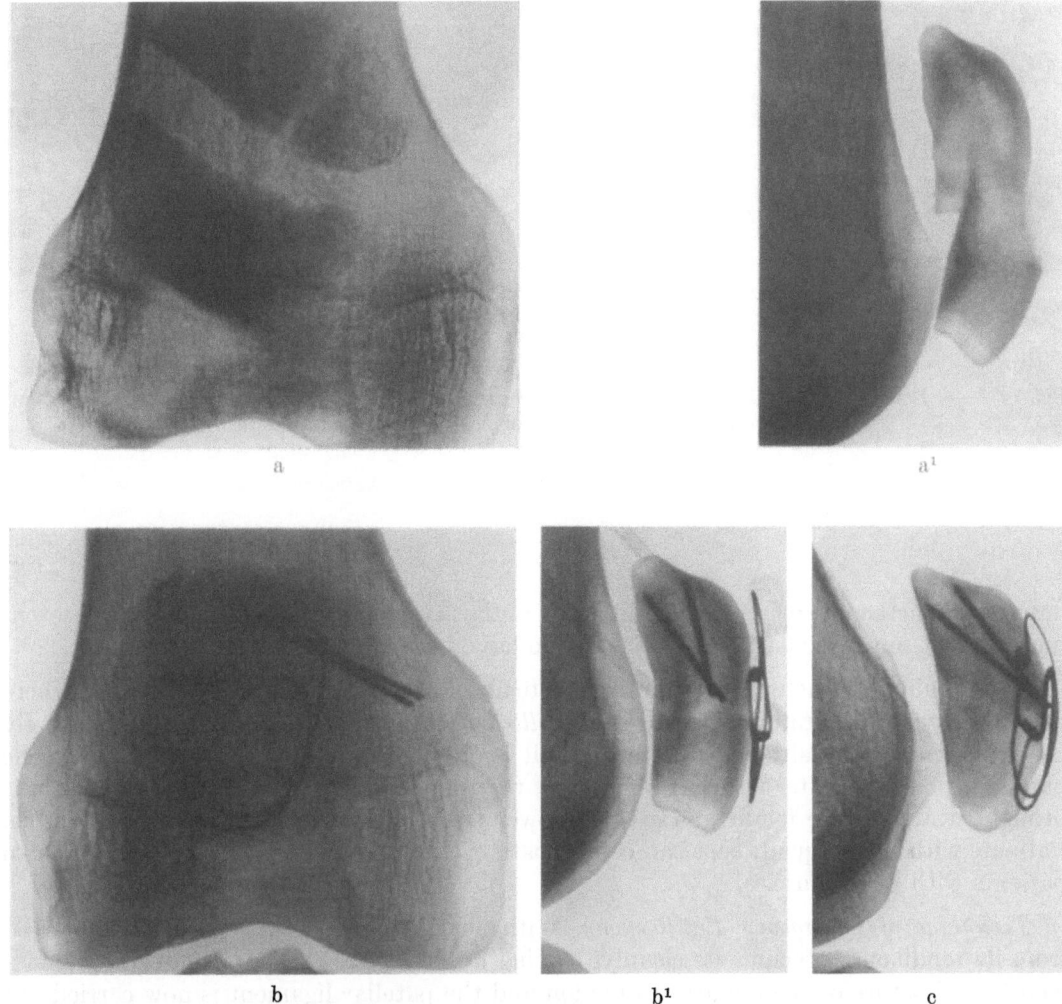

Fig. 162a—c. a and a¹ X-ray at the time of injury. b and b¹ Postoperative film. c At one year

Operative treatment. In exceptional cases with impending danger of dislocation exact reduction is secured and fixation maintained with cancellous screws. Active movements are begun at the third day and no plaster is used.

2. Simple fractures, with damage to the extensor mechanism and an intact articular surface: *Double traction absorbing wiring.* The patella is approached by a transverse incision and the articular cartilage examined, both on the patella and the femoral condyles. The patella should only be excised when there is a significant amount of damage to the articular cartilage, otherwise *a double anterior traction absorbing wire suture* is used, gaining a purchase only on the anterior Sharpey fibres (Figs. 161b and 162).

3. Comminuted fractures: A combination of KIRSCHNER wires and traction absorbing wires is advocated. The various fragments in a comminuted fracture are fixed with KIRSCHNER wires and an encircling wire inserted through the tendinous attachments to hold them together. A supplementary anterior circular wire is then applied and tightened up as much as possible in order to act as a traction absorbing wire. At the end of the operation the posterior surface of the patella must be examined very carefully from the side in order to

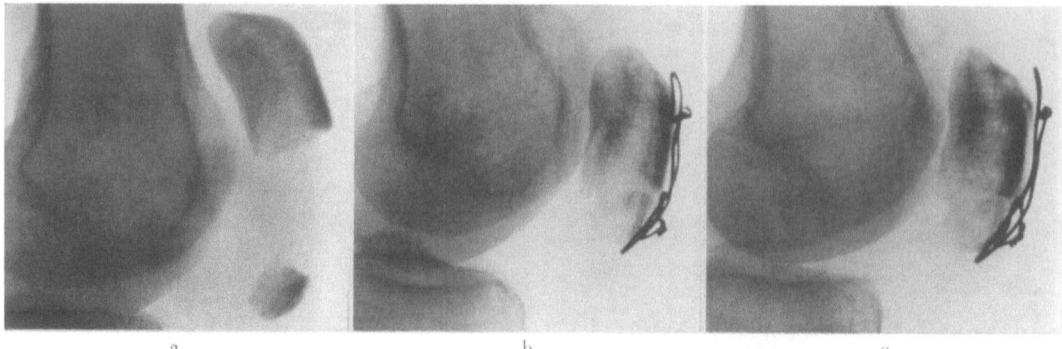

Fig. 163 a—c. Fracture of the patella with avulsion of the distal pole. a X-ray at the time of injury. b Appearance 2 weeks after internal fixation. c Appearance at 2 months

determine whether there is a significant lesion of the articular cartilage and if, after tightening the wire, any irregularities of this surface have been produced.

4. Comminuted fractures in which the articular surfaces cannot be restored, or where there is extensive separation of cartilage: *Patellectomy*. This operation has been increasingly used in recent years, although the final result is often considerably worse than when the patella is preserved after perfect reduction of the fragments. After excision the fulcrum is brought nearer to the femur and greater power is needed to keep the knee joint stable. Patients with strong quadriceps can compensate better for the loss of the patella than can patients with weak muscles.

Technique of Emergency Patellectomy. With sharp dissection the patella is removed from its tendinous attachments cleanly, leaving no periosteal or bony fragments behind. End-to-end suture of the quadriceps tendon and the patellar ligament is now carried out using braided nylon. A shortening of 3—4 cm. is thus produced, which is desirable in fresh cases. The tendon is closed in two layers, which gives a cosmetic resemblance to the patella, and synovial sutures using fine catgut are inserted at the side.

Postoperative Management. The knee is held in a flexed position and active exercises are begun on the sixth day. After the sutures have been removed a plaster cylinder is applied for three to four weeks. The main disadvantage of this operation is postoperative muscle atrophy, and in elderly patients with weak muscles the knee joint may become unstable especially while walking downhill or downstairs.

5. Fractures with lateral marginal fragments or comminution of the lower pole: *Partial excision*. If the whole separated fragment is excised, there is a risk of the tendon being reconstituted out of alignment. We therefore leave some bone attached to the Sharpey fibres, especially at the lower pole of the patella. Traction absorbing wiring is then used.

6. Old fractures. Patellectomy is more often indicated in these cases, though where there are two main fragments without much macroscopically visible damage to the cartilage, secondary traction absorbing wiring may be performed.

V. Fractures of the Forearm

1. Fractures of the Shaft of the Radius and Ulna

The conservative treatment of shaft fractures of the forearm bones in adults is difficult and experience shows that the results are not satisfactory. Closed reduction must take into account the complicated musculature of the forearm which in shaft fractures may produce lateral dislocation and angulation and sometimes rotational deformity. Immobilization of at least eight weeks in a plaster cast (Böhler, 1943) is needed, and this period may sometimes be extended to between ten and fifteen weeks before consolidation occurs. Perfect restoration of function can only be produced by anatomical reduction. There is no

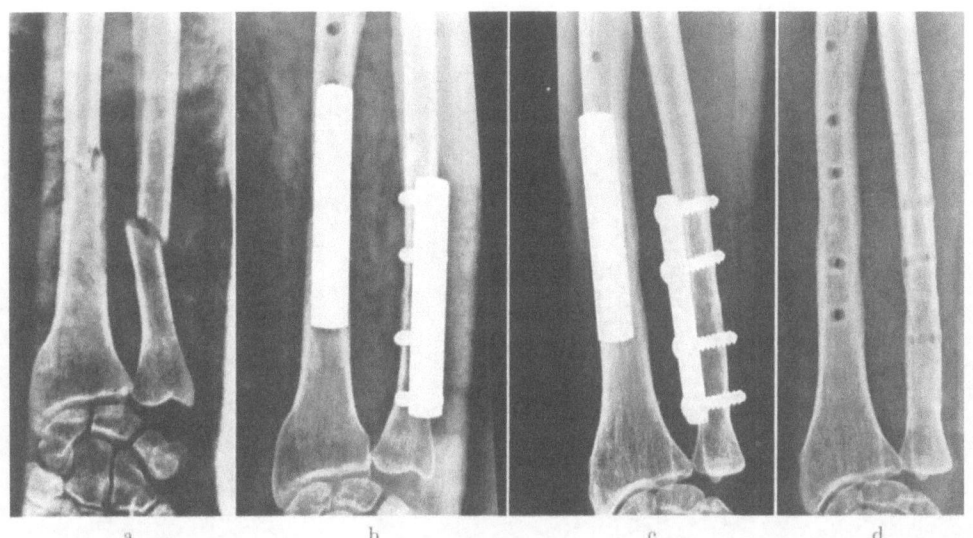

Fig. 164a—d. D. M., 56-year-old female. a Transverse fracture of the lower ends of both forearm bones. b Fixation of the radius and the ulna with a 4 hole compression plate to each. In such a case both bones must be fixed, even if one, as in this case, is not displaced. If this is not done, secondary displacement is very likely to occur. c Appearance 7 months postop. d Final result after removal of the plate

place for conservative treatment when there is interposition of soft tissues, when pointed bony fragments have become caught in muscle and when, in oblique fractures, a plaster cast cannot control the fragments. When only one of the bones is broken, nonunion may result, as the other bone makes the slight shortening which is necessary in conservative treatment impossible. In children, however, forearm fractures do well and as a rule therefore closed methods will be preferred.

Internal fixation can overcome the difficulties of closed reduction, and of the different operative techniques the use of compression plates deserves a special place. This method produces a high degree of rigidity so that plaster casts can be avoided and the arm restored to active use in a short time. Danis deserves the credit for having developed the technique of compression fixation for forearm bones to where it has become a very promising procedure.

a) Indications for the Choice of Method

Compression plate fixation is suitable for the treatment of fresh fractures as well as for nonunions. An exception is to be made for fractures near the joints as short epiphyseal fragments do not allow enough room for the application of a plate. Transverse and short oblique fresh fractures are well treated by this method. A nonunion is an excellent indication for internal fixation with compression, and the bone ends need not be freshened. Stability and compression leads to ossification in due time.

Selection of plate. For the transverse fracture a four or five hole plate is usually adequate, but if there are several fractures close together on the same bone it is better to fix them with a single longer plate. When fractures are widely separated, two short plates can be used. In a nonunion, more rigid fixation is obtained with a long six hole plate, and if there is an additional bone defect, a cancellous graft should be used as well.

Fractures of both forearm bones. Where both bones are broken it is safer to apply a plate to each bone as this gives excellent fixation and allows early postoperative movement without any plaster. The follow-up of our cases treated in this way confirm DANIS's findings.

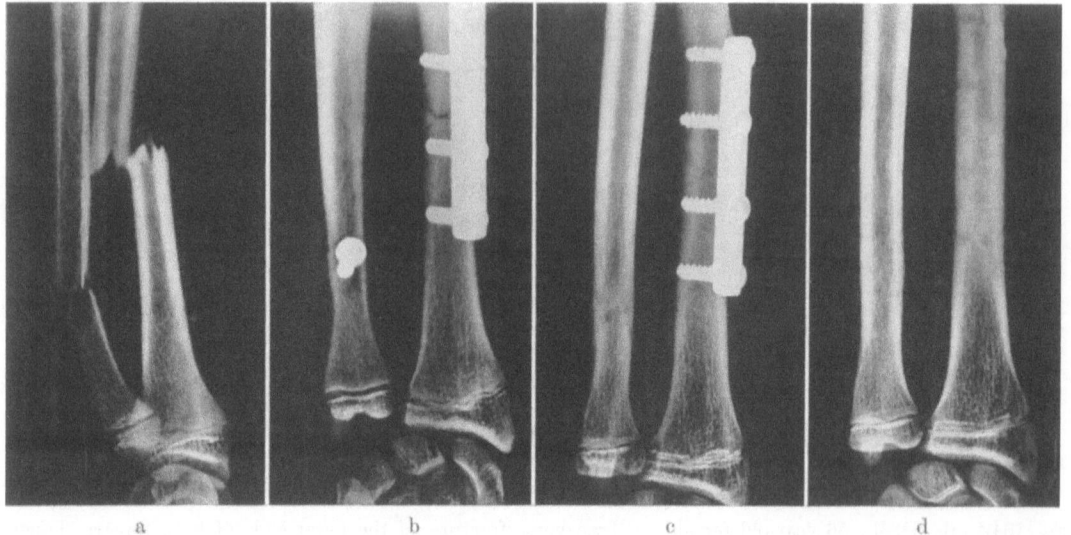

Fig. 165a—d. P. J. 19-year-old male. a Transverse fractures of the lower part of both forearm bones. b Treatment of the radius with a 4 hole compression plate and of the step fracture of the ulna with a single short cortex screw. c Appearance 6 months later after removal of the ulnar screw. d Final result at 1 year

Plates may be used in combination with medullary nails. EGGERS (1949), whose plate is well known, was one of the first to adopt this idea on a large scale (EGGERS et al., 1960). It has been suggested that the ulna should be plated and the radius nailed, following the concept that the ulna with its proximal fixed point is more subjected to rotational strain at the fracture site than the radius which can rotate at both ends. We have used this combination employing trifin nails (OBERHOLZER, 1946), RUSH pins or KIRSCHNER wires, whichever seem most suitable. Some cases of perfect union occurred even without plaster cast fixation, but others developed a pseudoarthrosis at the radial fracture. We therefore regard this combination as second best to compression plating of both forearm bones, which gives the greatest security against rotational instability.

b) Technique

A bloodless field is necessary in any form of internal fixation in the forearm as it allows full and careful examination of the injured parts, though operation without a tourniquet may be indicated when there is doubt about an arterial injury, or in cases with preexisting arteriosclerosis or BUERGER's disease. In general a tourniquet should not be left on for more than an hour to make sure that no damage is caused to nerves and blood vessels. When an operation is to be performed on the radius and then on the ulna at the same session, the tourniquet may be briefly loosened between the two procedures.

Time of operation. Both closed and open fractures of the forearm are treated primarily if there are no special contraindications. They are considered as "fractures of necessity".

Anaesthesia. If there is any reason against using a general anaesthetic, brachial plexus block may be used quite satisfactorily in forearm fractures.

Positioning. When the radius only is broken, the patient is placed on his back, but with fractures of the ulna, or both forearm bones, the prone position is better, as suggested by DANIS.

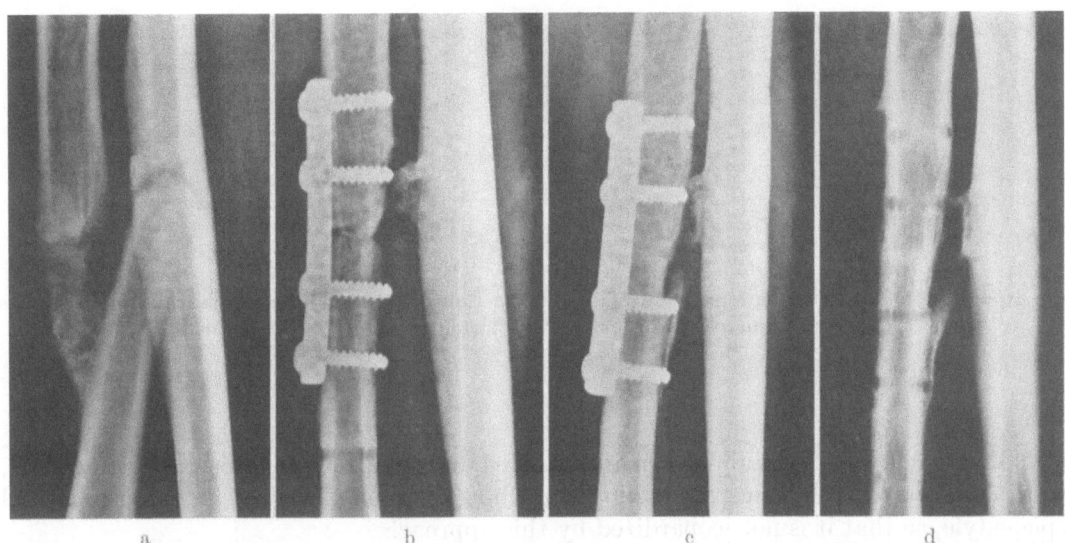

Fig. 166a—d. W. P., 31-year-old male. a Fracture of the shaft of the radius, united after conservative treatment with severe displacement. No rotation possible. b Same fracture after removal of the callus, reduction and fixation with compression plate. c Appearance 3 months after operation. d At 1 year, after removal of the plate

With the humerus abducted to 90°, the radius is accessible on supination and the ulna on pronation, and both can be reduced by traction. Screening with an image intensifier is easy in this position.

Approach. In general we recommend separate longitudinal incisions to expose fractures of the radius and the ulna. The soft tissues must be carefully treated in the forearm, especially to preserve the subcutaneous fatty tissue, for its function as sliding tissue. The incision is made not immediately over the bone but slightly to the palmar or dorsal aspect.

To expose the radius the following anatomical points must be borne in mind:

To expose the middle and distal thirds of the radius, longitudinal incisions are used (as indicated by BOURGERY). The incisions extend in the line between the head of the radius and the styloid process. Innervation of muscles is thus not impaired and access to bone is easy. The extensor carpi radialis muscle may be retracted to the volar side, the m. ext. dig. comm. dorsally.

In the proximal third the extensor digitorum, the extensor dig. quinti proprius and the extensor carpi ulnaris are innervated by branches of the deep branch of the radial nerve after it has penetrated the supinator muscle. At its point of exit from this muscle the nerve divides into a fan-shaped bundle of branches which, after a short distance, radiate into the above muscles. Any attempt to approach the radius from the radial side between the extensor carpi ulnaris and the extensor digitorum communis and dig. quinti proprius, may bruise or damage the nerve, especially as a large exposure is needed to apply the plate. A posterior approach between the extensor carpi radialis brevis and longus, or between the carpi radialis brevis and extensor digitorum communis also endangers the nerve. The safest mode of access is from the dorsal surface between the anconeus muscle and extensor carpi ulnaris. The anconeus is supplied by a muscular branch of the radial nerve which separates

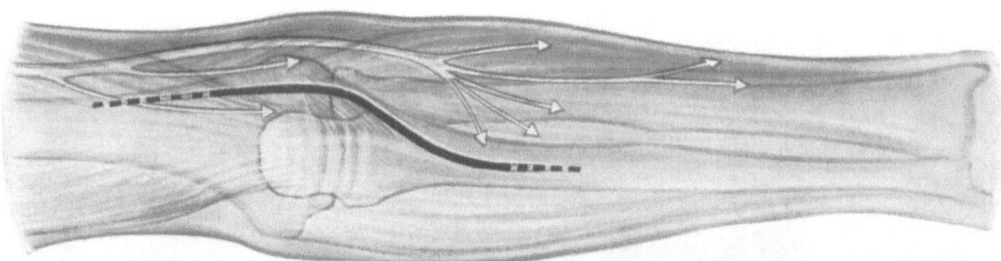

Fig. 167. Posterior view of the forearm. It shows the incision to expose the proximal third of the radius avoiding any injury to the deep branch of the radial nerve. See text for details

from the main trunk in the upper arm and, passing dorsally from the intermuscular septum, runs along deep to the triceps, crossing the elbow joint on the ulnar side of the lateral epicondyle, so that it is not jeopardized by this approach.

To expose the upper third of the radius a skin incision should therefore begin at the *lateral epicondyle*, curving along the edge of the anconeus towards the subcutaneous border of the ulna, three fingers distal to the olecranon and then down over the ulna. After dividing the fascia and the muscular insertions on the ulna, the extensors can be retracted in an *antero-lateral* direction to reach the interosseus membrane on the dorsal surface of the radius. This is rather a deep approach but avoids any damage to the radial nerve. It is also better for removing a plate as the nerve is more easily damaged if involved in scar tissue.

Approach to the ulna in its entire length is via an incision which passes from the olecranon to the wrist along the subcutaneous border of the bone, which is easily felt. The extensors are retracted dorsally and the flexors anteriorly. In fractures of the proximal third of both bones, the incision described for the radius will give adequate exposure of the ulna as well.

Reduction: After reduction and preliminary fixation, i.e. before final stabilization of one bone, careful reduction of the other forearm bone is advisable, as with too early fixation of the radius for example, serious difficulty in reducing the ulna due to ineffectiveness of traction might arise.

Application of the plate. The plate is applied most easily to the distal half of the radius on its lateral or dorso-lateral surface, to its proximal third on the dorsal surface, and to the ulna on its medial surface. It is sometimes helpful to flatten the bony surface with a chisel or to bend the plate slightly. Compression should be applied on the side of the longer fragment. The skin incision should be planned to allow for this.

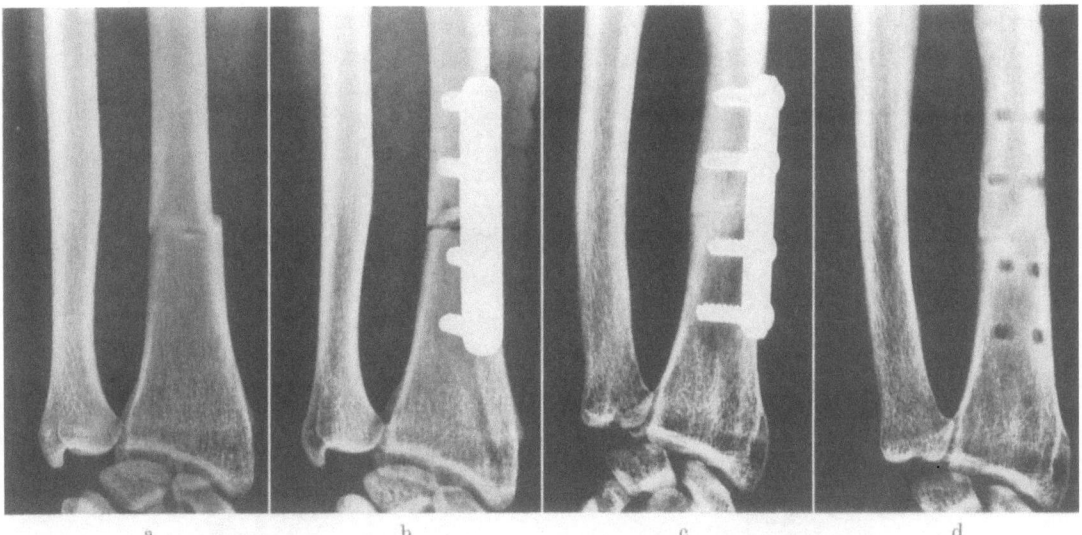

Fig. 168a—d. T. G., 31-year-old male. a Isolated fracture of the shaft of the radius at the junction of middle and distal thirds. An uncommon fracture in which conservative treatment often produces nonunion (HUGHSTON). b The same treated with a 4 hole compression plate. This is considered a "fracture of necessity" and internal fixation with a compression plate is the treatment of choice. c X-ray follow-up at 10 months. d Final result after removal of the plate

Selection of screws. The length of cortex screws should be determined with great care, as in the thin tubular bones of the forearm screws that are too short cannot hold the plate firmly, and too long ones may give rise to irritation and impairment of rotation.

Technique. The fracture is exposed and the fragments reduced with fine sharp hooks. To hold the reduction small HOHMANN bone levers are used, which are curved to fit the bone closely. Any rotational deformity is corrected. The compression plate, which has been selected according to the preoperative x-ray, is fitted to the bone and held to the short fragment with a cortex screw.

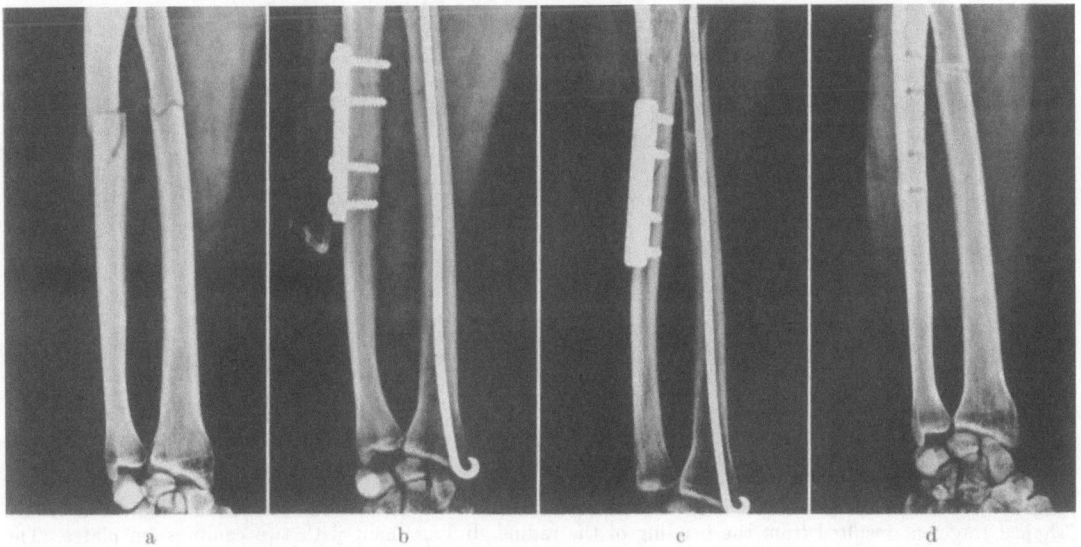

Fig. 169a—d. B. E., 19-year-old male. a Transverse fracture of the radius and ulna at the junction of upper and middle thirds. b Treatment of the ulna with a compression plate and of the radius with a RUSH pin. c Appearance 4 months postop. d Result after removal of the metal

11*

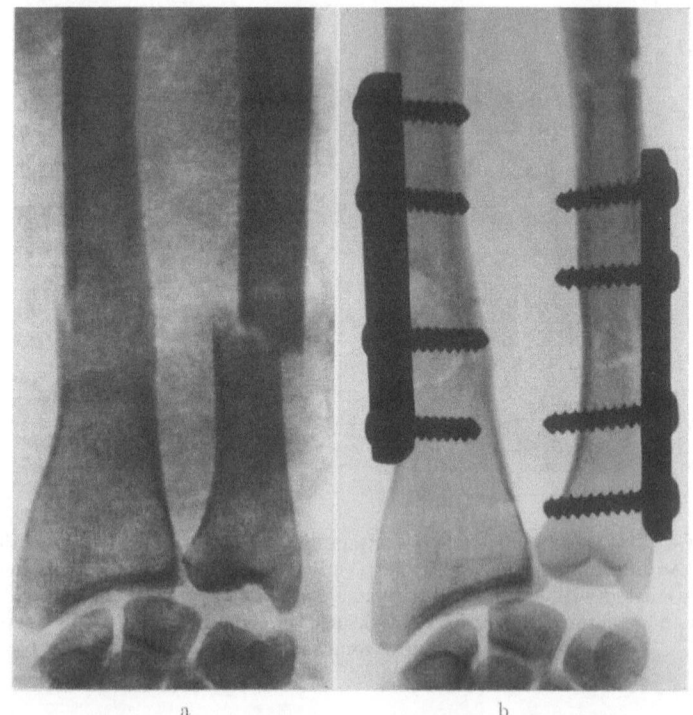

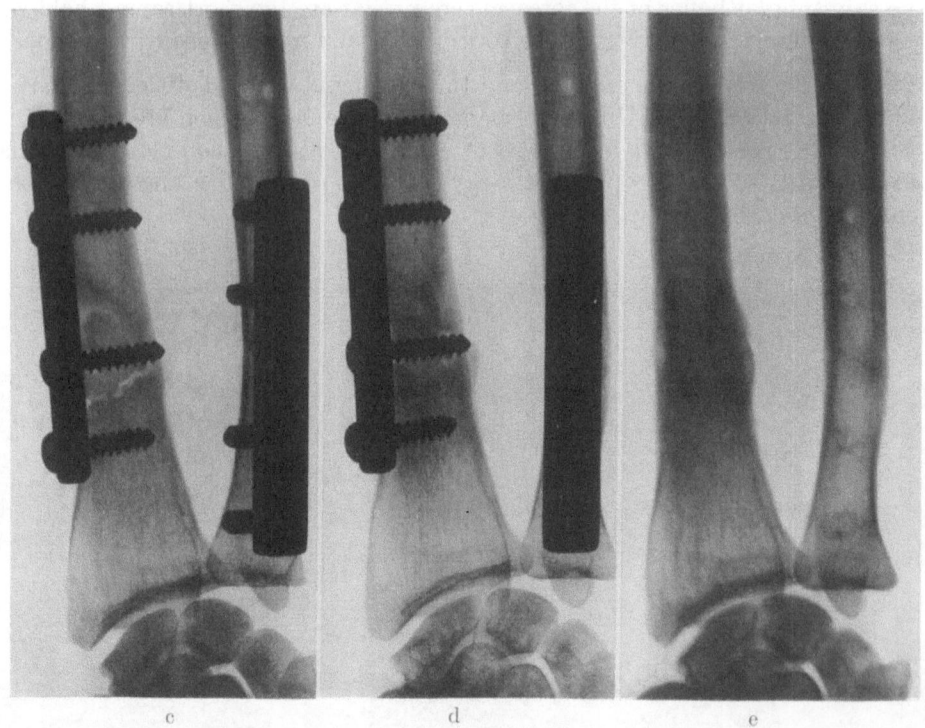

Fig. 170a—e. B. I., 33-year-old male. a Transverse fracture of the lower third of the radius and ulna. Wedge shaped fragment resulted from the bending of the radius. b Treatment with two compression plates. The radial fragment is fixed to the plate with one screw. The lowest screw is unfortunately too short. c After 4 weeks. d At 5 Months. e Final result at 1 year, after removal of the plates

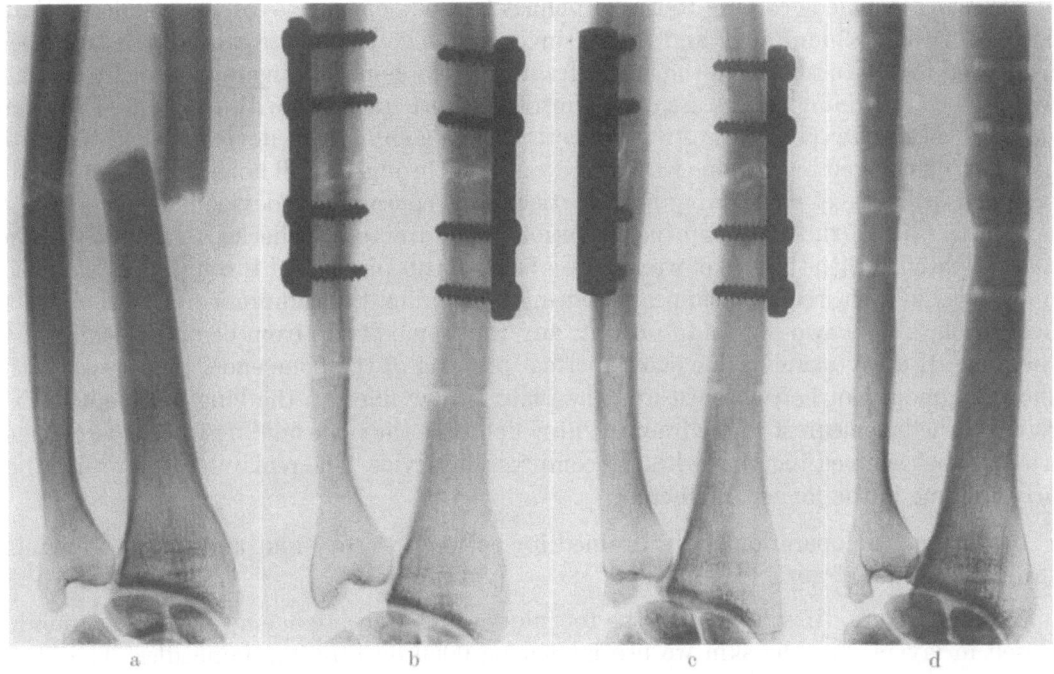

Fig. 171a—d. F. G., 21-year-old male. a Badly displaced fracture of the radius at the mid-shaft. Crack fracture of the ulna. b Treatment of both bones with compression plates. c 4 months after operation. d Final result, after removal of the plates

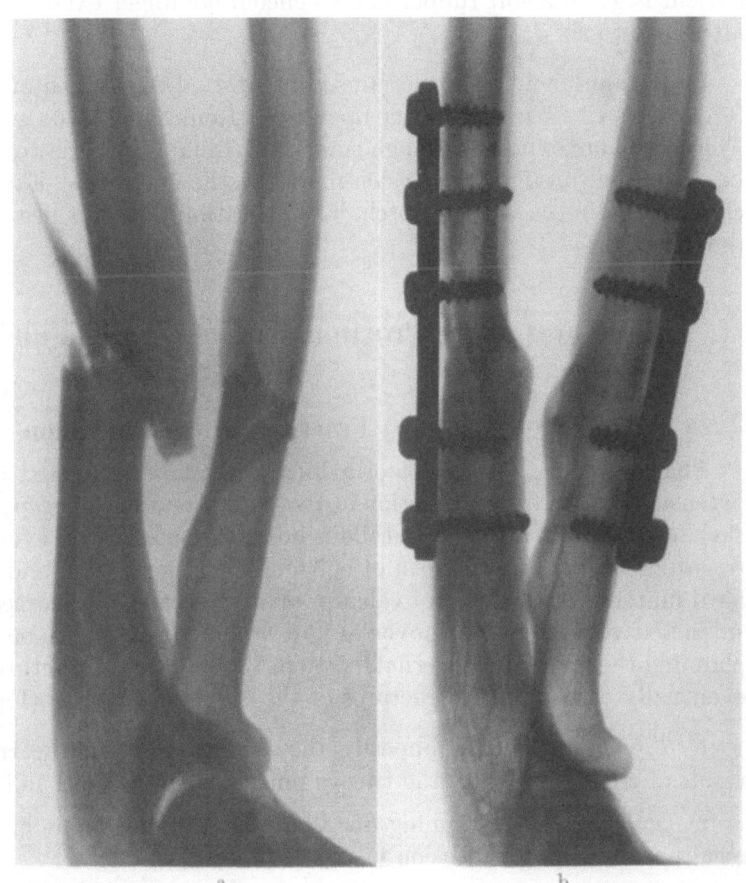

Fig. 172a and b. X. Y., 45-year-old male. a Fracture due to bending of both radius and ulna at the junction of upper and middle thirds. b At 1 year, before the removal of the two compression plates

Screwing is done according to the principles laid out on page 44 drilling holes in both cortices with a 3.2 mm. drill and then using a tap. The fragments are now reduced perfectly and the plate is fixed to the longer fragment by a bone holding forceps or by cerclage wiring. The remaining screws are driven into the short fragment with the help of the drill sleeve, every screw penetrating the far cortex. The compression device is then placed in position, being fixed to the bone with a screw passed through a drill hole, using the specially designed drill sleeve, penetrating both cortices. The compression device is hooked into its hole in the end of the plate and the reduction of the fracture rechecked. The compressing nut is tightened with the socket wrench or a STEINMANN pin passed through the hole in the nut until the fracture gap disappears. During tightening, the compression device must be held in place with two fingers to prevent any rotational strain from being transmitted to the bone. If x-ray examination shows perfect position of the bone ends, the screws in the short fragment can be tightened up. The plate is now fixed to the long fragment with a screw in the hole nearest to the fracture, at which time the bone holding forceps or cerclage wire can be removed together with the compression device. The remaining screws are then driven home in the longer fragment.

Drainage. The operation site is drained for between twenty-four and forty-eight hours through a Redon drain.

Wound closure. After removing the tourniquet and securing haemostasis, the wound is closed in layers. For the skin we use mersylene 0000 on atraumatic needles. The intracutaneous Donati suture leaves almost invisible scars. No plaster cast is ordinarily used.

Postoperative care: The arm is elevated for twenty-four hours and as soon as the patient has recovered from the anaesthetic, the fingers, wrist and elbow are moved actively. The patient is given a soft rubber ball to encourage finger exercises and is allowed to go home after four to six days.

Removal of metal. The metal used in internal fixation can usually be removed from the forearm 18 to 24 months after operation. Removing it too soon makes refracture likely. The screws are exposed through small individual puncture wounds and the plate itself can be extracted through the incision made for the end screw. Each of these small incisions is closed by a fine cutaneous stitch. The operation does not necessarily require admission to the hospital.

2. Fractures of the Proximal End of the Ulna and of the Lower End of the Radius

a) Fractures of the Olecranon

The olecranon, being part of a hinged joint, is subjected to considerable flexion and extension strains from the action of the triceps and biceps respectively. As elsewhere in the skeleton except in areas of cancellous bone, the sequence of events is that first the traction-resisting elements in the form of collagen fibres give way, and then the pressure-resisting hard material in the form of calcium apatite breaks. The forces to which the olecranon is subjected during active movement after operation must be taken into account when planning the method of internal fixation. Three types of fractures are common, all of which eventually combine with fractures of the coronoid process, (Fig. 173a to c):

1) *Transverse fracture* opposite the *deepest point* of the trochlear notch occurs as a result of a sudden pull of the triceps muscle, or of a direct fall on the olecranon itself.

2) *Oblique fracture* running distally from the mid-point of the trochlear notch, which results from a hyperextension injury of the elbow.

3) *Comminuted fracture* resulting from direct major injury.

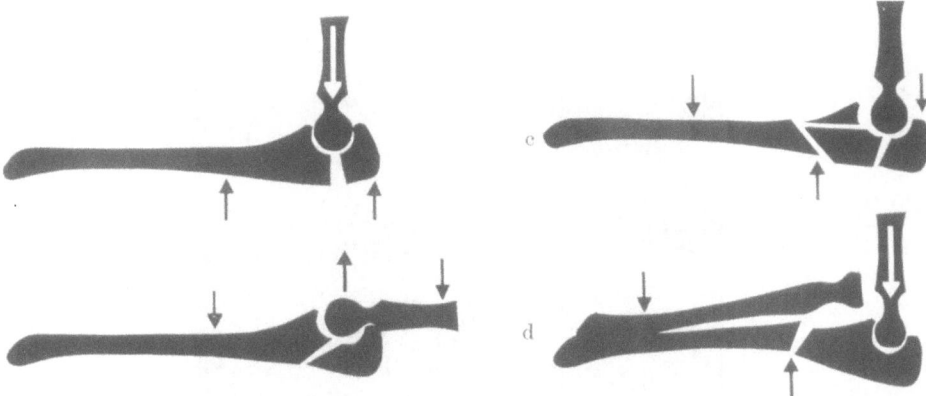

Fig. 173a—d. Types of fracture of the olecranon. a Transverse fracture. b Oblique fracture. c Comminuted fracture. d Monteggia fracture

Avulsion fractures of a small part of the tip of the olecranon attached to the triceps have the same mechanical features and can be treated the same way as transverse fractures.

As conservative management in olecranon fractures gives variable results, many methods of internal fixation have been advanced in the medical literature: simple wiring, and figure of eight wiring, (BERGER, BÖHLER, LISTER, ORAN, WATSON-JONES), longitudinal nailing (OSTLING), longitudinal screwing (CALLAHAN, HARMON, McAUSLAND) and LANE's plate (BECH, after ERIKSON, SAHLIN and SANDAHL). Internal fixation allows the elbow to be immobilized at 90°, which is a better position for postoperative treatment than the more or less extended position that is necessary in conservative management.

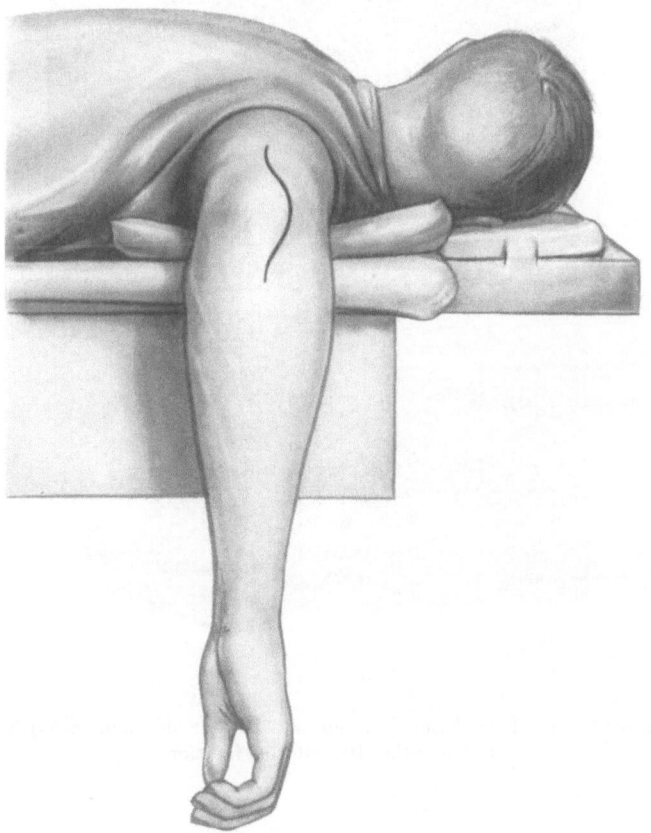

Fig. 174. Positioning and Skin Incision for internal fixation of the olecranon

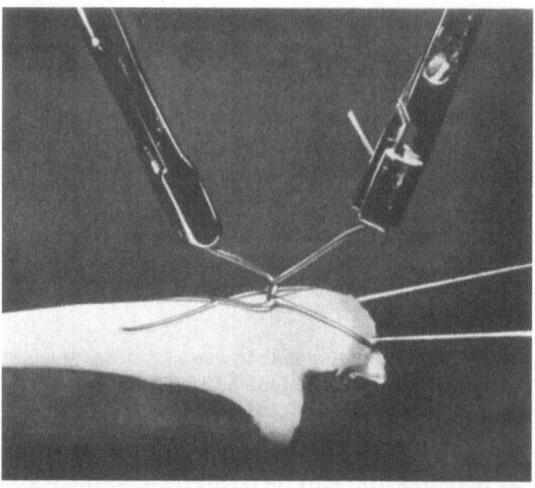

Fig. 175. Crossed pinning and figure of eight traction absorbing wiring (WEBER)

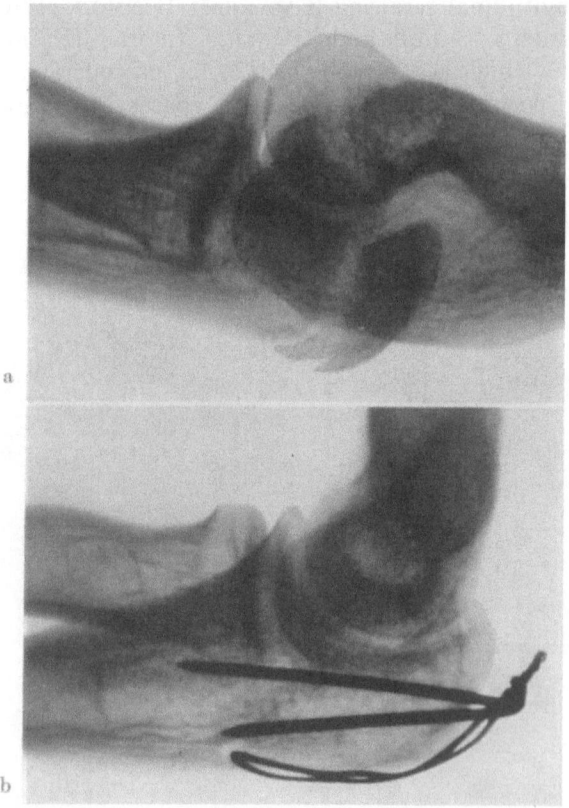

Fig. 176a and b. Transverse fracture of the olecranon in a 20-year-old man. a X-ray after the accident.
b 4 months after internal fixation

To avoid the need for any external support, we adopt the following procedure: The patient is placed prone with the elbow flexed at 90° over an arm table and the forearm hanging down. An S-shaped skin incision is made (Fig. 174). Internal fixation is performed using the tractionabsorbing wire held proximally over the ends of two KIRSCHNER wires as shown in Fig. 175 (WEBER, 1963).

1. Transverse fracture. An exact reduction is obtained with double hooks and two or four KIRSCHNER wires passed across the fracture in the longitudinal axis. A drill hole is made transversely through the edge of the ulna in the distal fragment and a 1 mm. wire is pulled through this hole, crossed over (figure of eight) and guided round the protruding ends of the KIRSCHNER wires. The wire is tightened up and then twisted, after which the ends of the KIRSCHNER wires are shortened and bent over to form small hooks. These are driven home over the traction absorbing wire (Fig. 176).

2. Oblique fracture. Reduction is achieved as above and is held either by axial KIRSCHNER wires or by a fine bone holding forceps. The oblique fracture can be stabilized with a single lag screw placed at right angles to the fracture line. A figure of eight wire is then applied as described above (Fig. 177).

3. Comminuted fracture. Here a clear view should be obtained of the articular surface of the distal fragment by opening up the fracture widely. With fine pronged hooks the fracture of the coronoid is first reduced and held with small bone holding forceps. A lag screw is then used, passing from the dorsal edge of the ulna. The other fragments are fixed one to the other by screws, hemi-cerclage wires or plates so that in the end it is virtually a two-piece fracture, after which the figure of eight wire can be used as described above.

In every case of olecranon fracture, the most important thing is to pass the figure of eight traction absorbing wire in addition to securing an exact reduction.

Our own experiments on the isolated ulna have shown that this method of internal fixation provides a resistance to flexion strains at the fracture site six times greater than that obtained by other fixation techniques. The superficially placed figure of eight wire takes up the distraction forces opposite to the trochlear notch of the ulna when bending the elbow. Traction forces are thus converted to compression in the fracture. Fixation with traction absorbing wiring, therefore, allows to forego the application of a plaster cast fixation.

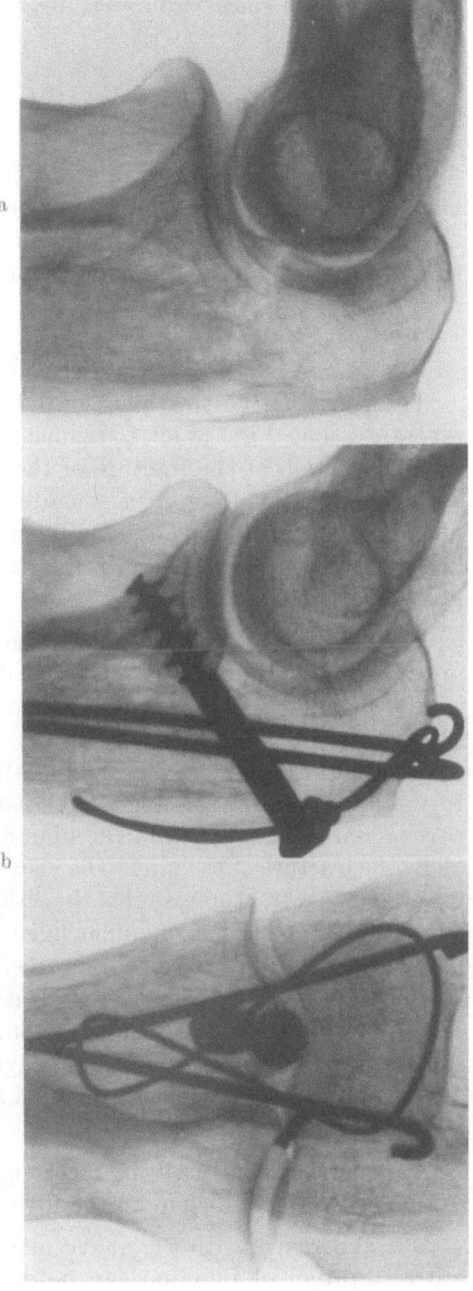

Fig. 177a and b. Oblique fracture of the olecranon in a 55-year-old man. a X-ray of the injury. b 4 months after surgery

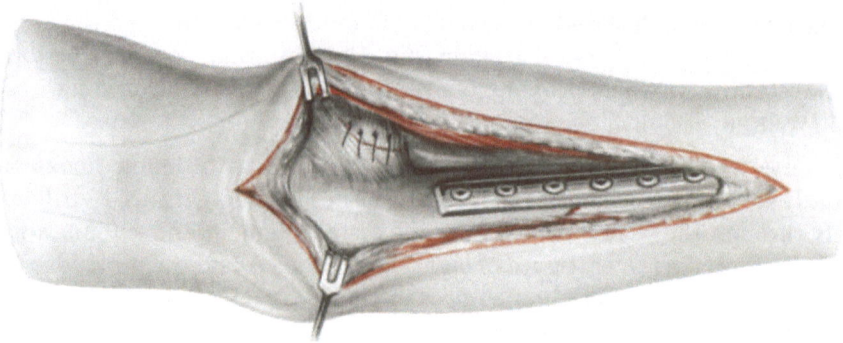

Fig. 178. Technique of internal fixation for a Monteggia fracture. Approach after SPEED and BOYD. Internal fixation with a compression plate. Suture or plastic replacement of the annular ligament

The wound is drained with a Redon suction drain for twenty-four hours and a plaster back slab is applied for a few days. *Active movements* are begun on the fifth day. The arm may be supported by a sling for about three weeks, and at four to six weeks the olecranon fracture has usually healed enough for full function to be regained.

b) Monteggia Fractures

The conservative treatment of a Monteggia fracture (Fig. 173d) is unsatisfactory for several reasons. First of all, to reduce the dislocated radial head it is necessary to secure an exact reduction of the fracture of the ulna. Then, because of the rupture of the annular ligament and the interosseus membrane, a closed reduction, even if accurate, is very unstable. The long period of immobilization which is then necessary until the ulnar fracture is healed almost always gives a relatively stiff elbow joint and considerable limitation of pronation and supination.

The outcome of a Monteggia fracture is considerably better if both components of this injury can be treated adequately and if long term immobilization can be eliminated. This is only possible by operative reconstruction.

Technique. Following SPEED and BOYD, the skin incision is made from the olecranon to the mid-forearm, running a little lateral to the subcutaneous border of the ulna. The periosteum is elevated from the ulna and the origin of the extensor muscles detached to allow the fracture of the ulna to be visualized. The fracture is reduced and fixed as described for other ulnar fractures, so that the dislocation of the radial head is reduced spontaneously. After this, only the torn annular ligament remains to be sutured or replaced by a plastic procedure (Fig. 178). In fresh fractures, the tear in the annular ligament is found to lie over the outer part of the radial head. The stumps of the ligament can then be sutured with some material such as 0 braided nylon. In delayed operation for this condition a primary suture may not be possible. In this event, a replacement, using a strip of fascia or skin guided through a drill hole in the ulna and round the radial neck, is sutured to itself near the ulna again.

A Redon drain is used for forty-eight hours and a plaster back slab for a few days. Active exercises are begun on the fifth day after operation.

Our experience with the above method has given good results, and with fresh injuries full restoration of function can be expected without any late joint stiffness (Fig. 179).

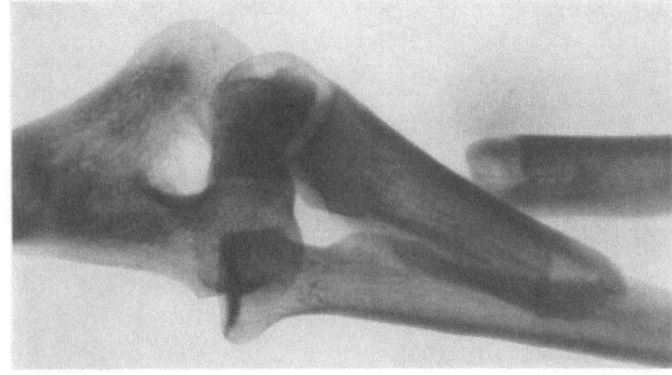

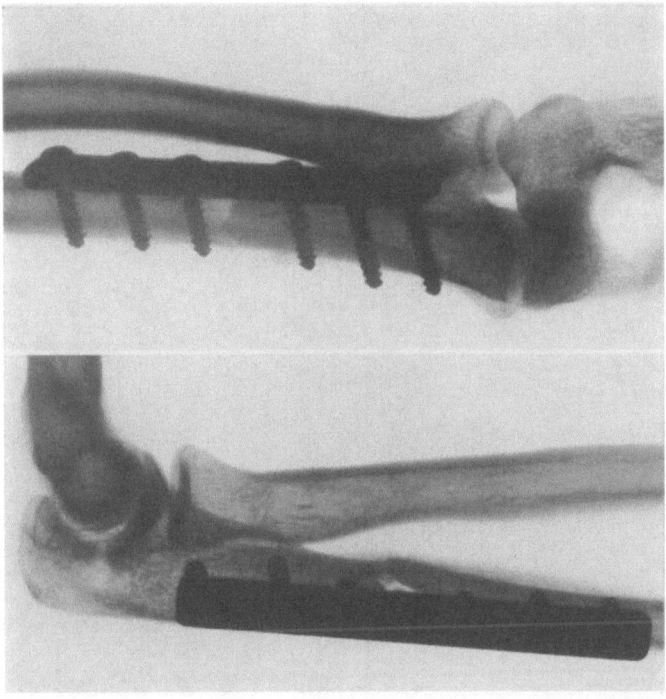

Fig. 179 a and b. Monteggia fracture in a 43-year-old man. a X-ray at time of injury. b 2 months after operation

c) Fractures of the Lower End of the Radius

In general we advocate a closed reduction and plaster fixation for typical Colles' fractures and radial fractures in the lower quarter. An axial deviation of less than 10°, except in special cases, is accepted, but even the slightest shortening of the radius compared with the ulna often gives pain in the distal radio-ulnar joint and limitation of supination. In some cases of unstable oblique fractures, or where there is much comminution, an excellent or even a good anatomical and functional result cannot be obtained with conservative treatment. In agreement with WILLENEGGER (1959), BOWLING and SAWYER (1962), we feel that internal fixation is indicated in the following cases:

1. Unstable oblique and comminuted fractures, especially in patients who depend for their living on a good and powerful wrist.

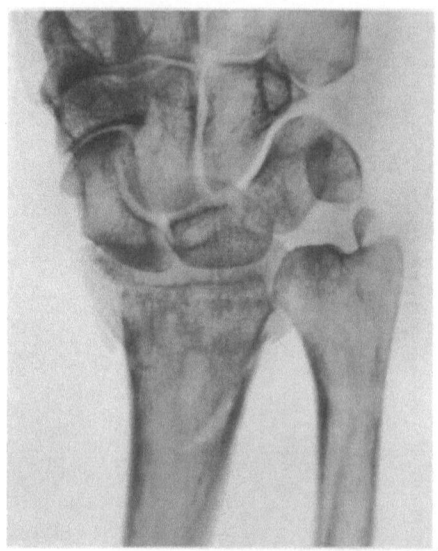
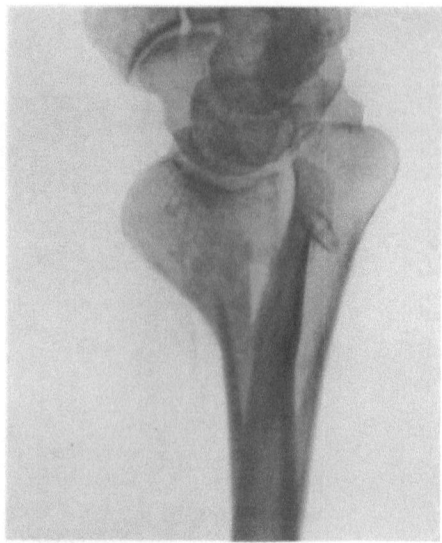

a

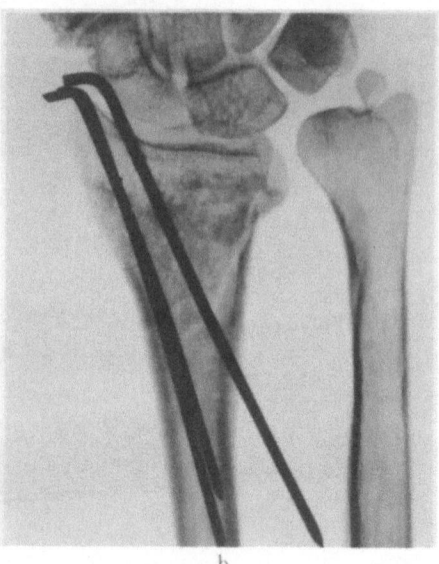

b

Fig. 180a and b. Unstable fracture of the lower end of the radius in a 62-year-old woman. a X-ray after injury.
b 4 weeks after closed reduction and percutaneous pinning

2. Unstable or irreducible fractures in adolescence when partial separation of the epiphysis
may produce uneven growth if union occurs without good alignment.

3. Compound fractures.

Technique

1. Brachial block anaesthesia is used except in children when a general anaesthetic is
preferable.

2. Closed reduction is performed using an image intensifier. An unstable fracture, having
been accurately reduced, is held manually and transfixed with two or three KIRSCHNER
wires. These wires are driven percutaneously by a machine drill from the styloid process of

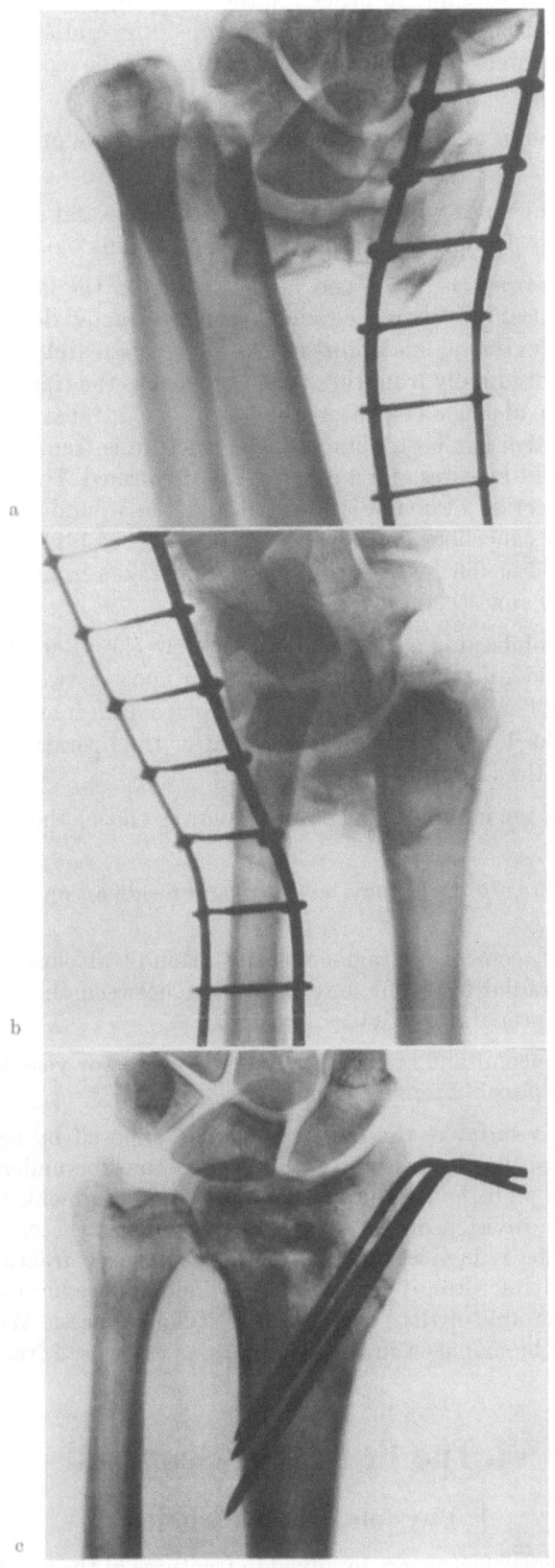

Fig. 181a—c. Compound fracture of the lower end of the radius in a 57-year-old man. a and b X-rays of the injury. c Postoperative result

the radius, across the fracture line to penetrate the cortex of the radius on the ulnar side. The wires are shortened so that only 2 cm. are left projecting, and a dorsal or volar plaster slab is applied. At three weeks the Kirschner wires can be removed and a new plaster slab provided for another two or three weeks.

3. If a good reduction is not obtained under x-ray control we proceed to *open reduction* as follows:

The patient lies on his back with the arm on an arm table and a tourniquet applied to the upper arm, which is possible when using a brachial plexus block.

An incision is made from the lower end of the radius on the lateral side for 5—6 cm. proximally. The superficial branch of the radial nerve is retracted dorsally and the tendons of extensor pollicis brevis and abductor pollicis longus are retracted anteriorly. The periosteum is split longitudinally from the styloid process to the fracture site. The fracture is reduced with the help of a small elevator which is inserted transversely into the fracture gap. When good reduction has been obtained, the fracture is transfixed with two to four obliquely placed KIRSCHNER wires and a check x-ray performed. The KIRSCHNER wires are shortened and bent, suction drainage is inserted and the wound closed. If there is any significant defect in the cancellous bone, which happens as a result of impaction during the injury, the defect should be filled with a cancellous graft taken from the crest of the ileum, in which case a general anaesthetic is necessary.

The fracture is immobilized in a volar slab for three weeks, after which the KIRSCHNER wires are withdrawn and a new plaster slab applied for another two to three weeks. If the wires have been buried, however, they may be left in place until fracture union is complete, but in any event not for longer than two months after the operation, to avoid irritation to the long tendons of the thumb.

A special indication for internal fixation of the lower end of the radius is a *compound fracture*. The reasons are:

1. The fracture is already open, may be soiled and needs an operative treatment anyway.

2. With severe displacement of fragments, any attempt at closed reduction will fail, because the proximal radial fragment may be caught between the tendons crossing the wrist and fibres of the pronator quadratus.

3. There may be concomitant injuries to tendons, nerves or vessels which need to be visually examined and possibly repaired.

If the skin wound is suitable, the fracture may be exposed by simply extending it, but if the wound is in an unsuitable position its closure may be undertaken first and the fracture approached by an orthodox incision. The proximal fragment, if button-holed into soft tissues, is freed by division of the dorsal retinaculum or the carpal ligament. Only then will the fracture be reducible. Both in a pure transverse fracture and in unstable oblique or comminuted fractures, it is advisable to hold this reduction with KIRSCHNER wires passed in the long axis of the bone from the styloid process. When the wound has healed, these cases can be managed in the same way as are closed fractures.

VI. The Fractured Scaphoid

1. Physiology and Pathology

Mechanical and vascular factors are involved in fractures of the scaphoid. It is the most mobile bone in the wrist, so that a fracture in it produces significant changes in the mechanics of the wrist joint. Under normal conditions angulation between the carpal bones follows the line from (A) to (B) (Fig. 182), but in fractures of the scaphoid the line runs from (A) to (C). In ulnar deviation, the fracture gap is widened and the distal fragment displaced radially (Fig. 183). A secondary movement of the intact scaphoid is that of palmar tilting during radial deviation, which produces a very typical displacement in the fractured bone (Fig. 184). Furthermore, palmar or dorsiflexion as well as all combined movements in the wrist and even finger movements are transmitted to the fracture.

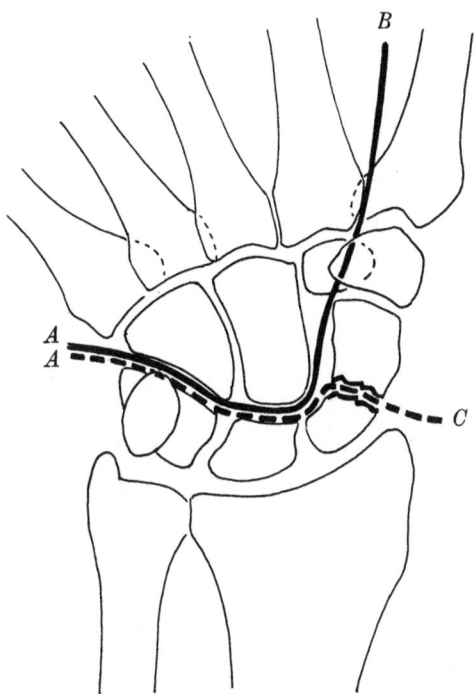

Fig. 182. Movement of the carpal bones during flexion, showing line of angulation. *A—B* With an intact scaphoid. *A—C* With a fracture of the scaphoid (after RITTER)

In spite of the efforts of various authors, the problems of the scaphoid blood supply have not yet been solved, as it is technically difficult to demonstrate the vessels angiographically. The vascular arrangements that are important in treatment (Fig. 185a and b) are as follows:

The main supply is from branches of the dorsal carpal branch of the radial artery. These fine vessels perforate the dorsal carpal ligaments, forming an arterial net that extends to the periosteum and into the bone.

An additional arterial supply is provided by a network of vessels coming along the lateral radial ligament and proceeding to the scaphoid tubercle. A third but variable supply, which may be important for the nutrition of the proximal fragment, comes from the ulnar side. It consists of small vascular bridges in the interosseus ligament and capsular connections between the lunate and the ulnar aspect of the scaphoid (LÜTZELER, 1932). The number of nutrient foramina in the scaphoid give a clue to the vascular phenomena that occur in this bone. The number is smaller in the scaphoid than in any other carpal bone (LOGROSCINO and DE MARCHI, 1938).

The points at which the foramina enter are in extraarticular areas and where the bone is covered with periosteum: a) a dorsal area tapering towards the ulnar side, b) a radial

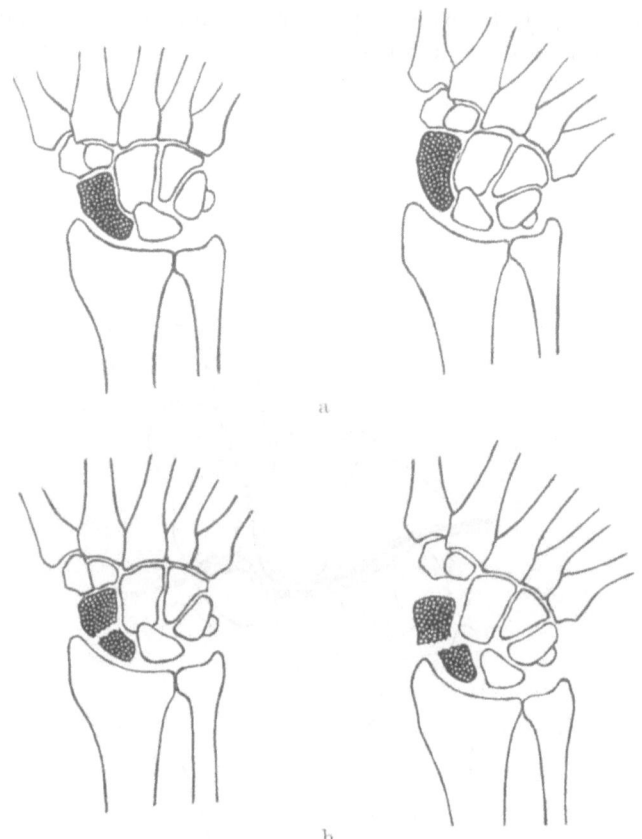

Fig. 183a and b. Movement of the carpal bones with ulnar deviation. a With an intact scaphoid. b With a fractured scaphoid (after RITTER)

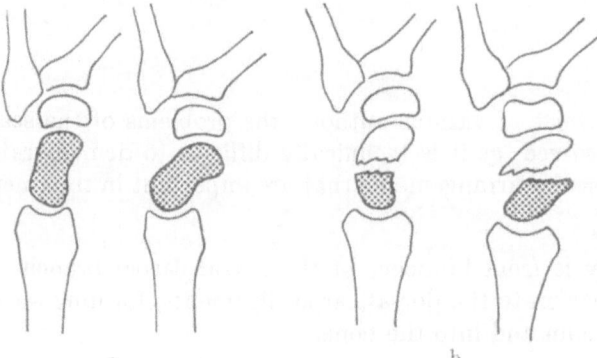

Fig. 184a and b. Palmar tilting of the scaphoid in radial deviation. a With an intact scaphoid. b With a fractured scaphoid (after RITTER)

area around the tubercle and c) a larger palmar area. In 10 to 20% of all scaphoids, the proximal intraarticular portion shows no foramina (OBLETZ and HALBSTEIN, 1938).

Scaphoid fractures can be grouped topographically into proximal, waist or distal fractures, or according to the type of fracture (Fig. 186).

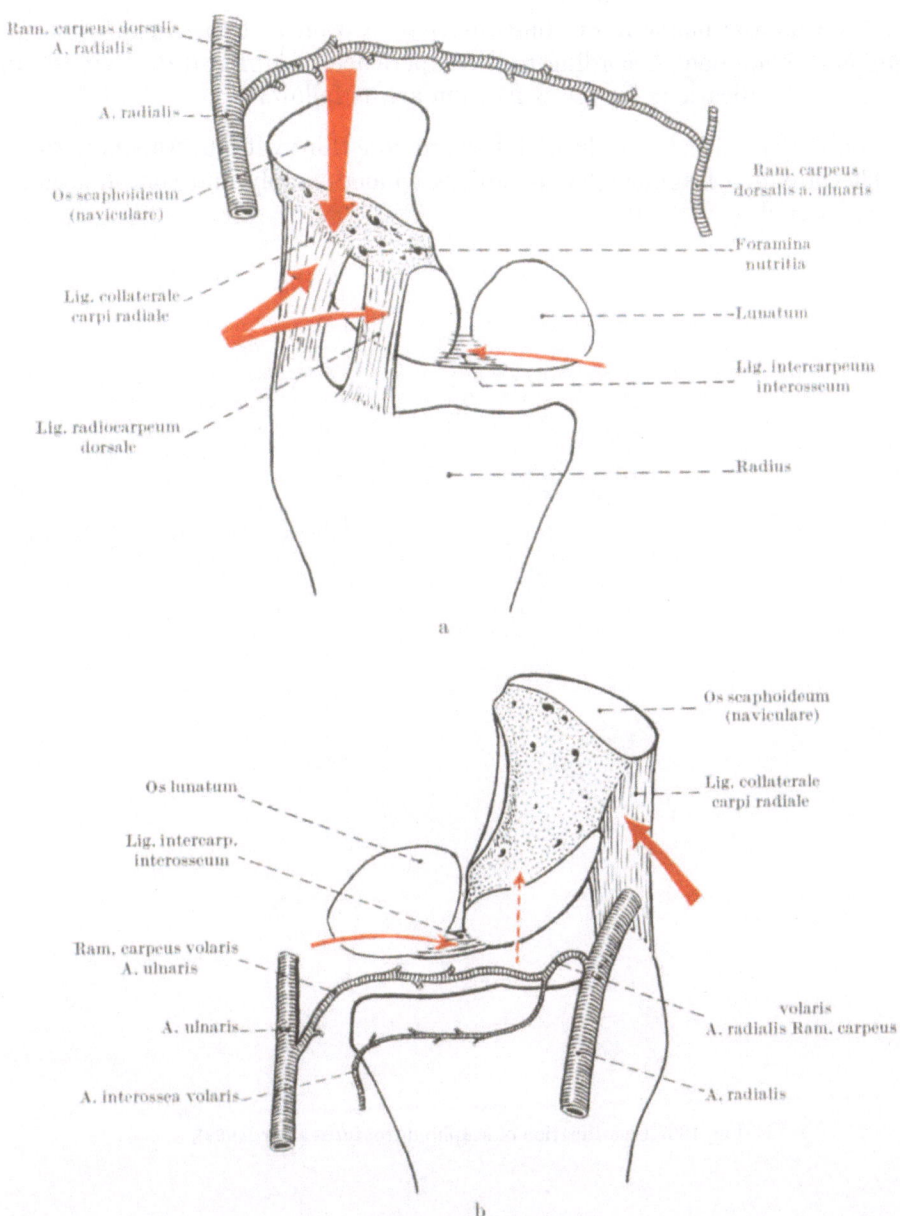

Fig. 185a and b. Arterial supply and nutrient foramina of the scaphoid. a Dorsal view. b Palmar view

2. Indications for Surgery

In reports of large series, union may be expected in 90% of fresh scaphoid fractures treated conservatively using special plasters. Operative treatment is therefore chiefly indicated for delayed union and nonunion. Here, surgical treatment, especially with screw fixation in a limited series of individual cases, has been so effective that a few authors have dared, in selected cases, to screw fresh fractures also. We feel that a cautious attitude should be adopted towards screw fixation of fresh scaphoid fractures and that it is indicated only in special cases: where there is a large gap at the fracture site and when for economic reasons the patient would have difficulty in following his employment in a long continued plaster cast. So for the moment we limit internal fixation to those cases where there is delayed union or nonunion. According to the experience of McLaughlin (1954) and our own, for these the indications for screw fixation are as follows:

a) Good indication: all cases in the distal and middle third without osteoporosis or osteoarthritis. The proximal fragment has a sufficient blood supply and consolidation can be confidently expected.

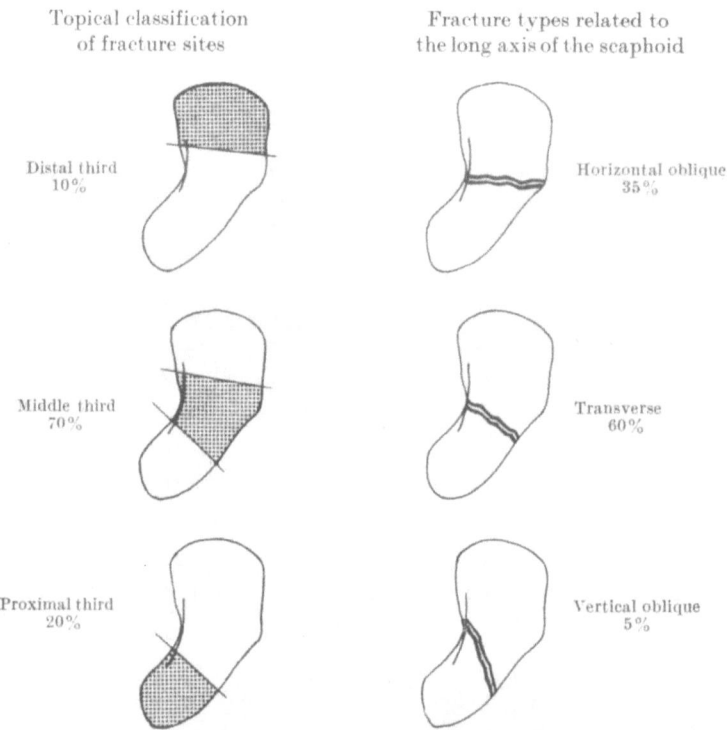

Fig. 186. Classification of scaphoid fractures after Russe

b) Relative indication: fractures of the proximal third in which the threads of the screw can be expected to grip the proximal fragment.

c) Poor indication: cases which have a very small proximal fragment. Here it is difficult to tap a thread in the proximal fragment, the alignment of the fractures surface is difficult to secure and a longitudinal split in the small fragment may be produced.

The presence of osteoarthritis means that little improvement can be expected by fixing a nonunion of the scaphoid. If, however, a fresh fracture occurs in the scaphoid, with pre-existing arthritis, primary screwing might be indicated because immobilization in a plaster cast would make the arthritis worse. It may also be necessary to resect the radial styloid if it is deformed by arthritis, but we have only needed to do this on two occasions in combination with screwing of the scaphoid. Since ossification occurs at the site of resection it is difficult to see what value this procedure has.

3. Screwing of the Scaphoid

a) General Considerations

Lag screwing of the scaphoid best fulfills the biological requirements of firm fixation. Rigid fixation can be obtained in properly selected cases when a good technique is used, and in this bone the advantage of absolute rigidity cannot be overestimated. Furthermore,

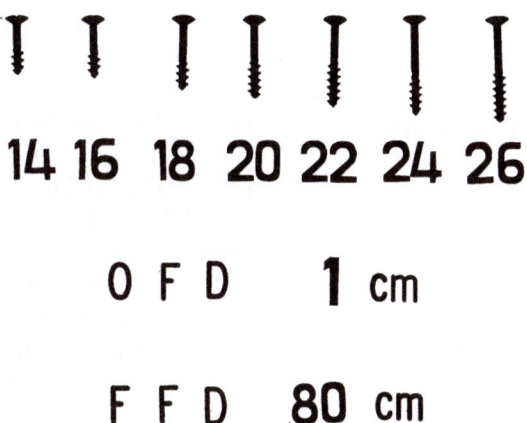

14 16 18 20 22 24 26

O F D   1 cm

F F D   80 cm

Fig. 187. Measurement chart (x-ray photograph) of the set of screws taken at measured distances
OFD = Object-Film-Distance; FFD = Focus-Film-Distance

accurate adaptation of the fracture ends and compression of the fibrous area in the non-union can be achieved with a lag screw, giving the best possible conditions for bone healing. The necrotic fragments have been cut off from their periosteal blood supply so that revascularization can only take place endosteally at the point of contact between the bone

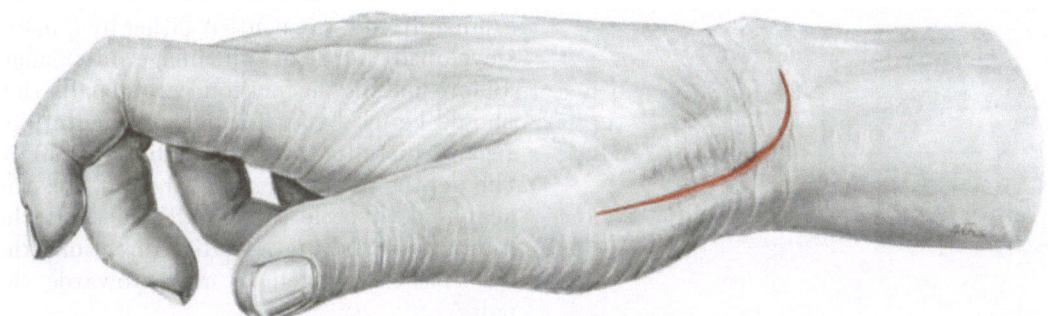

Fig. 188. Skin incision

ends at the fracture line, as in the subcapital fracture of the femoral neck. Thus, rigidity and compression are especially important in the scaphoid, which make fixation with a lag screw the treatment of choice for nonunion of the scaphoid. Furthermore, it allows earlier mobilization than does any other method. Experience so far suggests that fragments may be expected to consolidate finally whether they initially possess a blood supply or are dead, as long as the dead fragments can be rigidly fixed. The difference is chiefly in the length of time that may elapse, which may vary from months to several years in cases with a dead fragment.

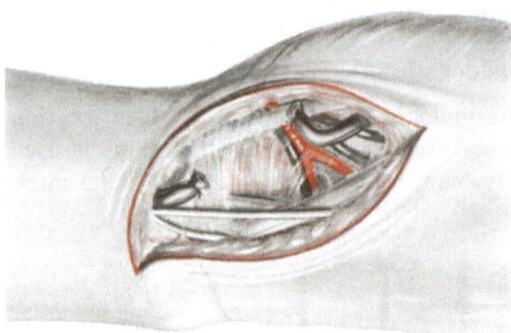

Fig. 189. Subcutaneous topography

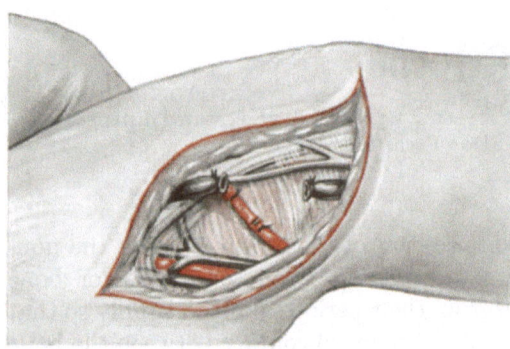

Fig. 190. Showing the anomalous course of the carpal branch of the dorsal radial artery

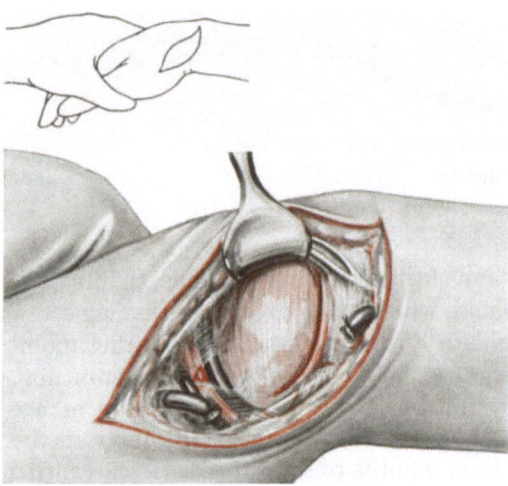

Fig. 191. Incision of the capsule

b) Preparation

For accurate diagnosis, two enlarged films should be taken in the anteroposterior projection and in the "fencing" position.

To determine the length of the screw (Fig. 187) a standard x-ray film of the whole range of screws gives increased safety (GASSER, personal communication). The set is photographed in such a way that the distance between the tube and the plate (Focus-Film-Distance FFD) is 80 cm. and the distance between the screw and the plate (Object-Film-Distance OFD) is 1 cm. The latter distance is approximately the same as when the screw is in the bone. For every operation, an a. p. view of the intact scaphoid on the opposite side is made with the same distance between the tube and the plate (FFD 80 cm.). To determine the length of screw needed, the standard x-ray photograph of the screw range is held in front of the viewing screen on top of the x-ray of the uninjured scaphoid. A screw is selected that will extend from the tubercle to the proximal end of the bone.

c) Operative Technique

General. General anaesthesia is used and a pneumatic tourniquet applied. It is best to have two assistants and facilities for intraoperative x-ray control, either by quickly developed films or an image intensifier. Before making the incision, careful palpation should be used to get a proper orientation; feeling distally from the radial styloid in the depths of the anatomical snuff box, the scaphoid tubercle can be identified. If the hand is flexed in a radial direction, the tubercle can be felt to move towards the palm.

Incision. Exposure is made according to MCLAUGHLIN's method. The curved incision begins over the proximal quarter of the thumb metacarpal, runs proximally between the tendons of extensor pollicis longus and brevis, across the anatomical snuff box and then curves medially to end where the tendon of extensor pollicis longus crosses the wrist joint (Fig. 188).

Subcutaneous topography. After elevation of the semi-circular skin flap in dorso-ulnar

direction (Fig. 189) a large vein and the
dorsal branch of the radial nerve usually
come into sight. The vein is ligated and
the nerve retracted gently towards the
ulnar side. Dissection brings the tendons
of the long and short extensors of the thumb
into view and at the distal end of the incision the radial artery appears deep to the
tendon of extensor pollicis brevis. It runs,
accompanied by its veins, towards the back
of the hand. All these vessels should be
carefully preserved. Occasionally an anomalous branch is found originating from
the radial artery, running transversely
across the snuff box towards the back of the
hand (Fig. 190). This may be present in between 10 and 15% of cases. If this branch
gets in the way, it can be cut without
concern; this will not jeopardize the blood
supply of the scaphoid.

Incision of the capsule. The capsule is
now approached (Fig. 191). Holding the
hand from above, an assistant bends the
wrist into palmar flexion of 30° and maximal
ulnar deviation. The scaphoid tubercle is
now in the centre of the field and can be
easily felt. This maneuver also pulls the
articular surface of the scaphoid away from
the radius towards the capsular ligament
producing a bulge in the capsule, thus
revealing the site of incision. The articular
edge of the distal end of the radius is found
by touch. Keeping in mind the importance
of vessels in this area, only a small, slightly
curved transverse incision is made. Any
enlargement that is necessary is made
towards the back of the hand, as extension
of the incision distally would jeopardize
the vessels, ligaments and periosteum of
the scaphoid. The joint between the
scaphoid and the capitate should not be
opened in the interests of the blood supply.

Inspection of the scaphoid. The exposed
scaphoid is now inspected. With traction
exerted on the hand in the correct position,
the proximal fragment and the fracture site
or nonunion can usually be seen quite well.
The fracture itself should be examined for
any signs of bleeding (indicating vitality),
for fibrous bridges, periosteal shreds as well
as any secondary change in the way of
density, cysts, decrease of the transparency

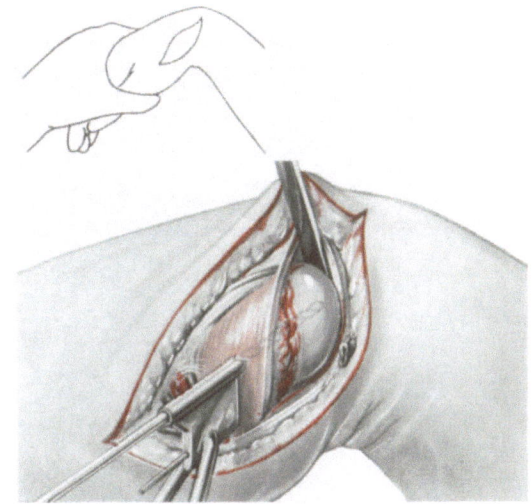

Fig. 192. Drilling

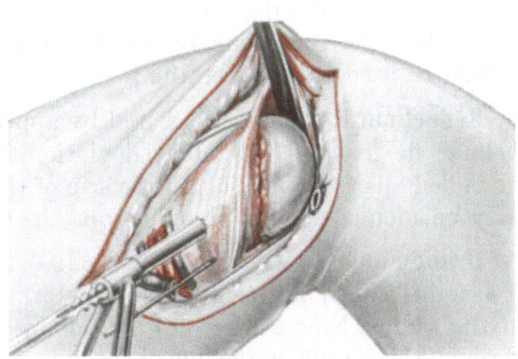

Fig. 193. Tapping

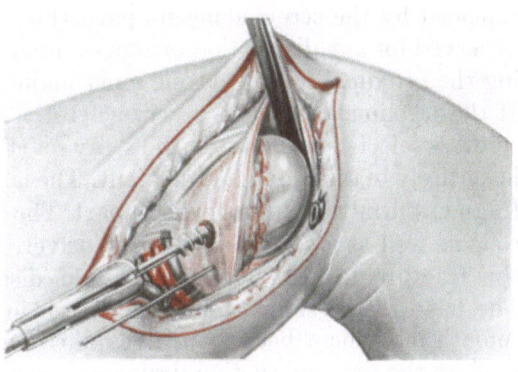

Fig. 194. Screwing

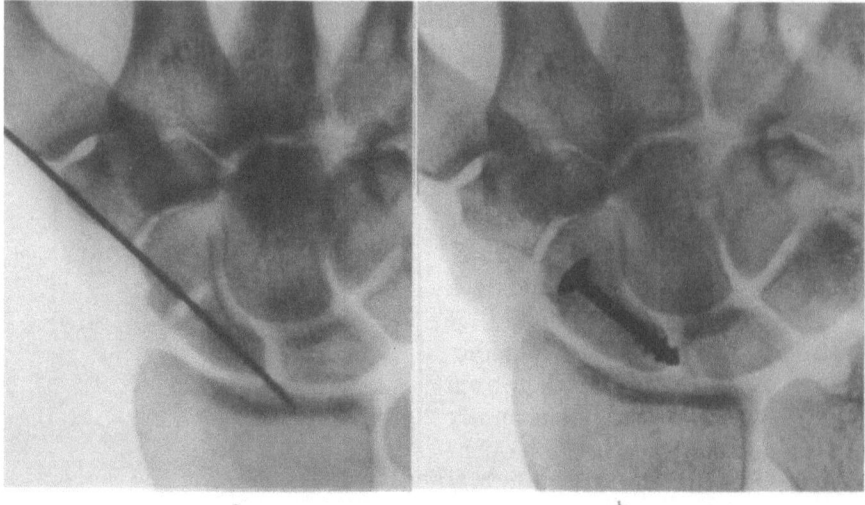

Fig. 195a and b. a Ideally placed guide wire in a 4 months old nonunion. b Disappearance of the line of non-union after compression with a lag screw

of the cartilage and the actual extent of the fracture itself. Special care must be taken not to displace the fragments by careless manipulation of the hand, and fine instruments should be used in this operation.

Reduction. Reduction is secured by applying traction again and pushing the hand into palmar flexion and full ulnar deviation. Under no circumstances should a nonunion be pulled apart. Depending on the size of the proximal fragment, a small shallow elevator may be adequate to secure reduction.

Drilling and screwing (Fig. 192 to 194). The assistant takes over the curette and holds it as a drill shield between the proximal fragment of the scaphoid and the articular surface of the radius. Now a wire of 1 mm. diameter and accurately measured length is driven through the capsule in the line of the axis of the scaphoid and, if possible, at right angles to the fracture line. An a. p. and oblique x-ray is taken to determine whether this wire is lying in the correct plane for the screw. The maneuver should be repeated until the wire is in the right position; it does not matter if the tip of the wire comes to rest beyond the end of the scaphoid (Fig. 195a). The capsule is now incised at the point of entrance of the wire for 2—3 mm. to allow entry of the drill. A second wire is introduced parallel to the first, so as to mark the direction and hold the fracture while the first wire is removed and replaced by the screw along its path (Fig. 192, 198b). During drilling the fracture line is observed for any distraction or sign of movement; especially when the drill tip is approaching the proximal fragment, one must make sure it is not just pushing the fragment away. If the proximal fragment is very sclerotic, it may be necessary to use a tap (Fig. 193). A screw is selected as shown in the x-ray set (Fig. 187). The threaded part of the screw should lie entirely in the proximal fragment. The last few turns of the screw will draw the proximal fragment firmly against the distal part. The instrument set for this operation includes guide rods as well as a self-holding screw driver, a drill sleeve and a tap. If reduction is exact, the fracture line or nonunion should disappear on tightening the screw (Fig. 195b). The head of the screw should be driven in flush enough so that it does not disturb the smooth movement between the scaphoid and the capitate. A few catgut sutures are used to close the capsule, suction drainage is arranged, a few subcutaneous sutures are inserted and accurate closure of the skin completes the operation.

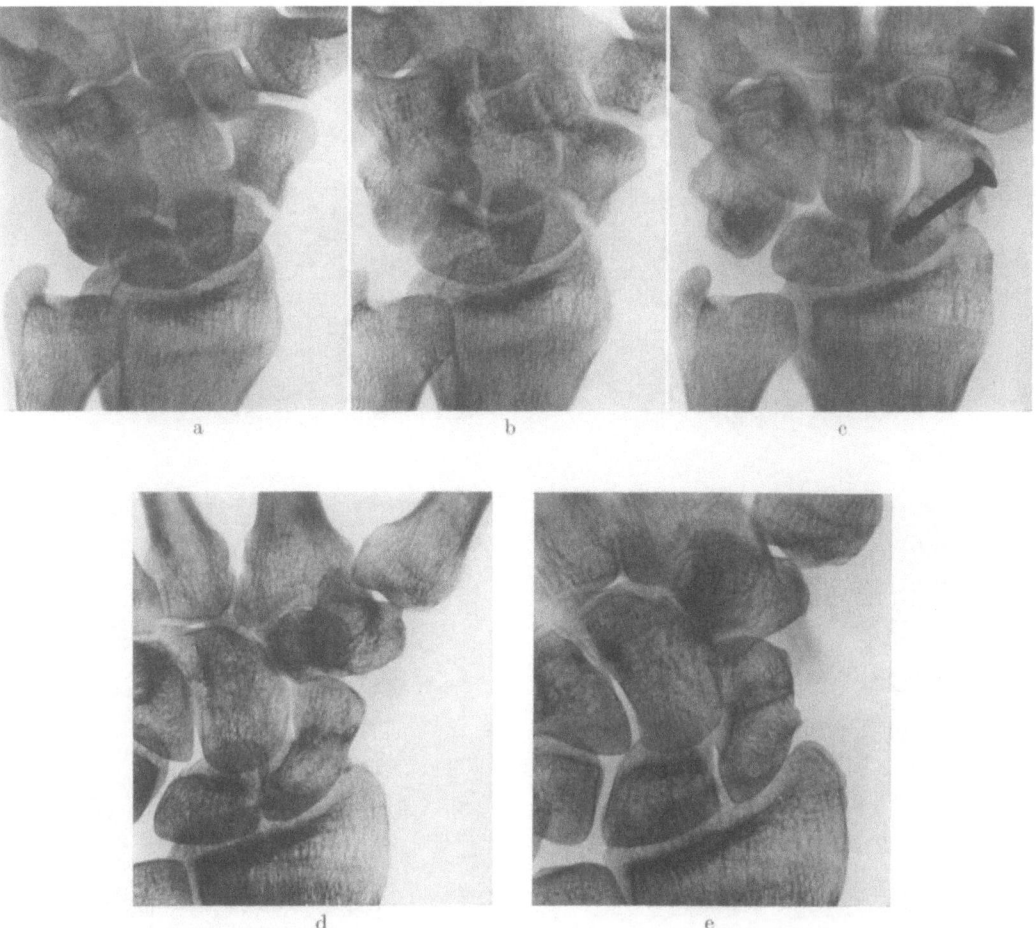

Fig. 196a—e. Good indication for fixation in an imminent nonunion. a X-ray at time of injury. b 11 weeks after the accident. c 4 weeks after screwing. d Appearance at 64 weeks. e Appearance at 185 weeks

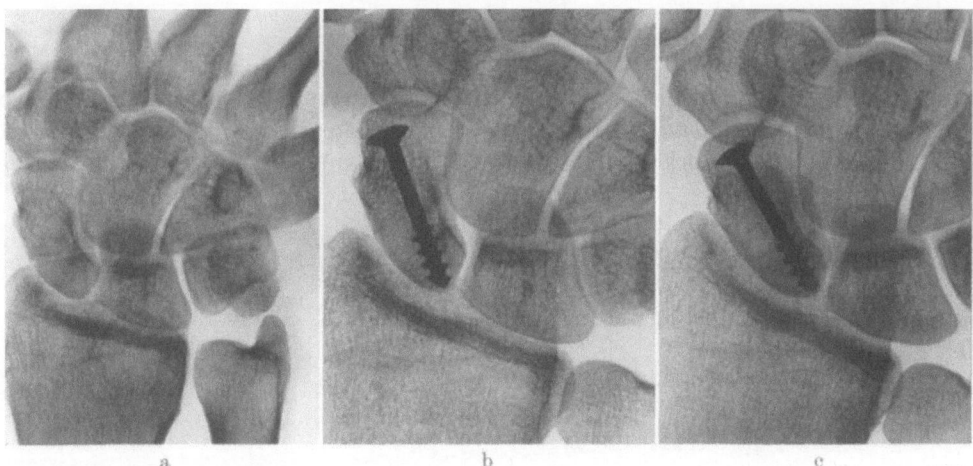

Fig. 197a—c. a 5¹/₂ months old nonunion providing a good indication for fixation. b At 5 weeks after screwing, ossification is evident. c Appearance at 1 year, no discomfort and full range of movement

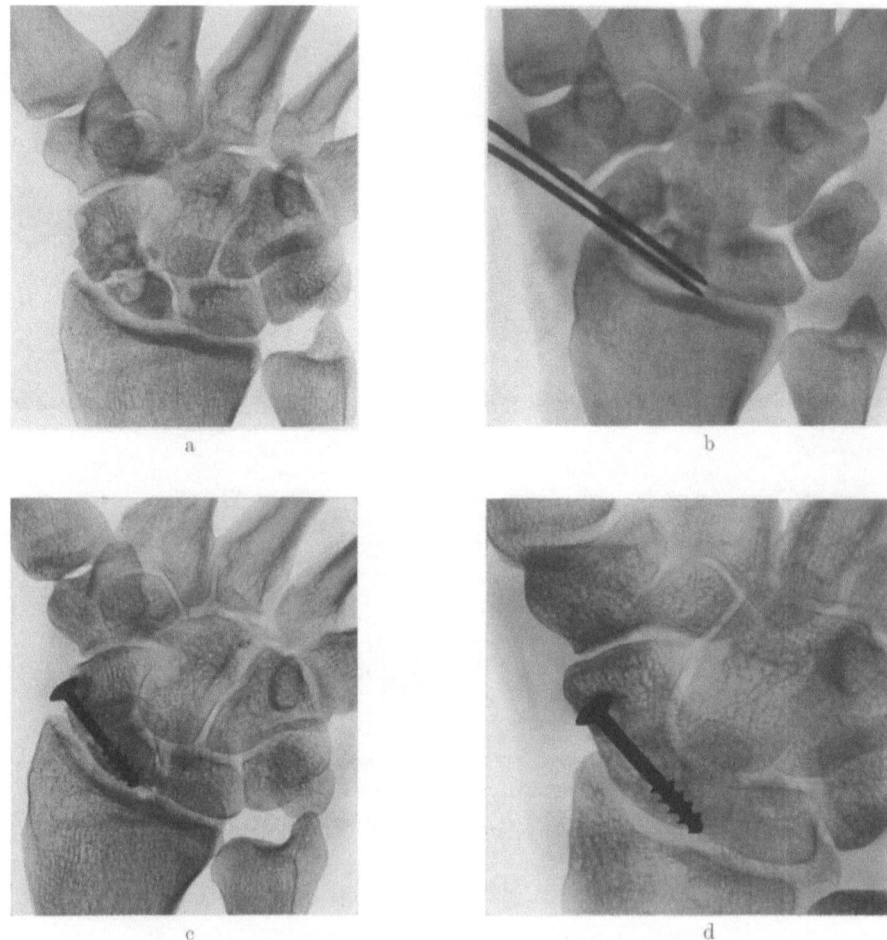

Fig. 198a—d. Successful screwing of a 7-year-old nonunion with necrosis of the proximal fragment. a and b X-rays taken during operation. c 43 weeks after screwing. d 92 weeks after screwing showing revascularisation of the bone. No discomfort and full range of movement

Postoperative management. In a properly selected case with rigid screwing, a palmar slab is all that is needed until the wound has healed. If the indication was only relative and fixation is not ideal, application of a scaphoid plaster for four to eight weeks is recommended. Heavy manual work should not be permitted until ossification is clearly visible on x-ray.

VII. Fractures of the Humerus

Most fractures in the upper arm, especially comminuted fractures and those of the neck of the humerus, are best treated *conservatively* for two reasons. First, because conservative treatment can be combined with early mobilization thus avoiding to a large extent the joint stiffness that follows prolonged immobilization; second, because access to these fractures is much more difficult than in the forearm or in the lower extremity. There are, nevertheless, *individual cases* in which only *operative reduction* can be expected to lead to full restoration of function. They will be discussed separately according to the anatomical sections of the humerus.

Anatomically, the humerus has a relatively wide medullary canal and a thin cortex in its shaft. The large cancellous mass in the head of the humerus lies partly beneath the articular cartilage or intracapsular and depends for its blood supply on capsular vessels, in the adult also on vessels from the metaphysis, while in children the nutrition is never supplied across the epiphyseal plate.

In the lower end of the humerus the medullary canal narrows down and disappears altogether at the level of the olecranon fossa, continuing in the form of a groove in the cortex that supports the condyles. The structure of the humerus itself influences the selection of technique for internal fixation. The wide medulla makes fixation by Rush pins or medullary nails difficult, since a nail that properly fills the cavity has such a large diameter that it damages the head of the humerus.

The relatively thick sheath of soft tissues round the humerus influences the operative technique; at the upper end, the well differentiated muscles inserted in the humerus require exact anatomical reconstruction of the bone if their function is to be preserved. Soft tissues must also be considered themselves while approaching a bone for internal fixation, and here the vessels on the medial side of the upper part of the humerus and the radial nerve in its spiral path are important. Exposure of the bone should take into account branches of nerves supplying individual muscles.

For all operations on the humerus it is important to have the forearm freely movable during the operation to facilitate accurate reduction and internal fixation of difficult fractures.

The incisions and approaches described below are suitable for internal fixation of all types of fractures occurring on the humerus:

1. Soft Tissues and Surgical Access to the Bone

a) Lateral Approach for the Shaft of the Humerus

The skin incision begins at the upper end of the delto-pectoral groove level with the clavicle, and follows the medial border of the deltoid in a slight curve to its insertion and thence in a straight line to the lateral epicondyle. The cephalic vein is retracted medially, but if necessary can be divided without ill effect. Dissecting in the interval between pectoralis major and the deltoid, and then between the biceps and brachio-radialis, the humerus is reached. The brachialis must be divided obliquely from above medially to below laterally. This can be done without interfering with its nerve supply as it is innervated by the radial in the upper and outer part and by the musculocutaneous in its lower and inner portion. The radial nerve is only encountered in the distal part of the wound lateral to the brachialis, having the brachio-radialis on its lateral side. Whenever the radial nerve is endangered by the incision or the type of fracture, it should be clearly visualized by dissection from an uninjured portion before the fracture is exposed or reduction begun. This is especially true when the tissues are difficult to identify as a result of hematoma,

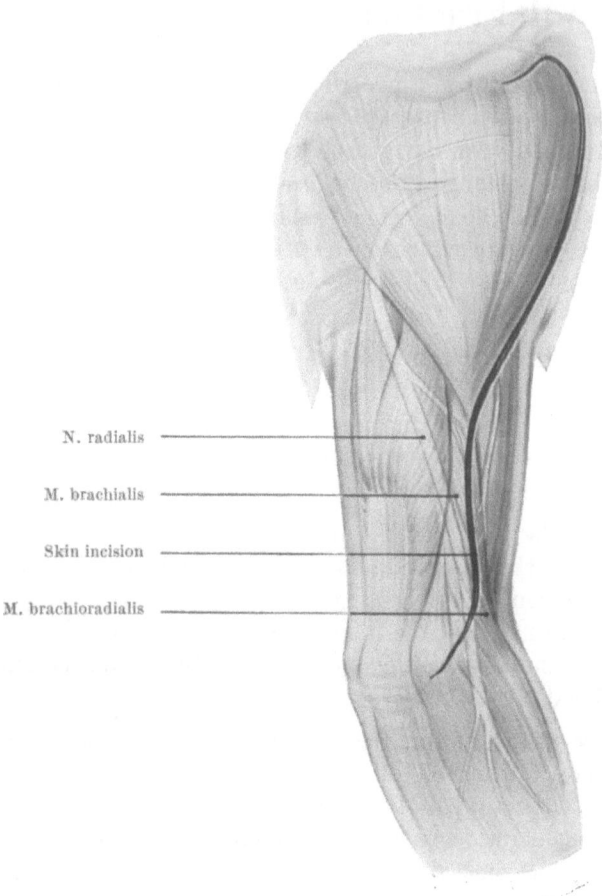

N. radialis ———

M. brachialis ———

Skin incision ———

M. brachioradialis ———

Fig. 199. Lateral approach showing the relations of the radial nerve and the muscles (see text)

edema or in later cases scar tissue giving rise to problems when a plate is being removed. In exposing individual fragments of the bone, care is taken to preserve the periosteum as much as possible.

b) Exposure of the Head of the Humerus

If the deltoid is not well developed, it can be retracted laterally with a HOHMANN lever, with the arm abducted so that an adequate view of the fracture is possible. If the muscle is thick or the fracture complicated, it is advisable to detach the clavicular head of the deltoid for between three and four cm. from its medial end and then to fold the muscle back laterally; as the axillary nerve enters the deltoid from above it will thus not be severed. Strong pressure with a bone lever against the under surface of the muscle should be avoided, and bone levers used at the very upper end of the humerus may injure the axillary nerve with their tip.

c) Exposure of the Medial Epicondyle

The incision begins eight to ten cm. proximal to the medial epicondyle, passing behind it and running down for five cm. towards the ulnar styloid. In operations on the medial epicondyle the ulnar nerve should always be visualized in its groove and it can then be followed proximally and distally. Its first branch to the flexor carpi ulnaris should be

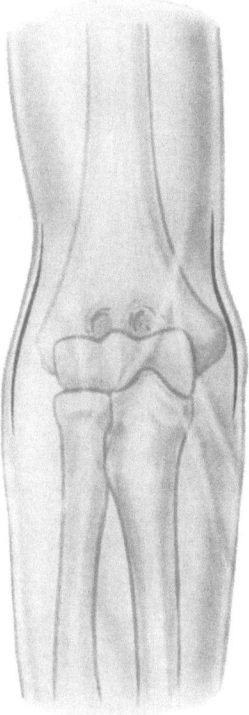

Fig. 200. Incisions to expose fractures of the condyles and supracondylar fractures

identified and preserved. If there is any danger of callus or wires used in internal fixation irritating the ulnar nerve, it may be transplanted anteriorly and buried beneath the flexor muscles.

An incision in the intermuscular septum prevents stretching of the nerve when the arm is extended. An accurate note of the position of nerves at the end of the operation should be made for future guidance when the time comes to remove the metal.

d) Posterior Approach to the Lower End of the Humerus

It is often necessary in fractures of the lower shaft of the humerus to decide early whether to approach it from the posterior or lateral aspect. A lateral approach can be extended downwards by curving the incision anteriorly towards the antecubital fossa. This will allow the fracture to be reached medial to the radial nerve, which is advisable especially when the brachial artery or the median nerve have been damaged.

If a more posterior approach is required to the fracture, it is advisable to split the triceps tendon from the olecranon upwards, continuing this split in a longitudinal manner in the muscle belly. The two halves of the muscle can then be retracted to reveal the shaft of the humerus. Using this technique the radial nerve is found a little below the middle of the shaft of the humerus, deep to the long and lateral heads of the muscle. If the lower end of the humerus is to be reconstructed, the muscle splitting incision of the triceps is not advisable as it does not allow a good exposure.

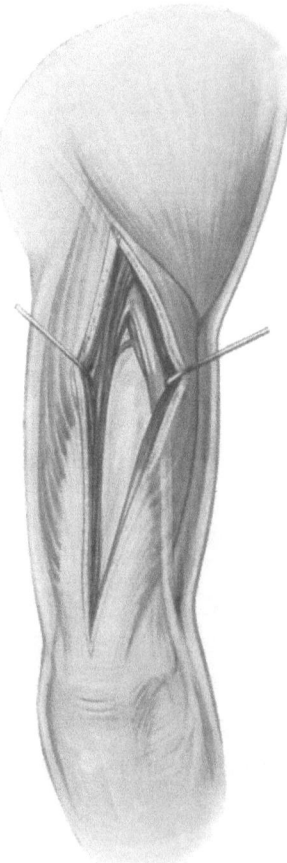

Fig. 201. Posterior approach to fractures of the lower end of the humerus. Note the radial nerve visible at the upper end of the incision (see text)

e) Closure of the Wound

Long muscles that have been split are closed by three to four catgut sutures, a Redon drain is inserted and the fascia, which in the upper arm is closely connected with the subcutaneous fatty tissue, is closed, thus loosely apposing groups of muscles.

2. Technique of Internal Fixation

a) Fractures of the Neck of the Humerus

Indication. Internal fixation is recommended when a fracture dislocation is present, when the head of the humerus has been destroyed, and less commonly in irreducible fractures of the head of the humerus and non union of the neck.

Materials. As the proximal fragment is short, a small T-plate provides adequate fixation. The T-plate which is 36 mm. long is curved to fit the circumference of the head and encompasses about a sixth of it. In addition it is slightly adducted, as is the neck of the humerus itself. The T-piece is fixed to the head of the bone with two cancellous screws,

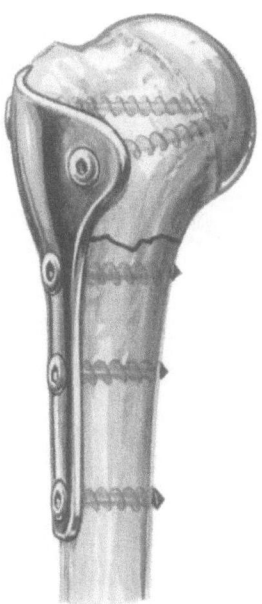

Fig. 202. T-plate for the neck of the humerus in position

while the 65 mm. shaft of the plate is adapted with three cortex screws. The compression device may be useful.

Operative technique. In the approach to the upper end of the humerus with the bone at its mid point of rotation, the lesser tuberosity is approximately in the middle of the field. Starring at the upper end of the tuberosity, lateral to the long head of the biceps, the periosteum is divided and elevated with a raspatory. Narrow bone levers are inserted subperiosteally from medial and lateral sides avoiding injury to the axillary nerve. The fracture is then reduced by traction, rotation and lateral displacement; if there is much abduction of the upper fragment, a fist placed in the axilla can be used as a fulcrum.

We do not elevate the periosteum widely round the head of the humerus as it may damage the nutrition of an already infracted bone and disturb muscle attachments. The plate is applied so that the T-piece bridges the bicipital groove and one cancellous screw is placed in the lesser tuberosity while another one gets a firm hold of the greater tuberosity. Care should be taken that the upper edge of the plate does not extend above the lesser tuberosity. The holes for the cancellous screws are drilled slowly and carefully so that it can be felt by the increased resistance that the far cortex has been reached. A depth gauge should be used to make sure that each screw is exactly the right length in this situation. The plate is then fixed to the shaft with cortex screws using the compression device.

All screws are tightened up, but if there is any comminution of the head of the humerus, it is better to omit the compression routine. The degree of rigidity is examined by moving the arm and it must be determined whether there is any obstruction to abduction due to the plate. Any larger individual fragments may be fixed back with cancellous screws in addition to the plate.

In segmental fractures involving small fragments with tendinous attachments it is desirable to hold these attachments with strong single sutures and to anchor them on the screws before the latter are tightened.

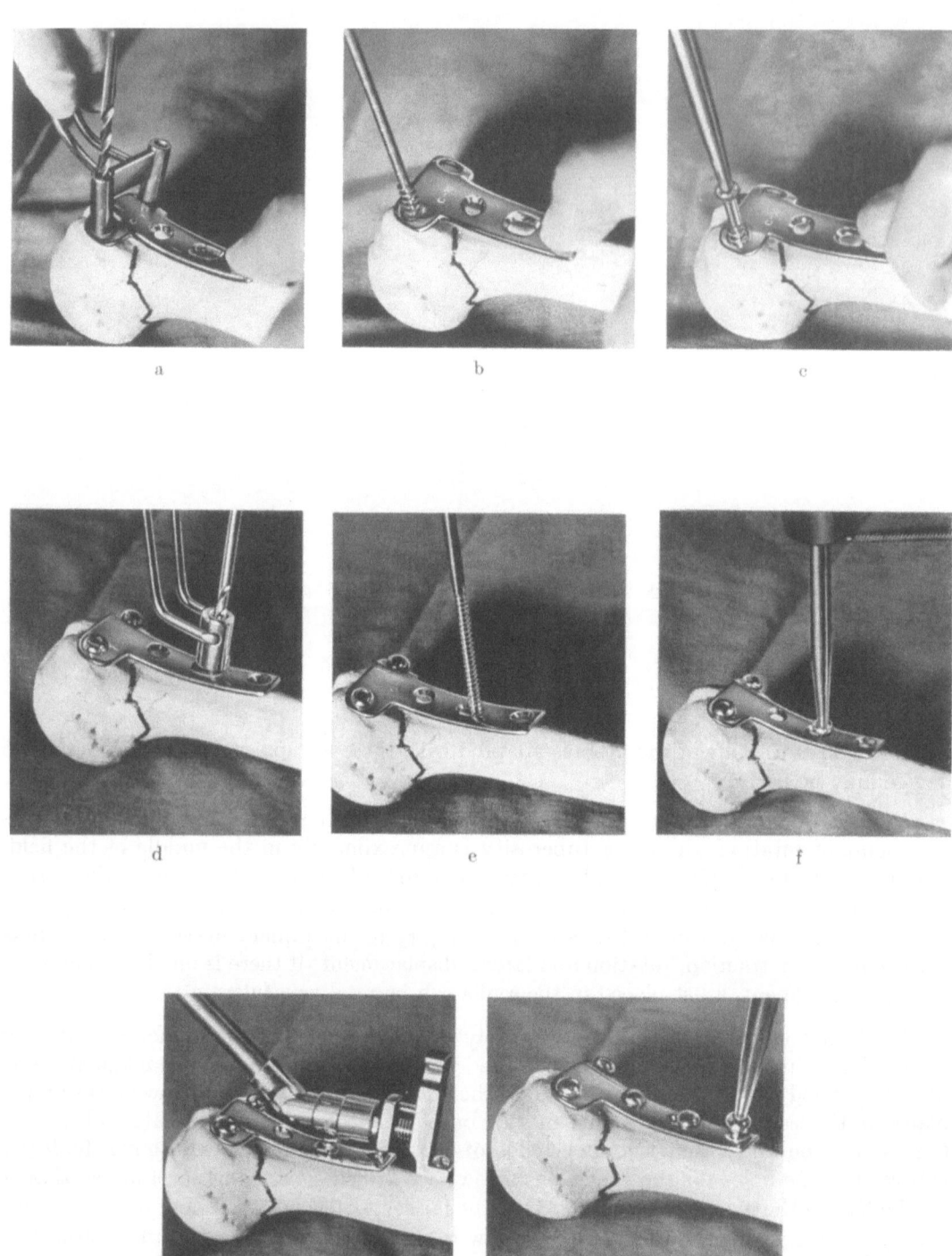

Fig. 203 a—h. Insertion of the T-plate: a Drilling the holes for the cancellous screws with a 3.2 mm. drill using the special drill sleeve. b Tapping the threads. c Insertion of the cancellous screw. d The hole for the first cortex screw is drilled using the sleeve to place it at the distal end of the oval hole in the shank of the plate. e Tapping the thread for this screw. f Insertion of the first cortex screw, at first loosely. g Tightening of the plate with the compression device to impact the shaft into the head of the bone. h The two proximal cortex screws are inserted and tightened. The compression device is removed and the final screw is driven home

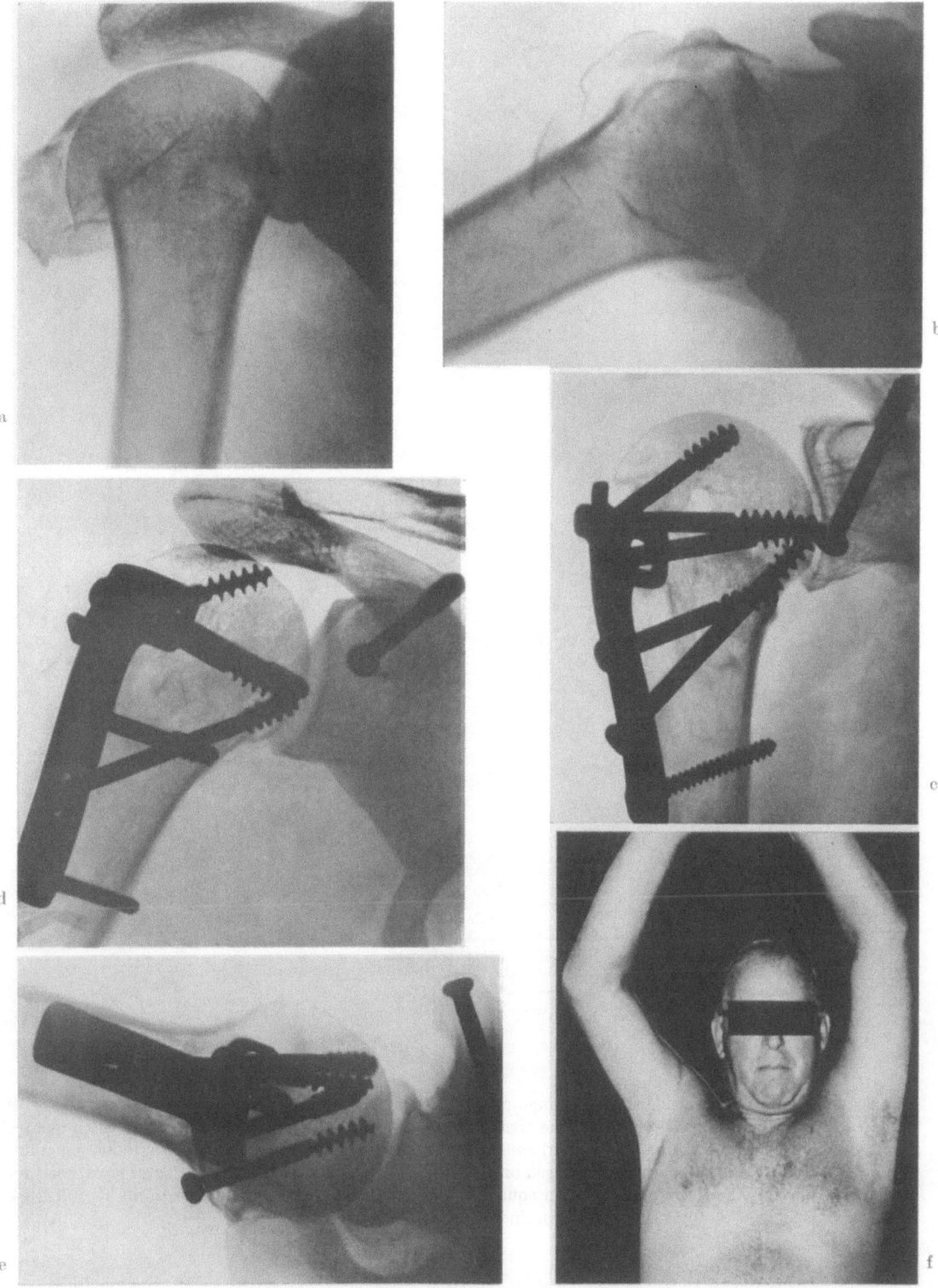

Fig. 204a—f. Sch. L., 50-year-old male. Skiing accident. a and b Displaced fracture of the head of the right humerus with comminution. c Reconstruction of the head of the bone with a cancellous graft achieving a good round surface. d 8 weeks postoperatively the head of the bone is of good shape and of firm structure. e 30 weeks after operation the axial projection shows only a small cortical spur anteriorly, otherwise there is normal structure and shape of the head. f Range of movement

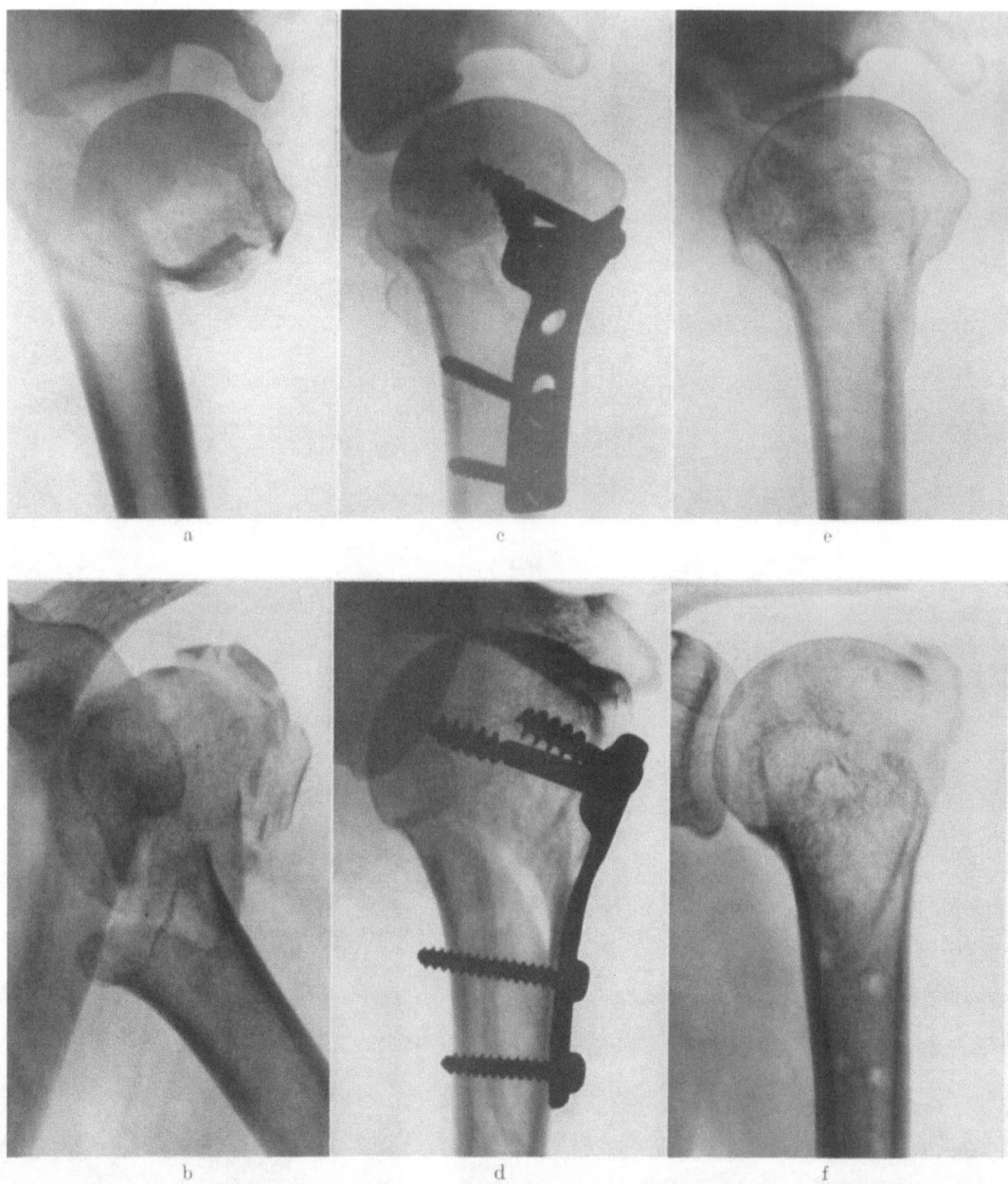

Fig. 205a—f. M. P., 39-year-old male. Skiing accident. a and b Fracture of the neck of the humerus with full displacement of the head, avulsion of the greater tuberosity and subluxation of the head of the humerus. c and d Internal fixation with a T-plate and assembling of the fragments with sutures. An abduction splint is worn for 10 days and the patient discharged on the 12th day. e and f Condition at 7 months: external rotation half normal, abduction and elevation equal on both sides. The patient was able to do his full work as a business man after 48 days

Radiography. This should always include antero-posterior and axillary projections. A first film may be taken after reduction and a final one before wound closure.

Postoperative care. On the evening after the operation or at least the next day, the patient may get up. If the clavicular insertion of the deltoid did not have to be divided, the patient need only wear a sling; if muscle insertion has been severed, the arm is placed in an

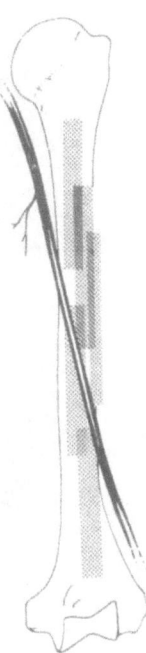

Fig. 206. The various positions of a straight plate on the shaft of the humerus showing the relations to the radial nerve

abduction splint for the first ten days. All joints are moved actively from the first day, but where the deltoid was divided, abduction is only done passively during the first ten days. Active external rotation is always performed by lifting the hand with the elbow supported and flexed to 90°. As soon as the splint has been removed, the patient may be discharged. He should only have had to spend ten to twelve days in the hospital.

b) Fractures of the Shaft

Open reduction of fractures of the shaft of the humerus may be indicated in compound fractures, in the presence of arterial or nerve injury, and in long oblique and segmental fractures extending down to the elbow. A rigid fixation can be obtained by the use of compression plates.

Technique. A lateral approach is used, but in special cases the posterior incision may be better, especially for fractures of the lower third of the humerus. Straight compression plates with four to six holes are used, fixed with cortex screws. In transverse fractures one must be on the alert for rotational deformity. Rotation will be found correct as soon as accurate reduction has been achieved, and it can easily be checked by seeing that the crest running down from the lesser tuberosity is continuous with the ridge extending up from the epicondyle. The plate is so placed as to avoid the area of the radial nerve, but if necessary it can be slid under the nerve and fixed there without damaging it. Interposition of viable muscle between nerve and plate, as a padding, is desirable in these cases. It is important to record the position of the radial nerve in relation to the plate and screws in such a case, and when the plate is removed facilities must be available to stimulate the nerve electrically.

In long oblique and comminuted fractures of the shaft, rigid fixation may be achieved only with an eight to ten hole plate, sometimes combined with a second (shorter) plate applied at right angles to the first. In rare cases, large gaps necessitate, in addition to the plate, a cancellous autograft.

Aftercare. No external fixation is needed and active mobilization of the whole extremity should be encouraged during the course of wound healing.

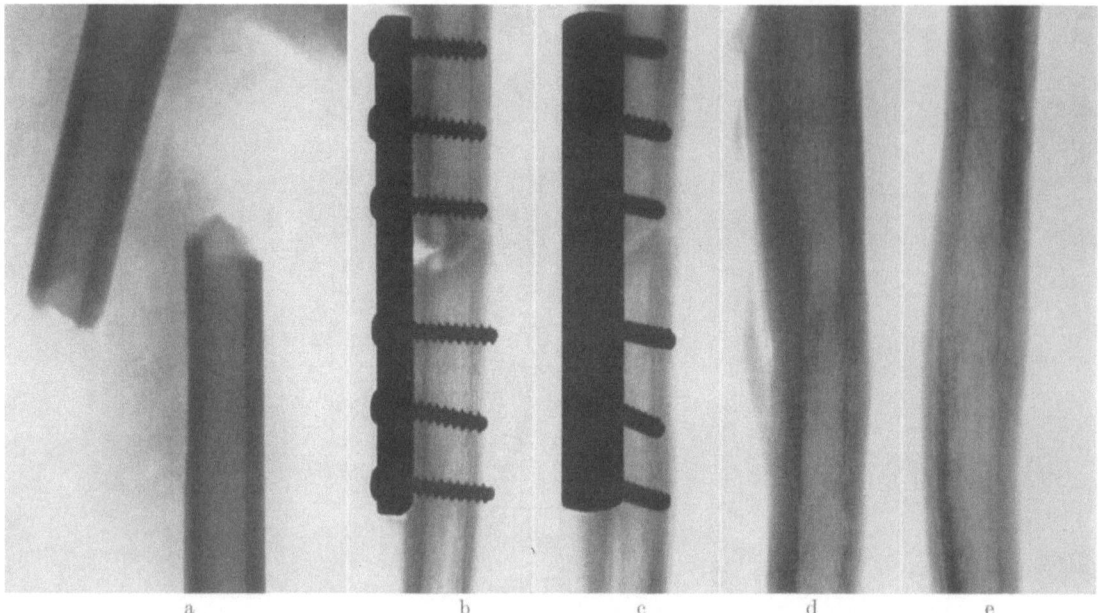

Fig. 207a—e. B. H., 15-year-old male. a Compound transverse fracture of the humerus, in the mid-shaft, severely contaminated, caused by a blow with a stone. Severe displacement, radial nerve intact. Emergency operation for internal fixation with a 6-hole plate. Immobilization for 10 days with a dorsal splint and hospitalization for 18 days. 4 weeks after operation the patient was able to work as an errand-boy for a bakery. b and c X-rays at 4 months: Little periosteal callus with bony union on the medial and posterior aspects, full function. 7 months after operation there was good ossification. At 12 months the plate was removed. Union was now complete and the function was equal to that on the normal side. The total period of disability, including the plate removal, had been 35 days. d and e End-result 15 months after the accident

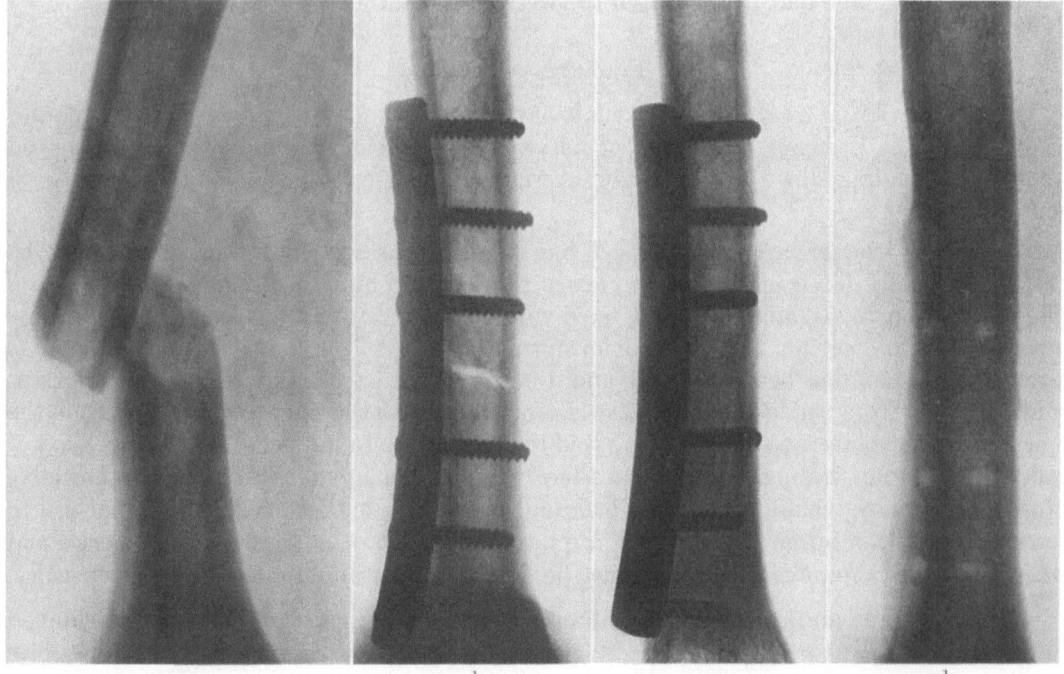

Fig. 208a—d. C. K., 25-year-old male. Tractor accident. a Transverse fracture of the humerus. b Internal fixation with a straight plate, bent a little at the distal end. Reduction was not entirely perfect, but rigid fixation was obtained. Patient remained in the hospital for 47 days. c At 8 months union was complete. d Condition at 15¹/₂ months, after removal of the plate. The patient had complained of a little pain when lifting heavy loads. Full range of movement without pain in shoulder and elbow joints

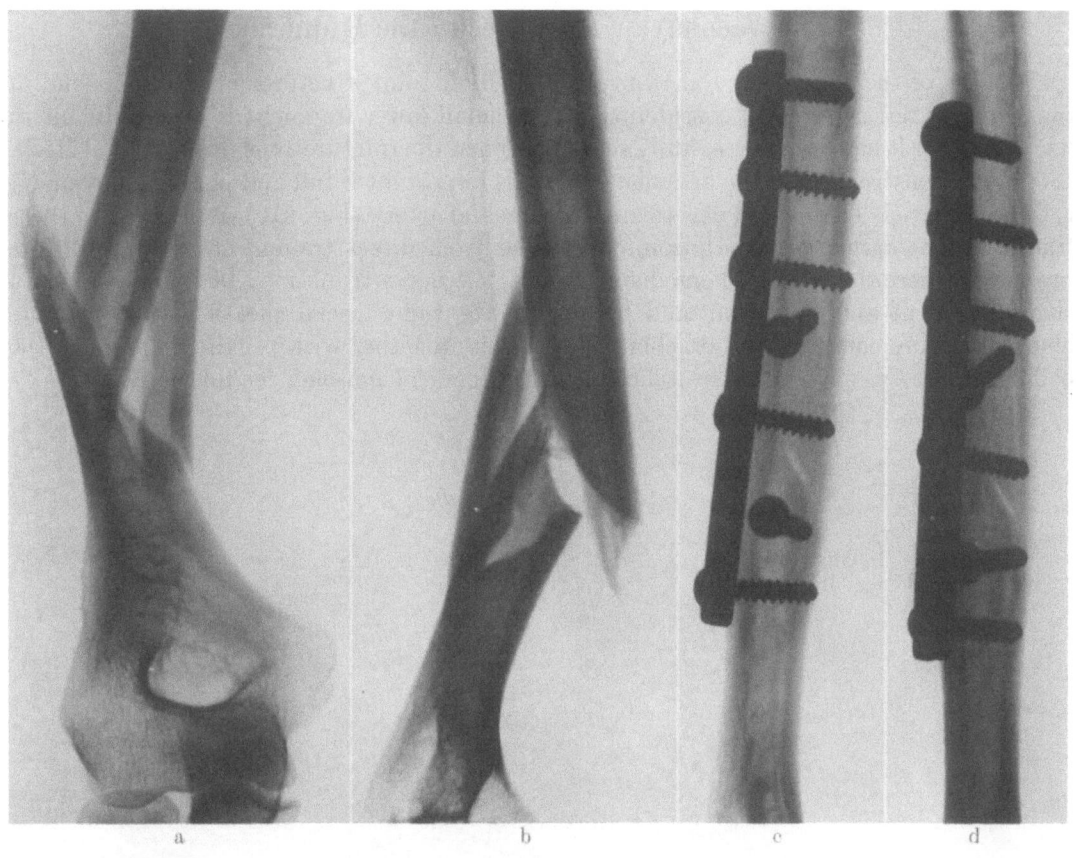

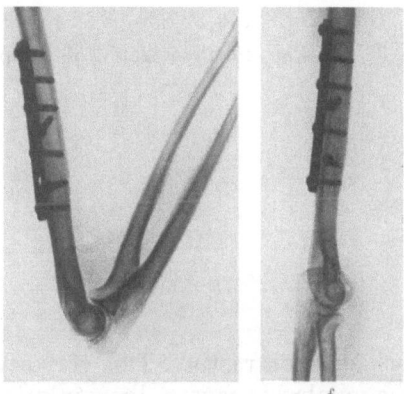

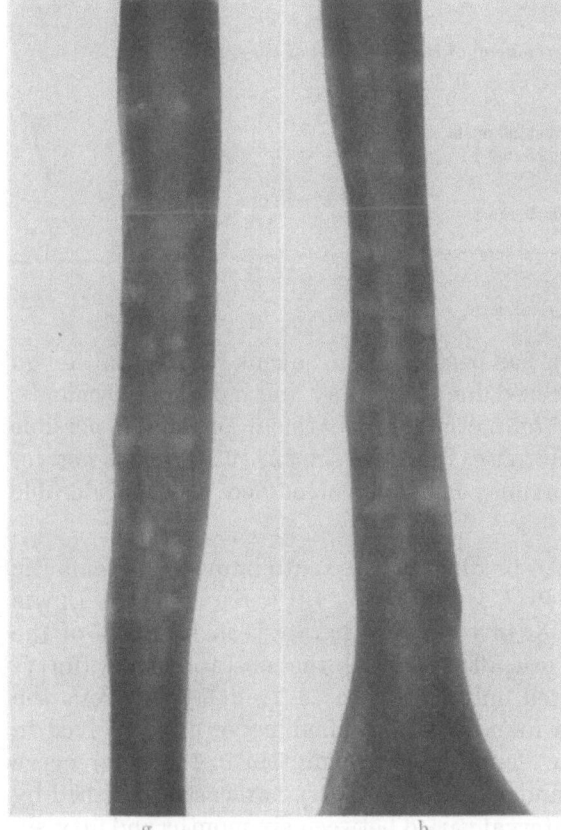

Fig. 209a—h. Z. C., 24-year-old female. Motor accident. a and b Long oblique fracture with a separate fragment between the middle and lower third. The radial nerve was intact. Internal fixation on the fourth day with a 6-hole plate with separate screw fixation of the loose fragment with 2 cortex screws. Reduction was not anatomically perfect but fixation was rigid. A plaster back slab was worn for 3 weeks, removed daily for exercises. Hospitalisation lasted 15 days. c and d Condition at 4 months showing good ossification. The toal disability was 105 days. e and f Functional status at 8 months: Rotations are free and the elbow range on the right is 50⁰ to 180⁰ (on the uninjured left 40⁰ to 180⁰). The patient was free from any discomfort. g and h Condition at 10 months, removal of the metal

3. Supracondylar Fractures of the Humerus

Because of the complicated anatomy of the elbow joint, fractures of the lower end of the humerus deserve special consideration. The small lower fragment is often difficult to fix, even after it has been successfully reduced. When the fracture runs into the joint itself, accurate reconstruction of the articular surface is important if full and painless movement is to be achieved. Three main nerves and the brachial artery (Fig. 210) are so close to these fractures that damage is not uncommon, either from direct trauma or by more diffuse pressure. Where there is bad bone displacement, the nerve trunk may be stretched over a sharp fragment and thus torn, and because of the tight fascial sheath even a fracture hematoma may compress the brachial artery. This, together with proximal spasm in the collateral vessels, may result in ischemia of the forearm muscles, leading to VOLKMAN's

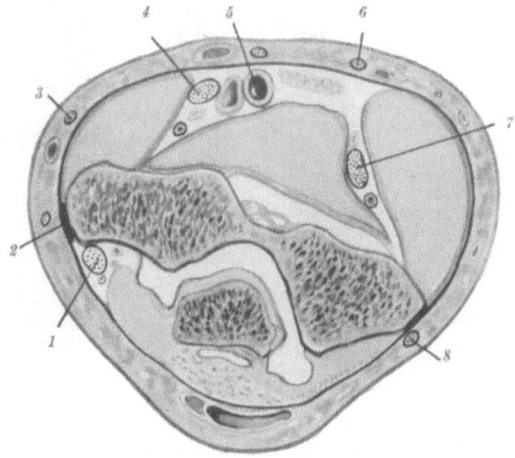

Fig. 210. Cross section of the upper arm at the level of the lower end of the humerus

1 N. ulnaris;
2 Septum intermusculare uln.;
3 N. cut. antebrach. uln.;
4 N. medianus;
5 A. brachialis;
6 N. cut. antebrach. rad.;
7 N. radialis;
8 N. cut. antebrach. dors.

ischemic contracture. This very severe lesion has become less frequent recently, although the number of severe elbow injuries has increased due to highway and industrial accidents. The improved results are probably due to better methods of treatment and so it is possible that the complication is largely iatrogenic (BÖHLER, 1961; LIPSCOMB, 1955). It has not yet been fully clarified whether neurogenic factors may not be involved here to a considerable extent.

Nerve lesions with this type of fracture can be differentiated into immediate traumatic paresis and delayed paresis (BERGMANN, 1949; CONSTENSOUX, 1918; HUNT, 1916). LEWIS and MILLER (1922) have described sixty cases of traumatic paralysis in fractures of the lower end of the humerus. The radial nerve was affected much the most frequently (forty-four cases) while the ulnar nerve was affected only in five cases. In delayed paresis the position was quite different, as the authors found that the ulnar nerve was involved in 94% of cases. The time between the fracture and the first symptom in the ulnar nerve varied widely (GAY, 1947; MURPHY, 1916) and in a series of forty-two cases published by the Neurological Clinic at Zurich the time interval varied between six months and fifty-six

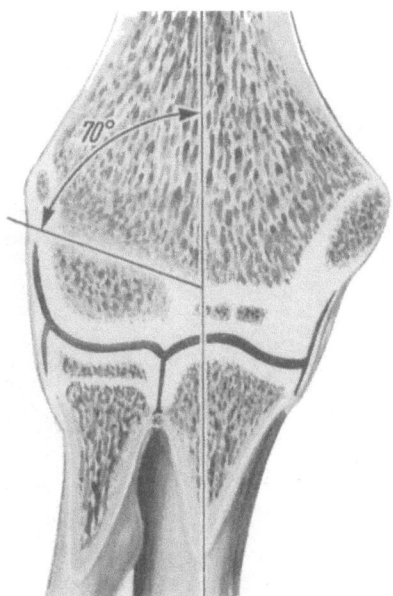

Fig. 211. Coronal section through the elbow joint showing the internal bony structure and the epiphyseal plate
(13-year-old girl)

years (MUMENTHALER, 1961). It is therefore perhaps not surprising that the patient may
not remember the fracture or the examining doctor does not think there is a causal connection (DRESSLER 1958).

If the bony elements of this injury are not well treated a pseudarthrosis or malunion
can occur, interfering with the function of the elbow joint. Young people who are still
growing are especially prone to bad late results if there has been direct damage to the
epiphyseal area, or when a separated epicondyle has not been properly reduced (Fig. 212).

A late ulnar palsy is most likely to occur after lesions of the lateral epicondyle with a
secondary valgus deformity. This is not thought to be due to an increase in the distance
which the nerve has to traverse, and the nerve does not become displaced as a result of the
deformity (MUMENTHALER 1958). It is rather because the joint between the ulna and the
humerus becomes unstable if it is unsupported on the lateral side by the head of the radius.
This results in thickening of the periarticular tissue in the same manner as in osteoarthritis
of the joint when an ulnar palsy may also occur (HENSELL 1953). When the nerve is
explored it is usually found to be embedded in thick fibrous tissue. As the joint itself has
suffered no primary damage, it may be assumed that the tissue reaction is produced by the
increased stress to which the joint is subjected without its lateral support. This should be
taken as a warning against resecting the head of the radius and the lower end of the ulna,
as the lateral instability produced may throw an excessive strain on the elbow joint by the
effect of gravity alone.

A typical complication of injury in this area is calcification around the joint, after injury
to its capsule. No other joint has so great a tendency as the elbow to deposit calcium in the
connective tissue and muscles. The treatment of the complications is discussed elsewhere.

The fractures of the distal humerus are so different in type and are so often complicated
by other injuries that no firm rules about their treatment can be laid down. The object of
treatment is to obtain proper reduction of the bone with congruous articular surfaces while

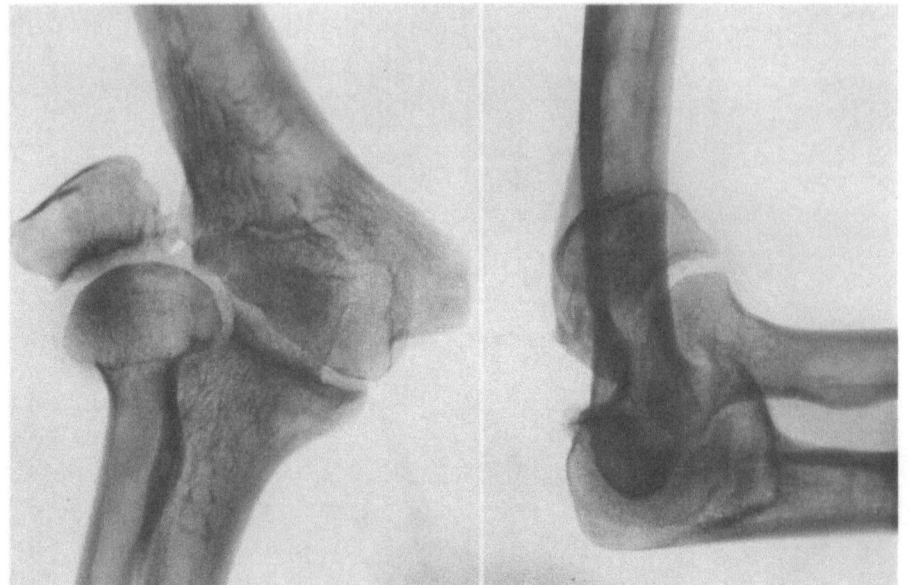

Fig. 212a and b. F. M., 37 years old. Fracture of the right lateral epicondyle at 10 years of age. After an injury to the elbow at 22 years of age, the patient suddenly experienced ulnar nerve symptoms accompanied by pain. There was a varying amount of severe discomfort which, over a period of 10 years, resulted in a 10% disability award. Thereafter, without special cause the symptoms increased; in consequence the patient had an anterior transplant of the ulnar nerve 10 years after the onset of discomfort

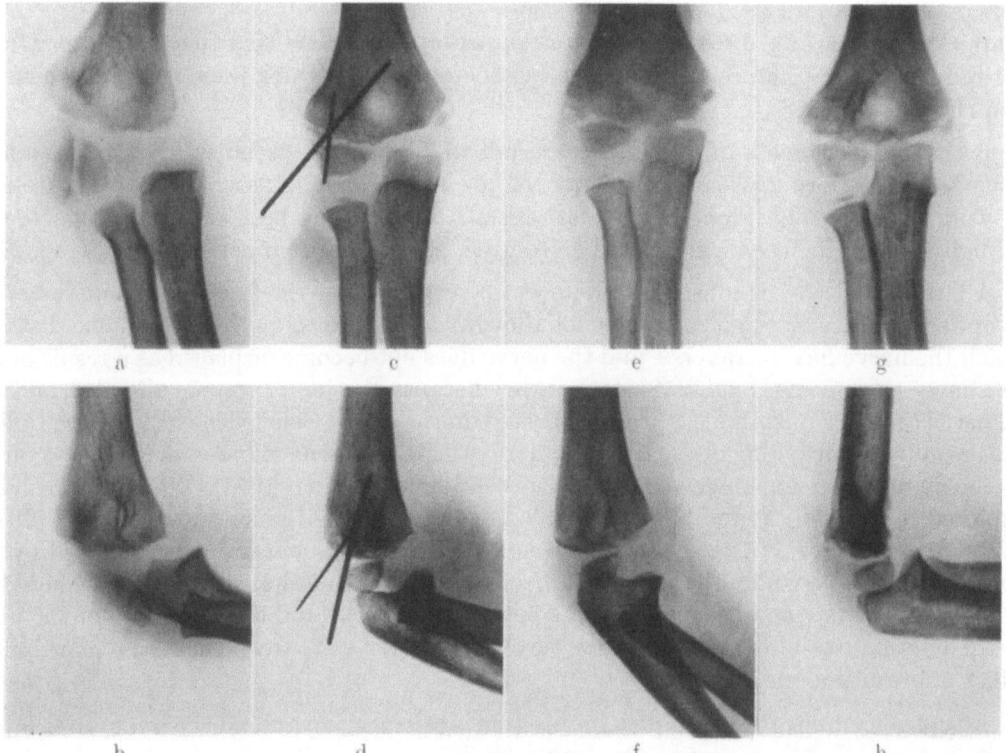

Fig. 213a—h. A. W., 6 years old. Patient jumped from a height of 2 meters, landing on the right elbow. a and b Fracture of the lateral condyle on the right, with severe displacement and rotation of the fragments. c and d Emergency open reduction and internal fixation with two crossed KIRSCHNER wires clipped off just beneath the skin, followed by a plaster splint. e and f 18 days after operation, the wires were removed and active movements begun. g and h At 4 months the function was almost normal but there was a varus deformity of at least 10°. Subjectively there were no symptoms

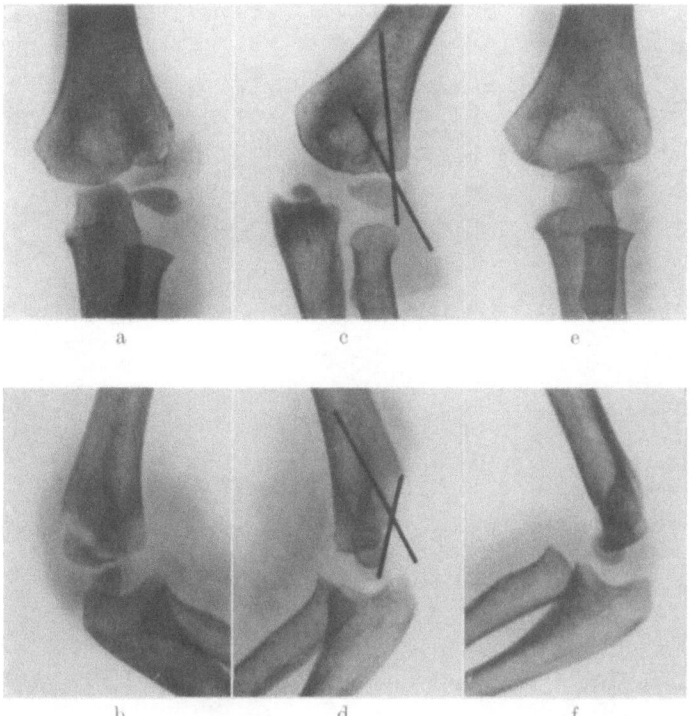

Fig. 214a—f. G. R., 4 years old. Fall on right elbow from a kitchen table. a and b Fracture of the right lateral epicondyle with moderate displacement. c and d Open reduction the day following the accident and internal fixation with 2 thin crossed KIRSCHNER wires. Immobilization in a plaster splint. The wires were removed 15 days after the operation. e and f At 4 months there was anatomical position, full power, joint movement equal to that on the other side and the fracture was not radiologically visible

maintaining full function. This is best done by rigid internal fixation, but the construction of the lower end of the humerus and the ease with which the epiphyses are injured impose some limitations on internal fixation methods which may need to be adapted to fit specific fractures.

Supracondylar fractures in children and adolescents. These are usually treated conservatively with either BAUMANN's technique (1960) using vertical traction or Dunlop traction as described by BLOUNT (1955).

If, besides the supracondylar fracture there is vascular disturbance or a nerve lesion, as may occur with a hyperextension fracture, surgery will be needed if reduction of the fracture does not improve matters.

Treatment of a fracture of the ulnar epicondyle depends on the size of the fragment and on neurological findings. An operative intervention must be taken into consideration, especially to diminish the chances of a late nerve lesion (SENGESSE, 1898). In children it is often difficult to assess the fracture properly on the x-ray and it is good policy to take a film of the opposite side. Varus or valgus deformity can be detected according to BAUMANN's "line of orientation" (1959): On a lateral x-ray of the elbow joint a varus deformity will show as an intersection of the epiphysis with the proximal ulna. This phenomenon is called "Signe de l'eclipse" (MARION, 1962). Internal fixation of the lateral condyle fracture is best done by using crossed KIRSCHNER wires (Figs. 213, 214); screws are seldom indicated,

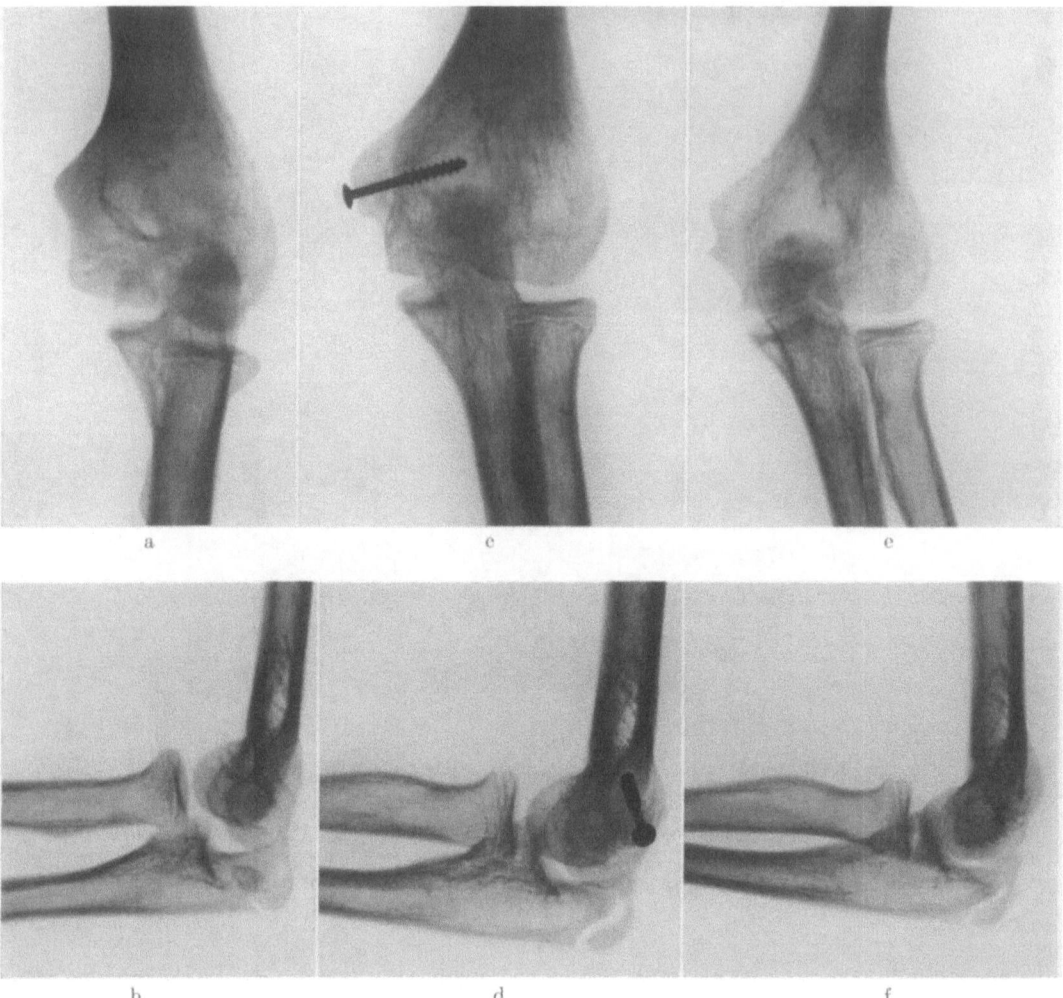

Fig. 215a—f. F. K., aged 15. Fall on the right elbow after jump over a garden fence. a and b Irreducible subluxation of the right elbow with avulsion of the medial epicondyle and a median and ulnar nerve palsy, but a range of movement equal to the other side. In this case a scaphoid screw was used instead of KIRSCHNER wires, since the fracture was 5 days old and because the pre-existing shortening made it difficult to hold back the avulsed fragment. c and d Condition 3 months after operation. The screw was left in place longer than usual to avoid any further scarring aggravating the ulnar palsy, which a further operation at a too early stage would have involved. e and f Condition 9½ months after the accident

as a screw in a small fragment can produce severe bone necrosis and KIRSCHNER wires do little damage to the epiphyseal plate. These wires do not produce rigid fixation, however, and a plaster splint will be needed for two to three weeks. In children and adolescents this plaster does not cause any stiffness and when removed the patient mobilizes his joints spontaneously without trouble. Small puncture incisions are used to remove the wires and then active exercises can be begun.

Supracondylar fractures in adults. There is a greater place for internal fixation in these fractures in adults, especially when the joint surfaces are involved, because conservative measures seldom produce good articular congruity. In older patients a stable internal fixation allows early mobilization and prevents stiffness in the elbow and shoulder. In these

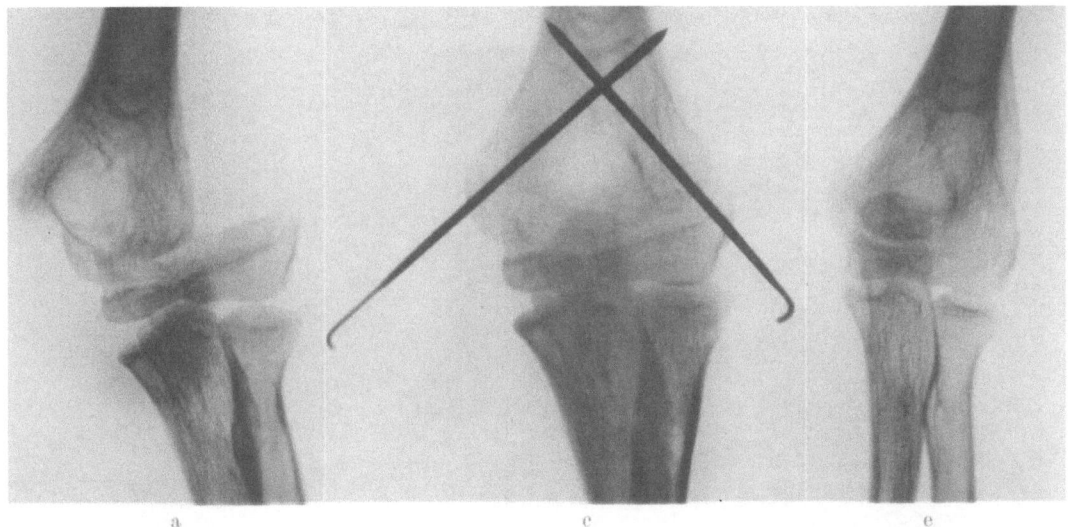

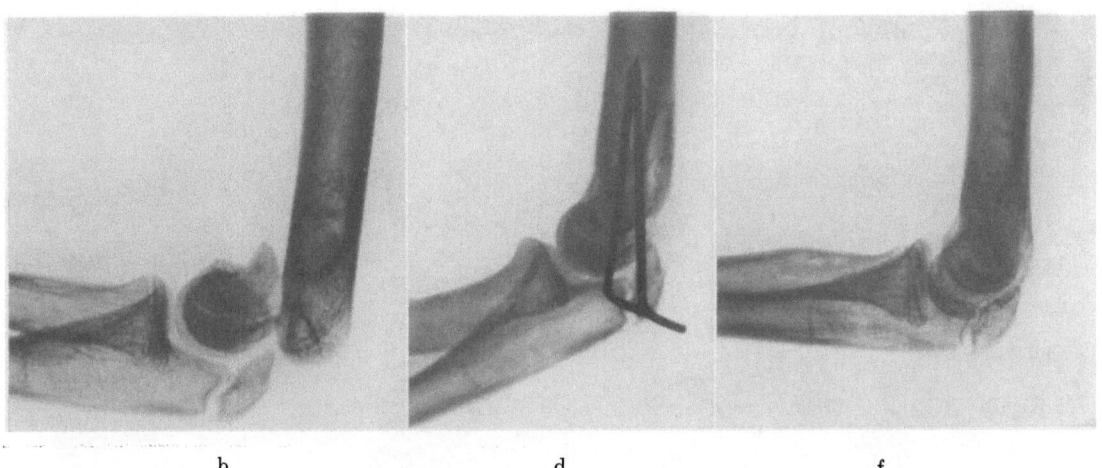

Fig. 216a—f. R. J., aged 13. Fall on the left elbow. a and b Emergency admission for supracondylar fracture on the left with early ulnar palsy. c and d The fracture was exposed by two lateral incisions. The ulnar nerve was tightly stretched over the proximal fragment. It was mobilised and transplanted anteriorly. The fracture was reduced and fixed with two crossed KIRSCHNER wires. A plaster splint was applied for $2^1/_2$ weeks, after which the wires were removed and movements begun. e and f X-rays at $4^1/_2$ months. There was no nerve palsy, flexion was limited by $10°$, as was supination. The patient was symptom free

fractures, we use either two plates without compression, or one plate combined with a lag screw inserted obliquely. In suitable cases two cancellous screws crossing each other can give good enough fixation.

In comminuted fractures with many small fragments, rigid fixation is not attempted but the joint surface is reconstructed using several KIRSCHNER wires, and a plaster may be necessary for three weeks as well. In severe cases where there is destruction of the joint surface, internal fixation should only be attempted cautiously and better results may be obtained with extension and early mobilization (BOCCANEGRA, 1961).

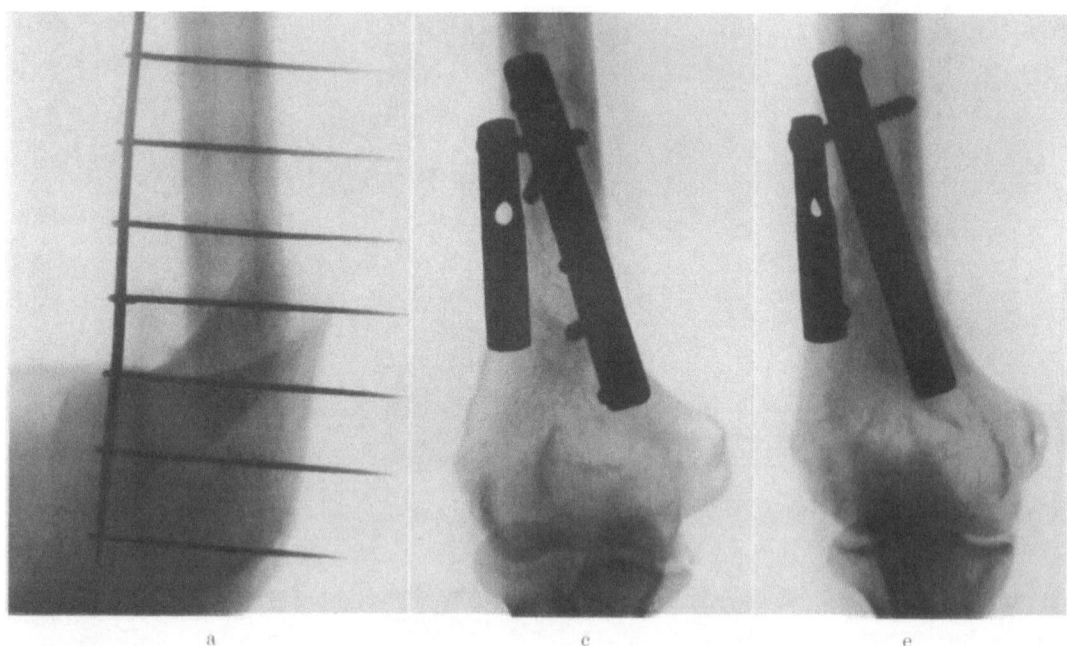

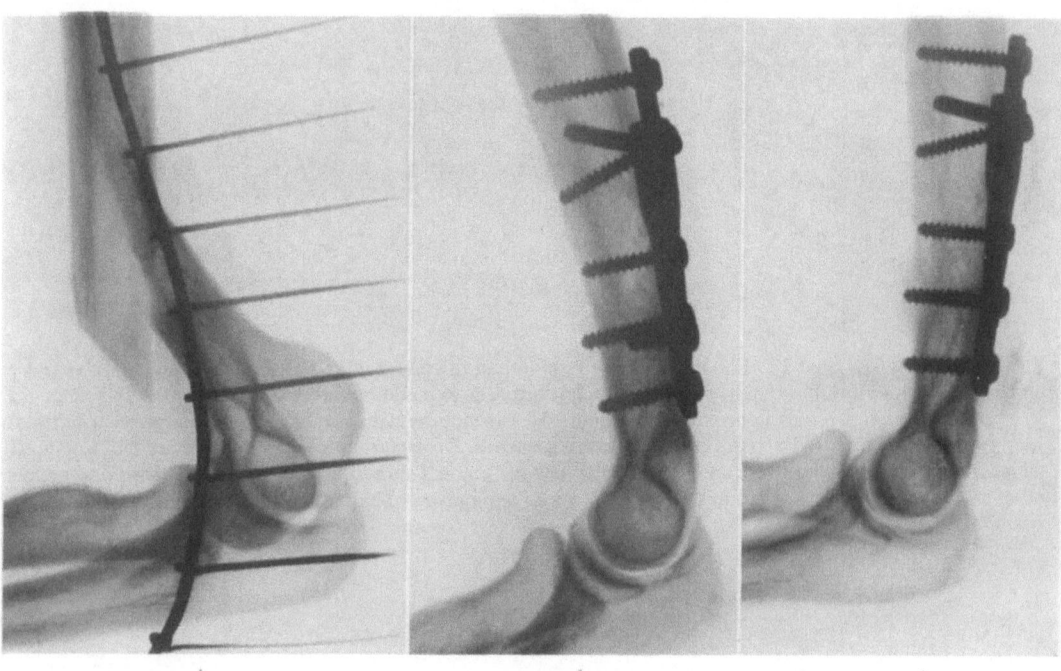

Fig. 217a—f. L. J., aged 78. Fall off a motor-cycle with no other vehicle involved. a and b Emergency admission with fracture of the lower third of the humerus on the left. No nerve or vascular involvement. c and d Operation the day after the accident. Posterior approach dividing the triceps at the junction between tendinous and muscular parts. Rigid internal fixation with 3-hole and 5-hole plates. No external support, active movements beginning on the 2nd day. At discharge 3 weeks after the accident, there was 10⁰ limitation of extension only, while all other movements of elbow, hand and shoulder were full. e and f At 4 months the fracture was united and the function remained full

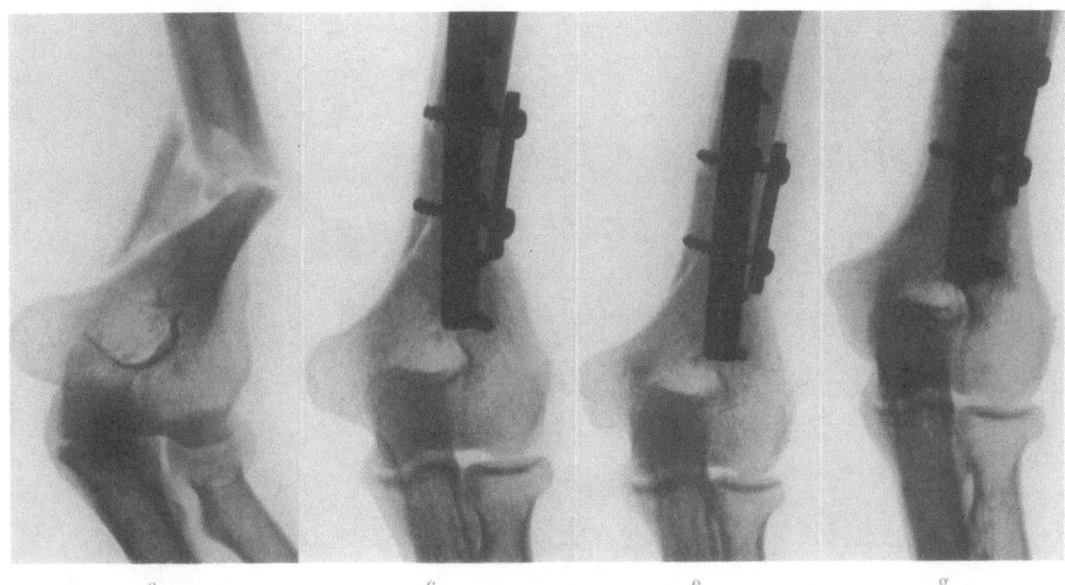

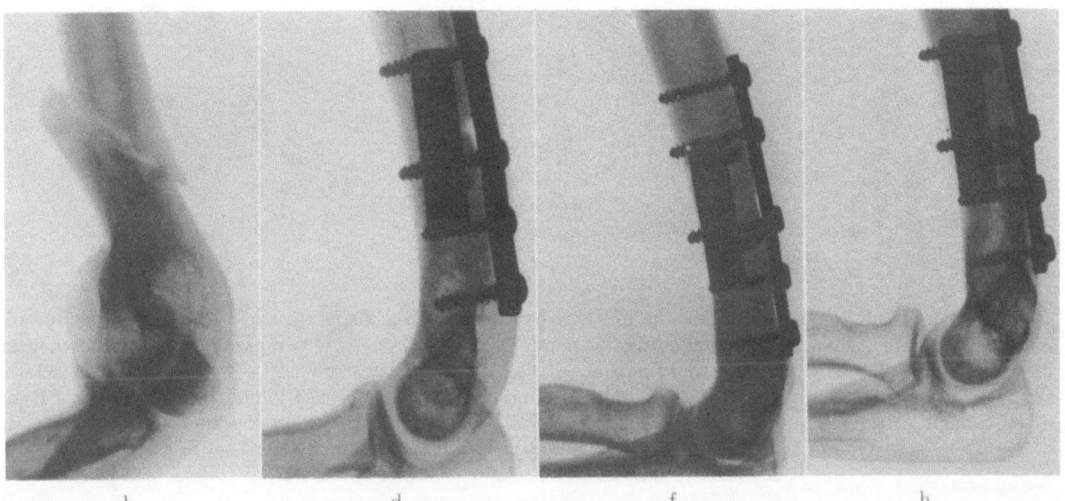

Fig. 218a—h. Di P. G., aged 23. a and b Patient was hit by a falling log in a building excavation. On admission he was in severe shock with multiple fractures of the right femur and the left humerus. c and d Because of the poor general condition, surgical treatment of the humerus was delayed until the 2nd day and the femur was fixed at 3 weeks with 2 plates. The humerus was approached laterally and a 5-hole and 2-hole plate applied. No external support. 14 days after operation the elbow could be fully moved without discomfort. e and f Condition 6 weeks after the operation. g and h At 4 months the range of movements in the elbow and shoulder was equal to that of the other side

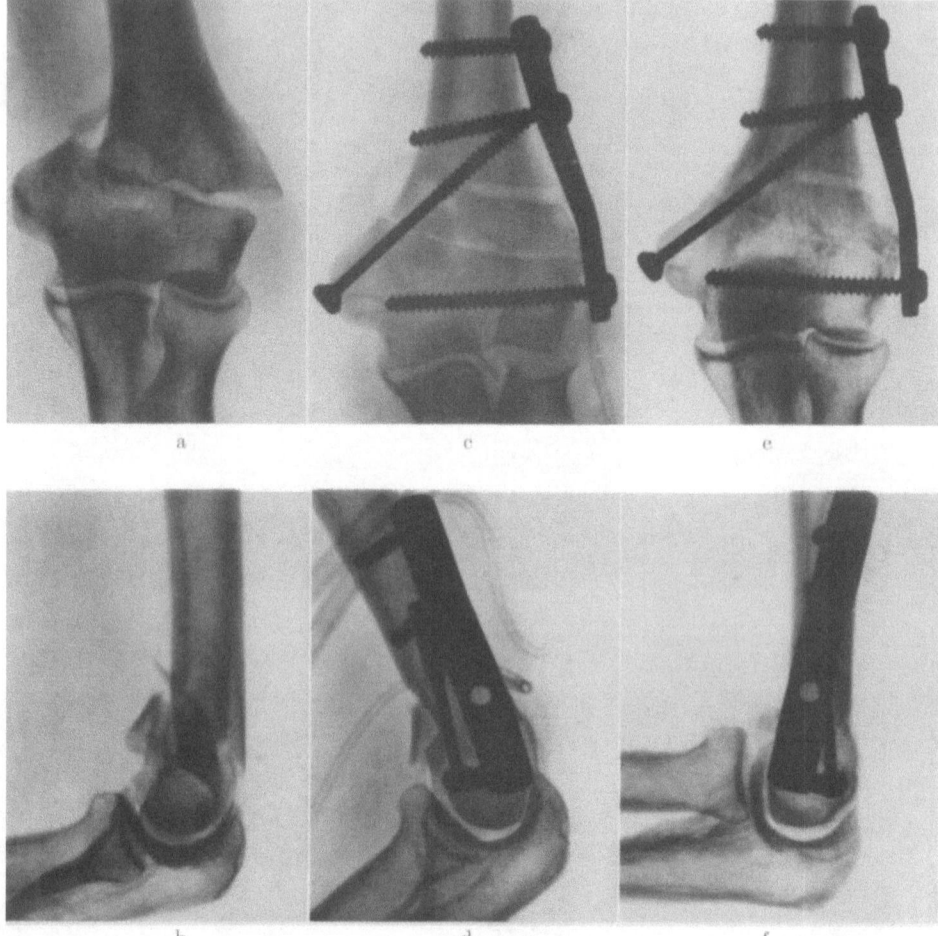

Fig. 219a—f. W. J., aged 78. Fall on the left arm by slipping on a carpet. a and b Supracondylar fracture of the left humerus. No nerve or vascular involvement. c and d Approach via two parallel longitudinal incisions on each side of the olecranon. Internal fixation with a long malleolar screw and a 4-hole plate. No external support, active movements after 2 days. e and f At 4 months diminished sensation in the ulnar fingers. Range of movement at the elbow was 160⁰ to 85⁰, supination was full and pronation was limited by 10⁰. In this patient the plate and screws will not be removed if the nerve signs subside

Approach. This depends on the type and situation of the fracture itself and on the presence of any neural or vascular complication. In children a medial or lateral approach gives adequate access, but in very low transverse fractures in adults and in Y-fractures, the dorsal approach is simplest and least dangerous.

With the patient prone, the skin is incised on the medial side, circumventing the olecranon to expose the ulnar nerve. The triceps is divided at the junction between its tendinous and muscular part and turned down, leaving its attachment to the olecranon undisturbed. The muscular insertion of the triceps is elevated together with the periosteum with a raspatory. If there is much involvement of the joint itself the olecranon can be removed with an osteotome and the triceps tendon turned backwards in a proximal direction. Before doing this a drill hole should be made through the tip of the olecranon into the shaft of the ulna, and a hole for a cancellous screw tapped out. This allows it to be accurately replaced afterwards.

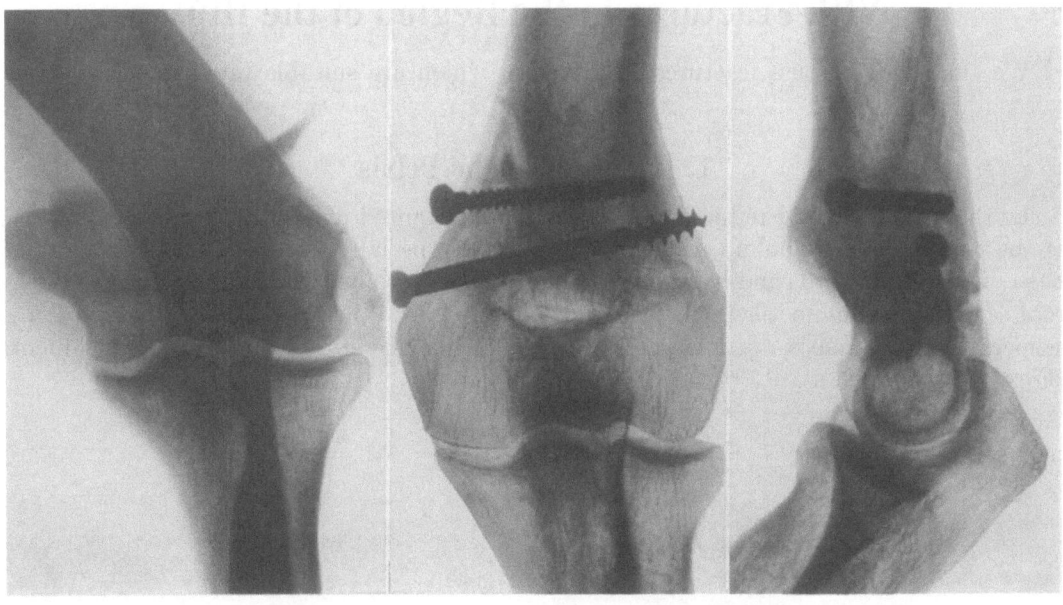

Fig. 220a—c. F. T., aged 64. a Patient fell onto his right elbow and was admitted as an emergency. He was an extremely fat and plethoric man, for whom external fixation would have been impossible. Immediate open reduction and fixation with 2 screws. Immobilization with a plaster splint until completion of wound healing, after which active movements were begun. b and c Condition at 4 months, extension, pronation and supination were full

A plate must be used that will not touch the olecranon fossa, as even slight injury here may prevent full extension. If a plate needs to be placed close to the ulnar nerve, or if the groove of the ulnar nerve has been injured through the fracture itself, it is better to transplant the nerve anteriorly beforehand, rather than to wait for a later paralysis.

The technique most commonly used is that described by NIGST (1953) and BATEMAN (1962). The whole flexor origin is detached from the epicondyle, and after the nerve has been transposed anteriorly the flexor origin is replaced over the epicondyle. To prevent any late neuritis the intermuscular septum should be removed from its attachment to the lower humerus, or the nerve has to execute a very sharp bend. The branch to the elbow joint is almost always too short and will have to be sacrificed, but the branches to flexor carpi ulnaris and to the flexor profundus may be lifted forwards with the back of the scalpel. The muscle origin may be reinserted with sutures to the epicondyle and no stitches are needed to fix the nerve in its new place.

After reduction of the fracture and temporary fixation, a check x-ray should also always be taken. When screws are used to replace the temporary Kirschner wires, a mild displacement of the lower fragment in a proximal direction may occur. An attempt should be made to place the screw at right angles to the fracture line. When a lateral approach is used to fix a detached lateral condyle, care must be taken not to injure the dorsal cutaneous nerve which perforates the fascia at this level and then runs towards the condyle as an easily visible branch. Even if a neuroma does not form after its divison, a troublesome area of insensitivity may be produced, so that primary suture is worthwhile if it is accidentally divided, or secondary suture when the plate is removed.

VIII. Fractures in the Region of the Hip

We shall only discuss fractures in this area which are suitable for internal fixation.

1. Fractures of the Pelvis

In the pelvis surgical reduction and fixation is required chiefly for avulsion fractures of the rim of the acetabulum, usually at the back, especially when the femoral head has been displaced upwards and backwards. Fixation may also be indicated in fractures of the roof of the acetabulum where the greatest pressure falls. When a posterior subluxation is suspected, an oblique x-ray is necessary to determine the size of any avulsed fragments (Figs. 221 b and 223 a).

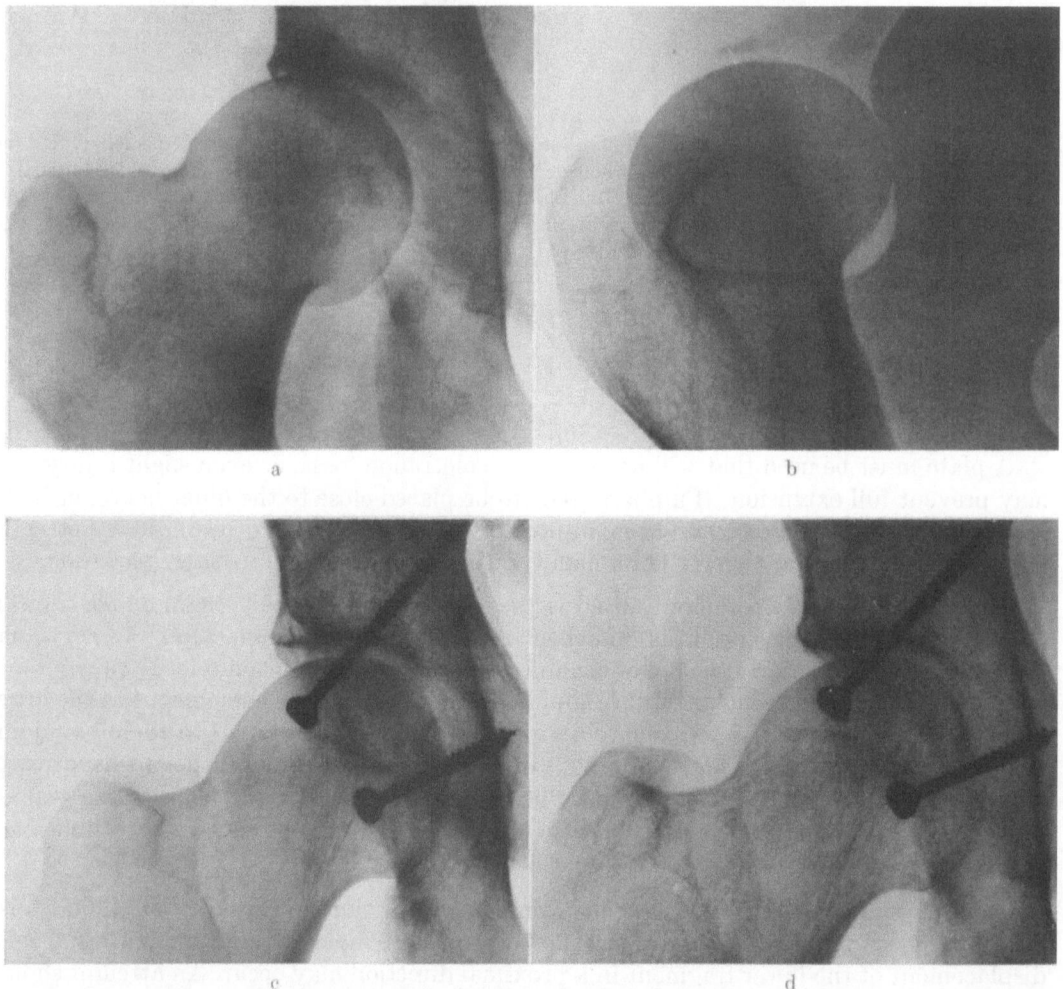

Fig. 221 a—d. Fracture dislocation with separation of two fragments on the posterior margin of the acetabulum. The fracture was reduced 5 hours after injury and fixed with two screws. The patient was able to get out of bed after 8 days and went home with two sticks on the 13th day. At six months the patient walked without a stick, with a slight limp. Hip movements were completely free except for slight limitation of rotation. a X-ray at time of injury. b Semi-oblique projection showing the extent of the dislocation. c X-ray following internal fixation. d At 8 months

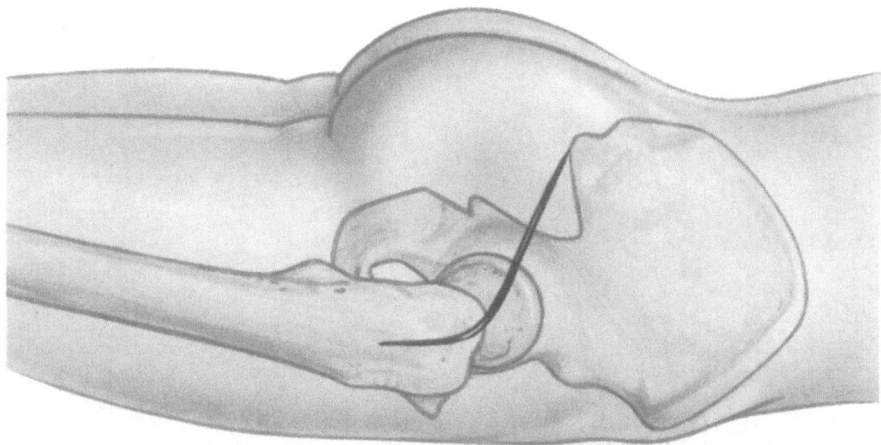

Fig. 222. Postero-lateral approach for internal fixation of the posterior margin of the acetabulum. Prone position in extension. Incision a finger's breadth below the posterior inferior iliac spine towards the greater trochanter and then a short distance distally

With the patient in the prone position, a postero-lateral incision is made as shown in Fig. 222, extending from the posterior superior iliac spine laterally to the greater trochanter, then down in the axis of the femur. The fibres of the gluteus maximus are separated by blunt dissection in the line of the incision and after exposure of the dislocated head of the femur, reduction is usually easily performed by extending the hip. Occasionally it is necessary to pull the shaft laterally at the same time, using a bone hook. Sometimes reduction is blocked by a fragment of the acetabulum lying within the joint, and this will have to be removed first. When reduction is complete and the surgeon is sure that there is no loose fragment of bone or cartilage in the joint, the roof of the acetabulum may be reconstructed, using thin Kirschner wires as a first step. For final fixation, screws are employed of the kind used for malleolar fractures (Figs. 221 c and 223 b). At one week, the patients can usually walk with the help of elbow crutches, but full weight bearing is allowed only after two to four months.

The same approach can be used for irreducible fractures of the acetabular floor, and to make sure of the safety of the sciatic nerve it should be exposed during the operation. A strong pull in the long axis of the leg reduces the fracture. A screw, driven in the distal fragment temporarily, or two screws on each side of the fracture may serve as a grip that helps the reduction maneuver. A small AOI plate or strong staples can be used to provide stabilization.

When such a fracture is combined with one of the neck of the femur, the problem is more difficult, but it is worthwhile to do an internal fixation even if large devitalized bone fragments have to be sacrificed. A Vitallium prosthesis is used only in an elderly patient. In younger people we always attempt reconstruction if there is any chance of a successful result.

2. Subcapital Fractures of the Femoral Neck
(Adduction Type Fracture)

Based on the pioneering work of FELSENREICH, SMITH-PETERSEN, and PUTTI, subcapital fractures of the femoral neck have been surgically treated in most clinics in the world. The fracture is either screwed, nailed or fixed with an on-lay graft (MOREIRA) or, in elderly

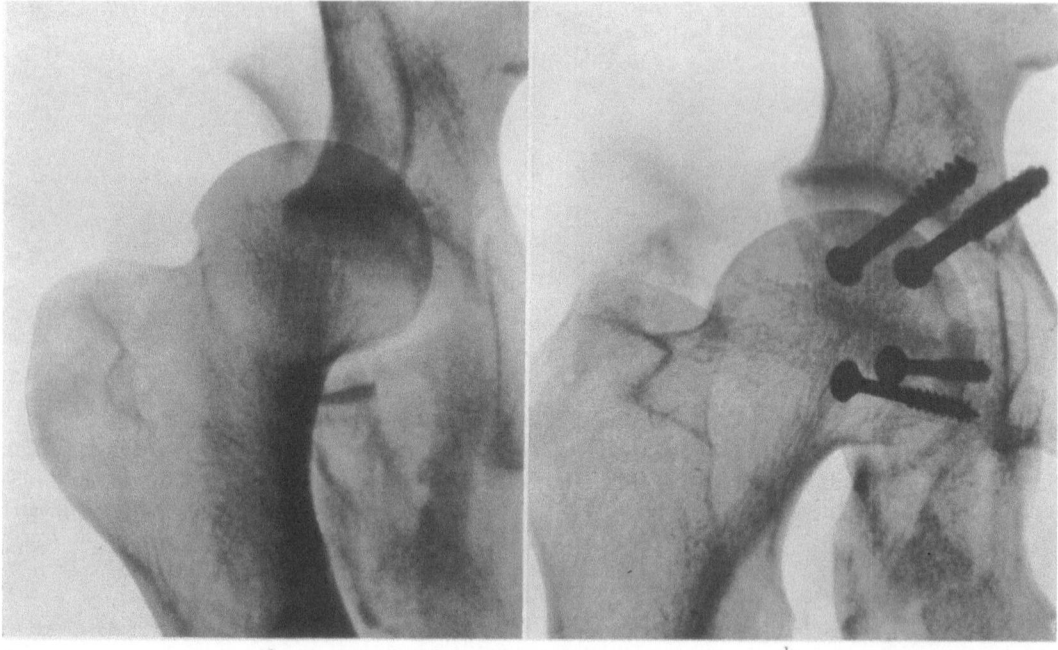

a   b

Fig. 223a and b. Fracture dislocation two weeks old with depression of the floor of the acetabulum. After reduction, internal fixation of the acetabular fragments with 4 screws. Active movements began at the second week and the patient was able to get out of bed at 4 weeks. a X-ray of the injury. b 1 month after reduction, healing with full movement

patients, the head of the femur is removed and replaced by a prosthesis. In these fractures the two important factors that vitiate results are *nonunion of the fracture and necrosis of the femoral head*.

Union of fractures of the neck of the femur can almost always be achieved by correct reduction, impaction and rigid fixation of the fracture, but the prognosis is always doubtful since the femoral head may collapse as a result of necrosis at any time up to ten years after the fracture. A good assessment of the value of this type of treatment therefore can be made usefully only at a five year review.

Necrosis of the femoral head depends on the state of the blood supply after internal fixation has been performed. The anatomy of the blood vessels of the femoral head has been known for 40 years and the more recent papers of JUDET and LAGRANGE (1955) have confirmed our knowledge in this respect. The three main vessels to the head of the femur are branches of the femoral circumflex artery. They run along the posterior surface of the neck of the femur in the synovial folds, and into the bone at the junction between the head and neck. On the anterior surface of the femoral neck runs a single artery coming from the ascending branch of the femoral circumflex artery leading to the neck only. There is therefore no anterior vascular supply to the head of the femur.

The incidence of necrosis of the head is increased if such arteries that have remained intact after the injury are destroyed by vigorous reduction maneuvers, or if a nail drives fragments of bone apart. With the hard cancellous bone that is present in the femoral heads of children and adolescents, the danger of distraction of the fracture by the nail seems especially great, and in fractures in this site we recommend the use of three or four

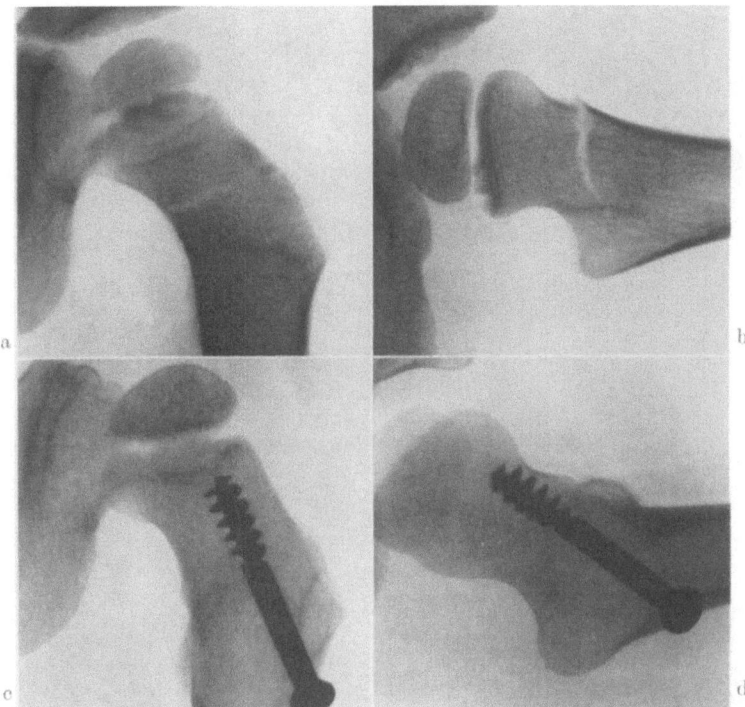

Fig. 224a—d. Basal fracture of the neck of the femur in a 7-year-old child. a and b After the accident. c and d 4 months after screwing. No necrosis of the head. Consolidation of the fracture

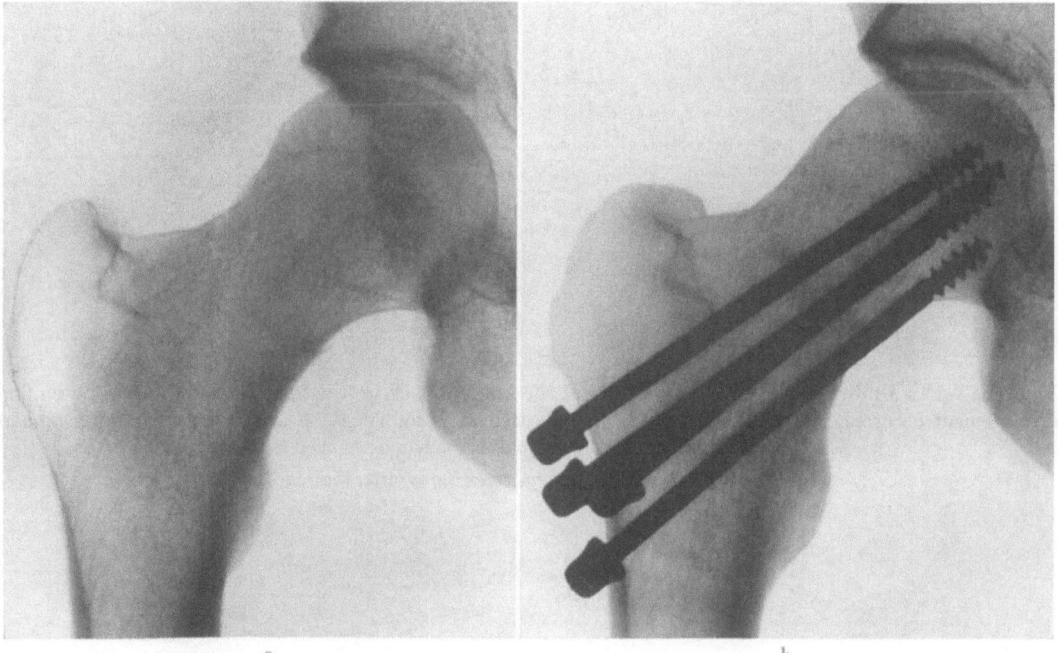

Fig. 225a and b. Screw fixation of a fatigue fracture of the femoral neck. a Before operation. b 6 months after operation

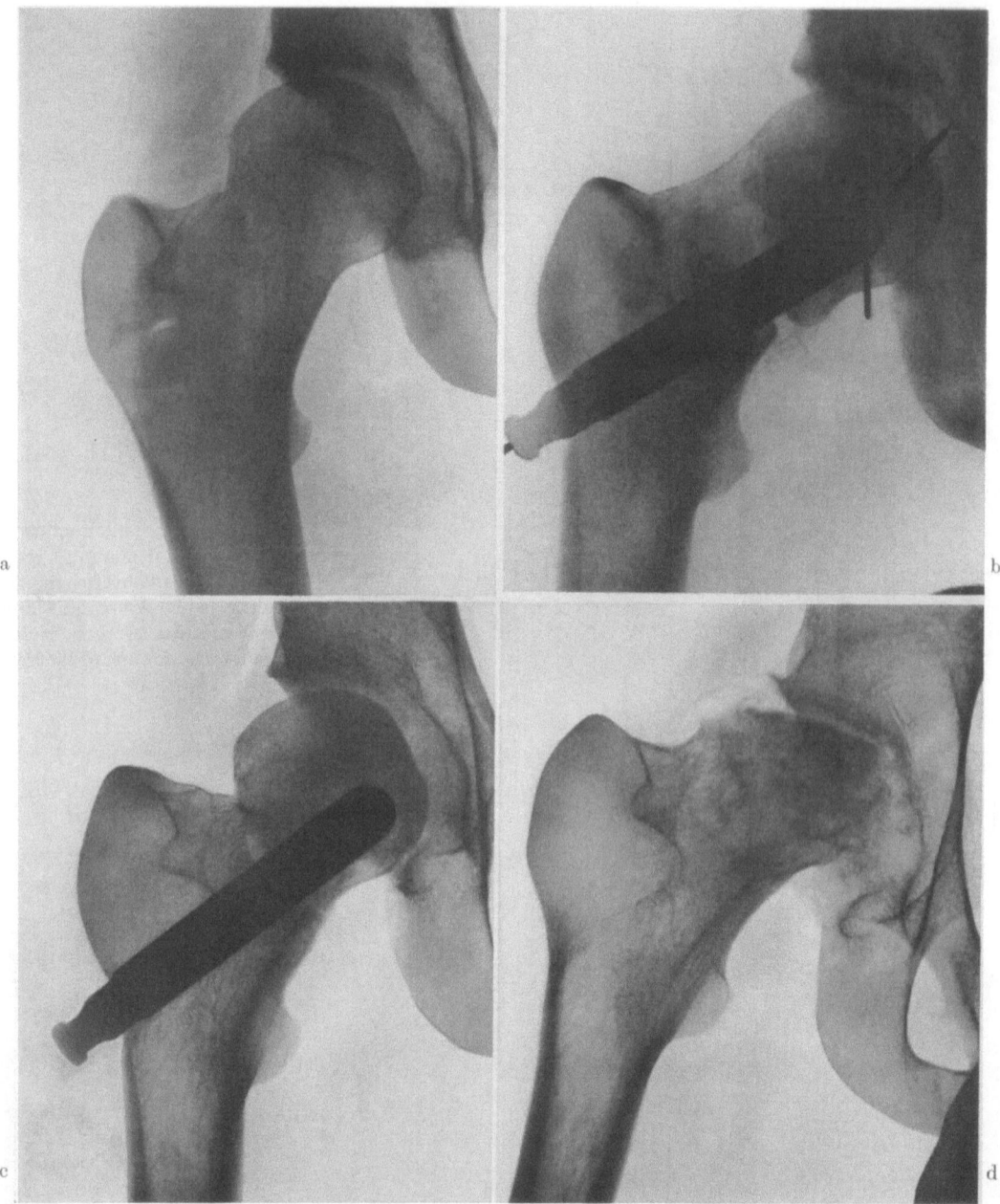

Fig. 226a—d. a Undisplaced subcapital fracture of the femoral neck in a patient aged 30. b During nailing displacement occurred. c At 6 months the result appeared satisfactory. d 2 years later the femoral head had collapsed and severe osteoarthritis had developed

In patients under 50 years of age screwing is better than nailing

long cancellous screws (Figs. 224—225). These screws need not be placed over the calcar femorale as is shown in Fig. 225b, but are better placed in the upper part of the neck since only in this position they can exert their maximal compressive force.

The necrosis of the head and nonunion do not have a causal connection, as could be shown by special x-rays (auto-radiographic studies). By means of auto-radiographs using P 32 we have been able to show in co-operation with BESSLER, that on the one hand pseudarthrosis of the femoral neck can occur with a necrotic or vascularized head of the femur, and on the other hand fracture union is possible even with a necrotic head. In one case (Fig. 227) revascularization extended 1 cm. beyond the fracture site. At the junction between dead and live bone, however, a comminuted area developed suggesting a pseudarthrosis, and in this case histology confirmed the radiological findings. M. E. MÜLLER's "Radio-ischiometer" has proved effective in the diagnosis of early aseptic necrosis of the femoral head (Fig. 229).

The rigidity obtained depends on the quality of reduction, the technique of internal fixation and the impaction of the fragments

In subcapital fractures correct alignment and impaction of the fragments, is needed rather than exact reduction. In adduction fractures of the femoral neck there are not only small separated fragments, especially in the dorsal part, but the cancellous bone which is porotic in elderly patients is impacted as in fractures of the lower end of the radius. If both cortices are placed in exact apposition, the head tilts off downwards and backwards (Fig. 230a). If the axis of the calcar is brought to lie above the lower cortex of the femoral head, an even worse displacement occurs and pseudarthrosis is almost unavoidable in spite of perfect nailing. A similar result occurs when the anterior surface of the neck of the femur is not applied to the femoral head (Fig. 230c).

Consequently, a reduction into a position of the femoral head with slight valgus and anteversion should be sought so that the extended calcar curve runs below the femoral head and an extension of the upper surface of the neck runs into it, when viewed in an axial x-ray (Fig. 230b). The valgus displacement must be slight or it may occlude any vessels supplying the head on the upper surface. Also it will throw an increased strain on the femoral head, the lever being shortened markedly by shifting the center of the femoral head closer to the gluteal muscles, therefore producing pain and later osteoarthritis.

Internal fixation with screws is useful only in young patients who have dense and well vascularized cancellous bone here. In older patients with porotic bones, the threads of the screws can destroy the few remaining vessels without giving good support to the fracture. After some unhappy experience with individual screws (after PUTTI and REIMERS) and with four-quadrant screws in older people, we have abandoned this technique and reverted to nailing. Many different nails have been developed since SWEN JOHANNSON, SMITH-PETERSEN, 1937, and BÖHLER, 1957. The most rigid nail is without doubt the one developed by LAING (1961) of H-section, but it is so large as to jeopardize the nutrition of the femoral neck and is also very difficult to introduce. The U-section nail we have chosen allows the femoral neck to be gripped and held, as though by a fork, in its caudal part, and the strength of the U-blade-plate is almost equal to that of a nail with H-section.

Before driving the nail, its track is cut with a special chisel which is introduced near to the fracture line and gives a powerful leverage on the distal fragment. The nail is driven in until its tip ends up about 0.5 mm. from the surface of the head and *the fragments are impacted* to accelerate the healing of the fracture (BÖHLER, 1957). The amount of impaction needs to be skilfully judged, and in elderly patients 1—1^1/$_2$ cm. must be allowed when choosing the nail of right length. Impaction is done with the help of a slotted hammer placed between the lowest point of the greater tuberosity and the point of entrance of the nail. The end of this hammer is then struck with another one.

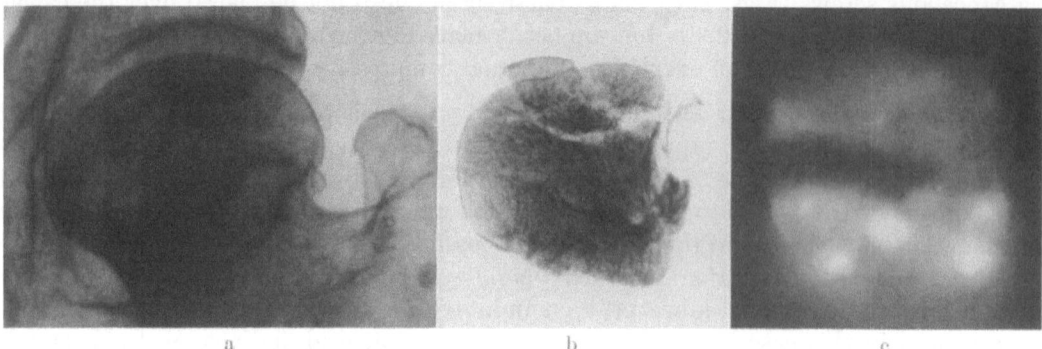

Fig. 227a—c. Necrosis of the femoral head two years after an impacted abduction fracture. a X-ray before operation. b X-ray of the resected head of the femur: There is infraction and fragmentation of the weight bearing parts. c Auto-radiogram shows significant radioactivity for 1 cm. above the ossified fracture, but no activity in the middle of the head. Infiltration of the collapsed bony parts with radioactive synovial fluid
(after BESSLER and MÜLLER)

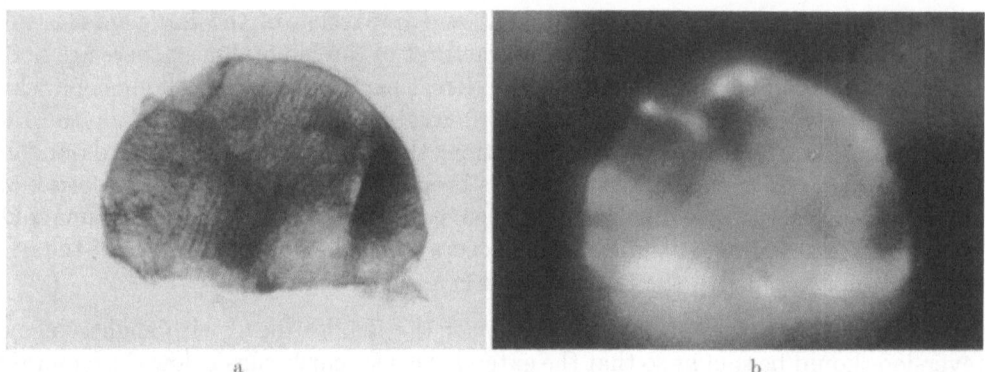

Fig. 228a and b. 6 months old nonunion of the femoral neck. a X-ray photograph. b Auto-radiogram of femoral head. Sclerosis of the upper and outer part of the head above the nail canal. Elsewhere an osteoporotic cancellous structure. Much radioactive material in the whole femoral head. Slightly less radioactivity around the fovea capitis and in the upper and outer quadrant

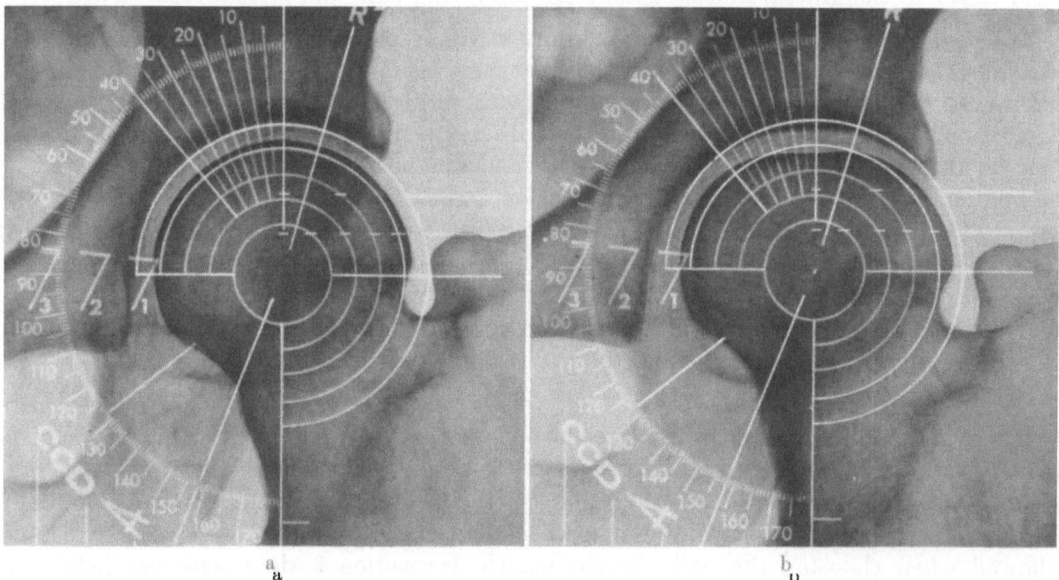

Fig. 229a and b. a Normal circular contour of the femoral head. b Early collapse with slight loss of the circular structure. Diagnosis with "Roentgenischiometer" (BESSLER and MÜLLER)

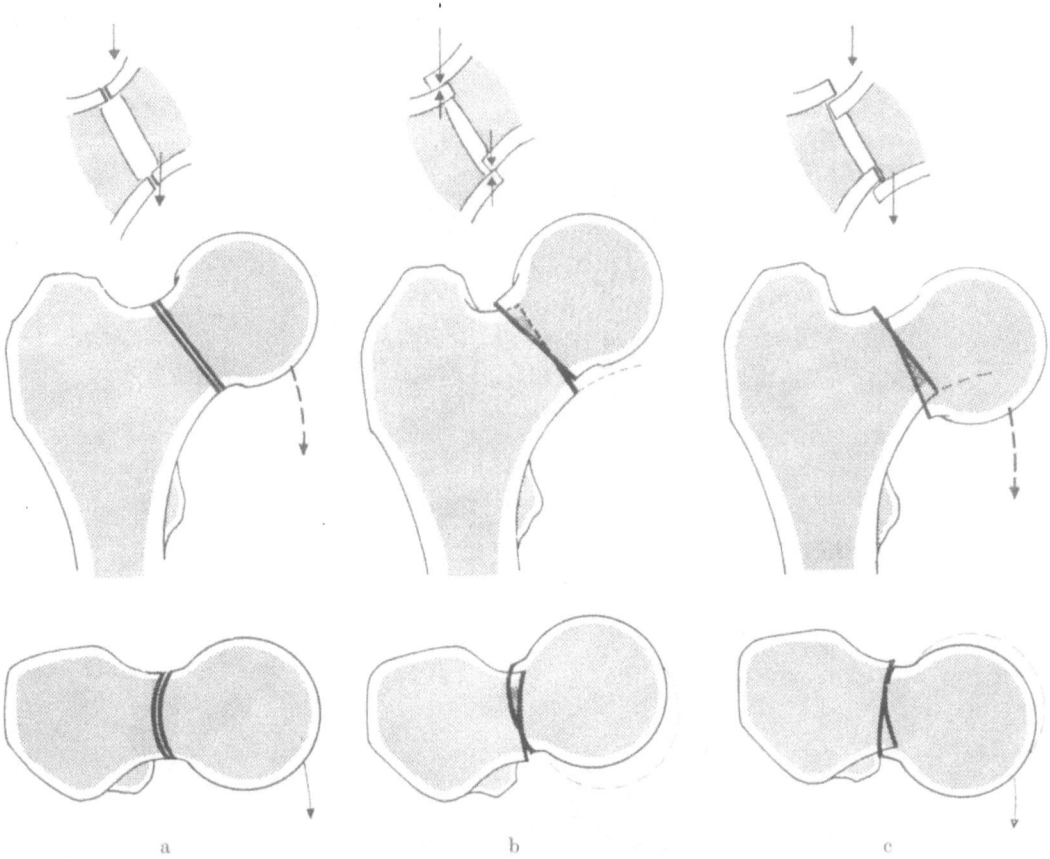

Fig. 230a—c. In elderly patients instability must be expected in an adduction subcapital fracture, depending on the reduction and the softness of the cancellous bone (comparison with 2 overlapping wooden frames after McElvenny). a With exact reduction there is a tendency towards tilting, since the cortex is firm but the cancellous bone is soft. b Ideal reduction in slight valgus. Extension of the lower part of the femoral neck passes below the head of the femur. In an axial view there is slight over-correction of internal rotation. c Inadequate reduction in both directions. Later slipping cannot be prevented by internal fixation

In femoral neck fractures we advocate *open reduction under direct vision*. Using the small curved Hohmann retractor the soft tissues can be pushed aside and the tip of the instrument brought to lie over the anterior acetabular margin which gives a good view of the fracture. The retractor should never be placed inside the joint as the articular cartilage would be damaged, nor should it be placed too deeply on either side of the femoral neck (Fig. 231 b).

The vessels supplying the femoral neck are not injured by the advocated approach, and reduction under direct vision preserves the soft tissues. In practised hands this approach is successful as a rule at the first attempt. X-rays are taken, although the accuracy of reduction and any possible distraction during nailing can be observed directly. Postoperative complications are unusual, and we feel that open reduction using an ordinary table without a pelvic support allows a shorter operating time and is therefore less traumatizing than the difficult procedure of blind nailing. The x-ray control of blind nailing procedures is always somewhat uncertain and a surgical assessment of an apparently good blind reduction may show that the femoral head may be rotated 30° or more about

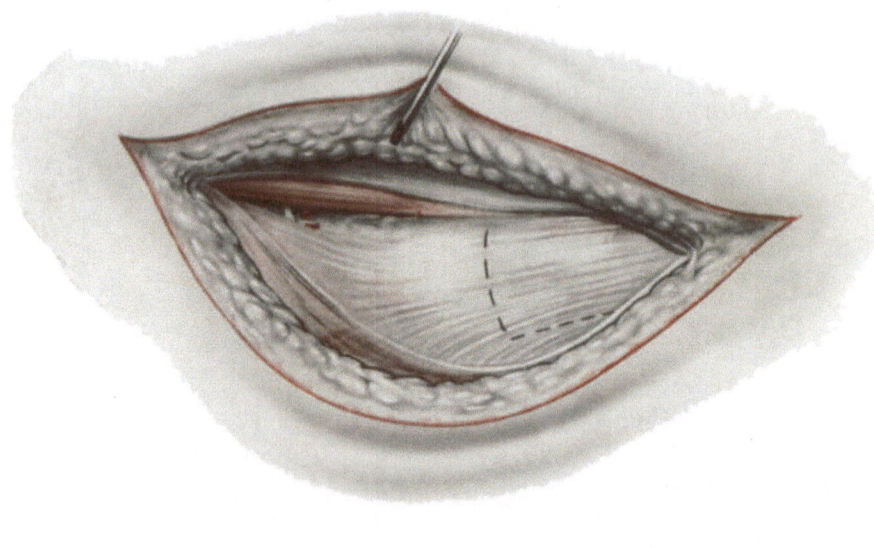

a

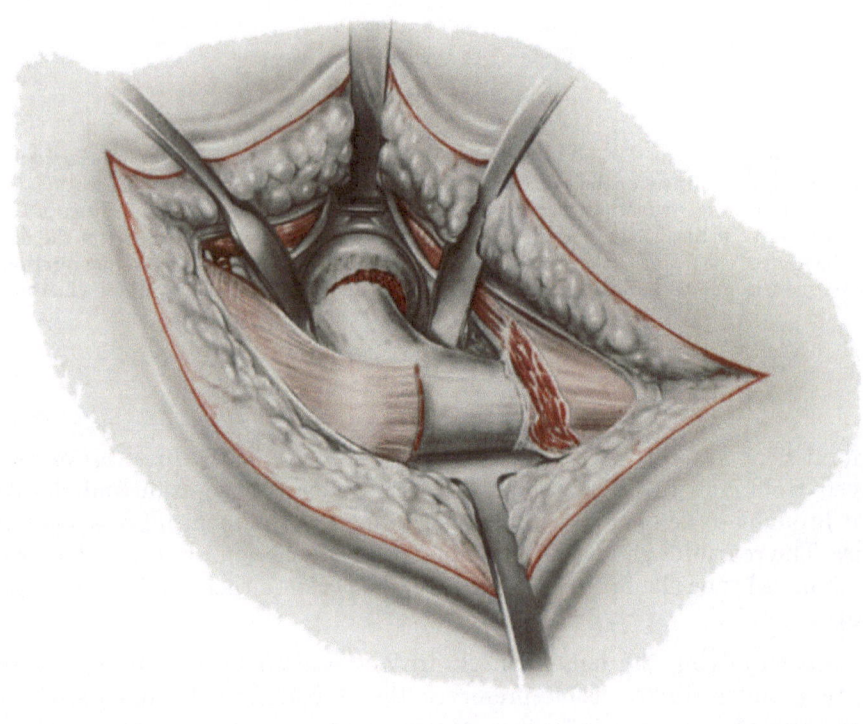

b

Fig. 231a and b. Technique of open reduction of subcapital fractures of the femoral neck. a After a curved incision through the skin and fascia above the greater trochanter, the proximal insertion of the vastus lateralis is incised in the shape of an L and retracted. Dissection proceeds between the glutei and tensor fasciae femoris. b After longitudinal incision of the capsule and retraction of its outer incision, 4 Hohmann levers are inserted; the uppermost is the most important, its tip being engaged with the anterior border of the acetabulum its own axis. It should not be forgotten that a fracture of the femoral neck, with a distal spur which gives the best prognosis as far as avascular necrosis is concerned, can be accurately reduced only under direct vision. The hard spike on the distal fragment is usually so well embedded into the cancellous bone that only a strong pull on the femoral neck with a bone hook placed over the lesser trochanter, while adducting and externally rotating the leg, can free it. If this fracture is carefully reduced (MÜLLER, 1957) a good result can be expected since the vessels supplying the femoral head are undamaged.

Timing of the Operation

Surgery should be undertaken after a thorough examination of the patient on the day of the accident, if possible. Although most patients are in poor condition, delay and the so-called "building up preparation", is shown by experience to increase the risk of the operation (JUDET, 1952) especially in elderly patients, and the motto "motion is life, life is motion" is applicable. As soon as these patients can move their legs without pain it is surprising how quickly they recover. The danger of irreversible necrosis of the femoral head also increases with every day that passes. We therefore aim to establish reduction of the fracture so as to allow the circulation of the femoral neck to join that of the femoral head within the first eight days.

Technique

Open reduction and internal fixation of fractures of the femoral neck, is shown in Fig. 231. The patient lies on his back on an ordinary operating table with an x-ray cassette under the buttocks. A curved incision of between 15 and 20 cm. begins midway between the anterior superior iliac spine and the tip of the greater trochanter. It runs over the greater trochanter and 8 to 10 cm. in the line of the femoral shaft, the fascia being incised in the line of the skin incision from below upwards. Between the muscles of the upper and lower thigh a small pad of fatty tissue is found on the anterior surface of the inter-trochanteric line; from this point the blunt dissection proceeds towards the anterior superior spine between the tensor fasciae latal and the glutei down to the anterior surface of the capsule. In the course of this dissection two blood vessels run into the tensor fasciae latae. The blood vessels are divided, but not the nerve to this muscles. The origin of vastus lateralis is freed and the posterior edge of this muscle is identified and detached for a distance of 8 to 10 cm. after division of the vastus lateralis at the level of the lower border of the greater trochanter on to the capsule.

With a raspatory the muscles are elevated towards the medial side until the whole anterior surface of the region of the greater trochanter is exposed. The capsule is now opened longitudinally from the femoral neck to the margin of the acetabulum. A stay suture is inserted into each capsular flap and a curved bone lever can now be introduced between the femoral neck and the lesser trochanter. A second retractor is slid in on the upper surface of the femoral neck just medial to the great trochanter and a third lever with a long narrow end can be passed medially along the femoral neck under the capsule until its tip hooks over the margin of the acetabulum. The fracture can then be well seen and it is only rarely that any further incisions are needed. Any collapse of the neck or head of the femur, together with any loose fragments of bone on the anterior surface can now be observed.

The track for the blade can now be cut, starting 3 cm. distal to the lower edge of the great trochanter with the aid of the 4.5 mm. drill and the cannulated chisel, which is driven in until its tip almost reaches the fracture site.

After determining the position of the head of the femur, reduction is carried out under direct vision. If the head is rotated relative to the neck, the fracture can be reduced only after correcting the rotation with an elevator while lateral traction is exerted, using a bone hook against the calcar. The muscle should be fully relaxed with the help of muscle

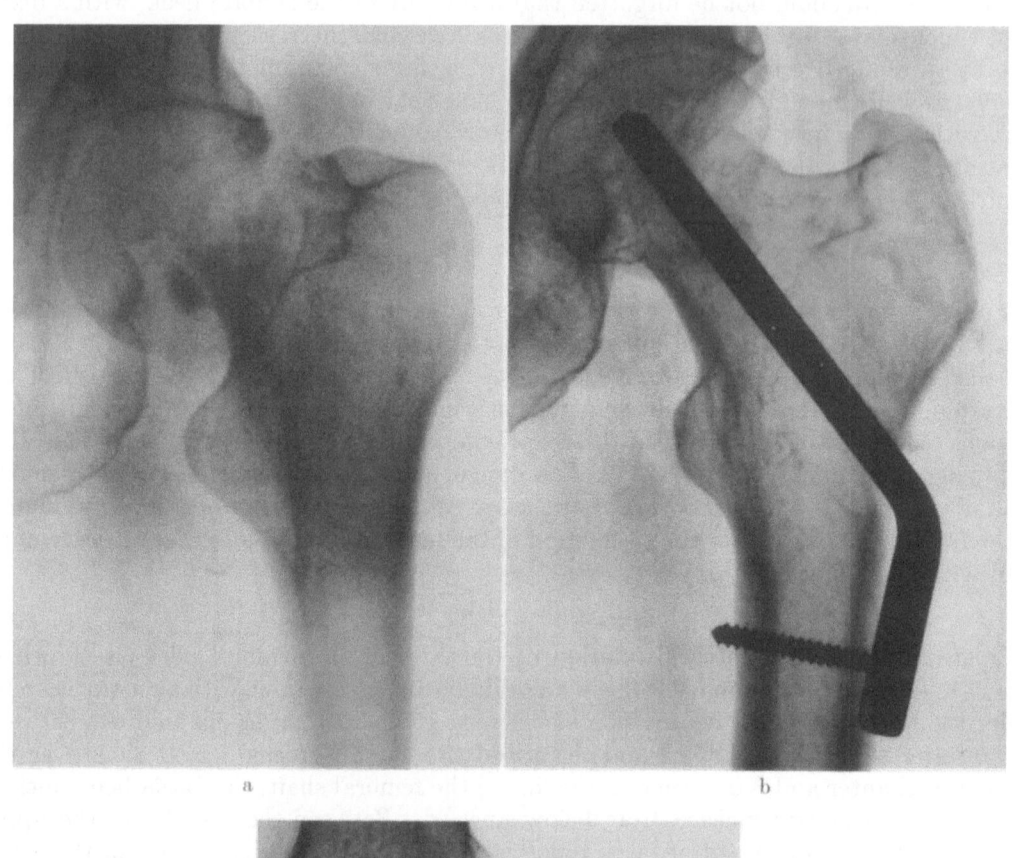

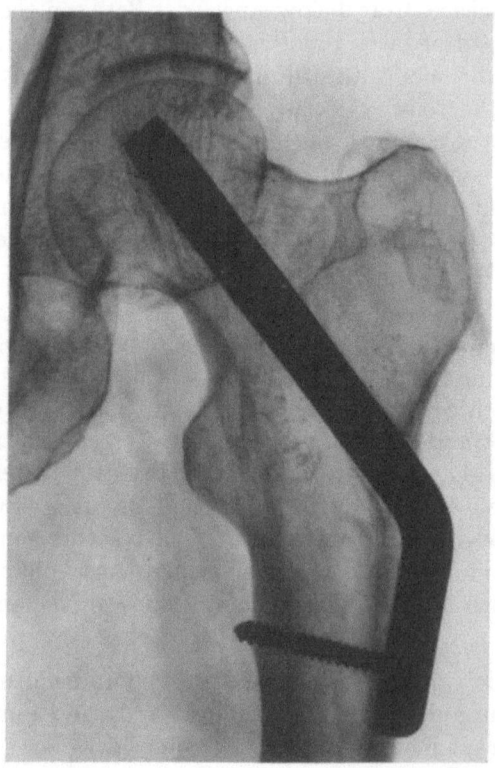

Fig. 232a—c. Subcapital fracture in a patient of 68. a After the accident. b 4 months after open nailing.
c 1 year later

relaxing drugs, allowing strong extension, adduction and external rotation. As soon as the fragments are disimpacted they are aligned in their correct relationship, and the leg is then brought into full abduction and internal rotation. Extension can now be discontinued. Two KIRSCHNER wires are introduced to hold the femoral head, and while the leg ist slowly externally rotated, the security of the reduction can be observed with special attention to the caudal and anterior aspects. If all seems well, the special cannulated chisel is driven in further, through the fracture site. At this point, if there is any doubt about the quality of the reduction, radiographs are taken in two planes.

In estimating the right length of the blade-plate, the distance is first measured between the entry point on the shaft of the femur and the fracture line. $2^1/_2$ to $3^1/_2$ cm. are added to this length according to the diameter of the head. The special chisel is now withdrawn and the selected blade-plate inserted, after which the fracture is impacted, using the slotted hammer as described above.

X-rays are now taken in an antero-posterior and lateral view with the thigh flexed at 90° and abducted to 30°. The lower leg is flexed at right angles and lies parallel to the table. The x-rays are interpreted according to the principles shown in Fig. 230a, b and c. If the blade-plate is well seated, the plate is screwed to the shaft of the femur after the fracture has been impacted again. The wound is closed in layers and two Redon drains are inserted. The gluteus medius and the vastus lateralis are repaired and the skin closed with nylon sutures.

Postoperative Management

The patient is nursed with the leg in a foam rubber splint in slight internal rotation and abduction with the foot elevated about 20 cm. and the knee slightly flexed. After twenty-four hours knee and foot exercises are begun; breathing exercises, especially in elderly patients, are instituted from the first day. At 48 hours the drains are removed, and anti-coagulants are started on the fourth day. The patient can put his legs over the side of the bed on the sixth day and between ten days and two weeks walking is allowed without weight bearing on the affected side. If an x-ray at four months is satisfactory, weight bearing can be allowed, but each case must be judged on its merits. Early ambulation after internal fixation of a subcapital fracture is advocated, but always without weight bearing.

As very old patients cannot always tolerate a long period of non-weight bearing, necrosis of the femoral head has to be expected in over 35% of the cases. A prosthesis often has to be inserted when necrosis of the head of the femur occurs or a pseudarthrosis develops. We thus have adopted a policy of replacement of the femoral head primarily with a

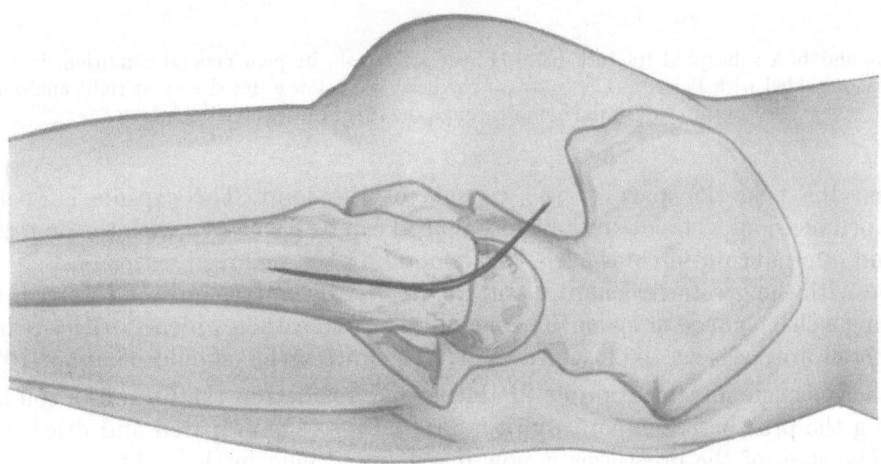

Fig. 233. Skin incision for the insertion of a MOORE's prosthesis with the patient lying on his side

prosthesis of the MOORE, THOMPSON or EICHER model in patients who are over 75 years of age or in poor general health. This allows them to get out of bed after the seventh day as a rule. Recently, improved fixation of the prosthesis has been affected by using polymerized methylmetacrylate as a cement (CHARNLEY).

It is important with these prostheses that enough bone is removed to allow the tip of the greater trochanter to lie slightly above the middle of the prosthetic head (Fig. 234b), as any greater length of neck will unduly stretch the muscles in the region, producing premature wear of the articular cartilage of the acetabulum at the point of greater pressure, and osteoarthritis will supervene.

Technique of Insertion of a Moore or Thompson Prosthesis

The patient is placed lying on his side and the skin incision begins from a point midway between the posterior iliac spine and the tip of the greater trochanter, curving down to a point a hand's breadth below the greater trochanter. The fascia is incised and the muscle fibres of the gluteus maximus are separated. The external rotators are divided,

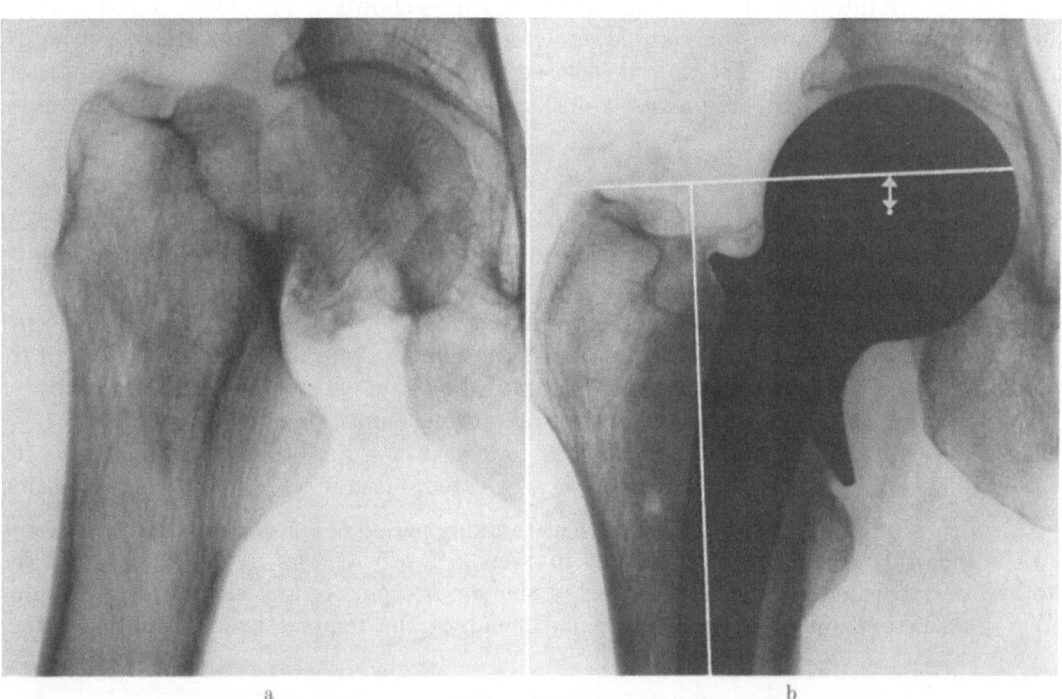

a   b

Fig. 234a and b. A subcapital fracture in a 71-year-old female in poor general condition. b A THOMPSON prosthesis embedded with Palacos. The centre of the head lies below a line drawn at right angles to the axis of the shaft of the femur through the tip of the greater trochanter

revealing the posterior part of the capsule of the joint. The capsule is opened with a T-shaped incision, whereupon the femoral head can be dislocated with the help of a broad lever and internal rotation of the leg. The femoral neck is removed with an osteotome at its junction with the greater trochanter and the lesser trochanter, and the former is hollowed out, using a sharp gauge or spoon. The medullary canal is then widened with a reamer until the selected prothesis can be inserted easily. The antetorsion should be about 10°.

The acrylic cement, for example "Palacos", is prepared in the form of a roll and after removing the prosthesis temporarily, it is pressed into the prepared and dried medullary canal. The stem of the prosthesis is now inserted and held in the right position until the cement has set. Any excess methylmetacrylate is removed while it is still soft. The prosthetic head is then replaced in the acetabulum by extension and external rotation, after which the capsule is closed and two fine polythene drains inserted. The wound is closed and the limb placed in a foam rubber splint.

3. Pertrochanteric Fractures

Internal fixation of these fractures makes it possible for the patient to sit up after five or six days and to get out of bed soon afterwards, and he can be discharged from the hospital after four or five weeks. Pertrochanteric fractures usually unite readily under conservative treatment. Recent statistics, however, show that the operative mortality is less than that with conservative treatment which involves prolonged immobilization. In cases treated by operation, decubitus ulcers, joint stiffness, dislocation and long periods of rehabilitation are almost unknown.

Internal fixation of a trochanteric fracture must be so rigid that the patients can get out of bed early. This may be difficult with porotic bones or comminuted fractures; sometimes the hollowed out femoral neck has to be filled with an acrylic preparation. Blade-plates with a fixed angle and the same U-section as those used for the femoral neck have proved effective.

Timing of the Operation

The operation should be done whenever possible on the same day, or at the latest on the day following the accident, but if for any reason a few days must elapse, skeletal traction is established with a KIRSCHNER wire inserted through the tibia two finger's breadths above the ankle joint.

X-ray and Reduction

To judge the length of the required plate, a film of the whole pelvis is taken before operation with the uninjured leg held in internal rotation.

As the cancellous bone is always impacted in trochanteric fractures, we aim to engage a spike of the calcar into the shaft, so that reduction alone will produce some rigidity (Fig. 235). If this spur is brought to lie medial to the shaft, the blade-plate will have to carry the whole weight of the body and metal fatigue may result in a fracture of the blade-plate.

Technique Used in Simple Pertrochanteric Fractures
(see also Page 61 and Fig. 77)

First, the point of entrance of the nail into the shaft is determined from the x-ray taken at the normal side with the selected plate superimposed. As a rule the operation is performed under general anesthesia, but in rare cases local anesthesia can be used. In these cases, the fracture site should also be infiltrated with the solution. An ordinary table or an orthopedic table may be used. Reduction can be held by extension, abduction and internal rotation. A 15 cm. skin incision is made in a straight line distally from the tip of the greater trochanter. Fascia is divided and the bone approached from behind the vastus lateralis retracting the muscles medialwards so that the whole intertrochanteric region can be exposed. The vastus lateralis is divided close to the major trochanter. A small bone lever is introduced over the femoral neck, medial to the tip of the greater trochanter and a broader retractor placed against the calcar femoralis to allow palpation of the lesser trochanter.

The reduction is examined by sight and the fragments impacted. If reduction is inadequate it should be improved with an elevator and a bone hook, but further manipulation may be needed using first extension with adduction and external rotation, and then abduction and internal rotation. The fracture is temporarily fixed with KIRSCHNER wires, using the triple drill guide. A guide wire, or a 3 mm. drill is introduced from the point below the greater trochanter, directing it along the anterior surface of the femoral neck towards the anterior edge of the head, not entering the neck of the femur and only slightly cranial to the calcar.

A hole is drilled in the femoral shaft through the triple drill guide with a 4.5 mm. drill, ca. 3 cm. below the narrow point of the great trochanter and widened with a router so that it will accept the blade. It is widened at its lower end to accommodate the plate in a curve so that the bone is not split when the implant is driven home. The special cannulated chisel is now driven in parallel with the guide wire 2—3 cm. beyond the fracture line and an x-ray is taken in the a. p. and lateral views with the hip flexed to 90° and abducted to 30°.

A plate of the correct angle with a blade of the right length is now introduced so that its tip comes to lie about 15 mm. from the surface of the femoral head and the plate is held to the femoral shaft with a clamp. With a 3.75 mm. drill a hole is made in the trochanter parallel to the plate for the cancellous lag screw which has 32 mm. of its length threaded. This screw should be between 7 and 9 cm. long. A check x-ray is taken in the same views as before.

Postoperative Management

Exercises for the quadriceps and foot are started on the first day. For the first four days the leg is rested in a position of slight internal rotation. After this the patient may sit on the edge of the bed and as soon as walking is comfortable he may be discharged.

Comminuted Trochanteric Fractures

Commonly, both trochanters are broken off. If the lesser trochanter can be easily reduced after reduction of the main fracture, it can be fixed with a cortex or cancellous screw, but is otherwise left alone. The detached greater trochanter may present a more difficult problem.

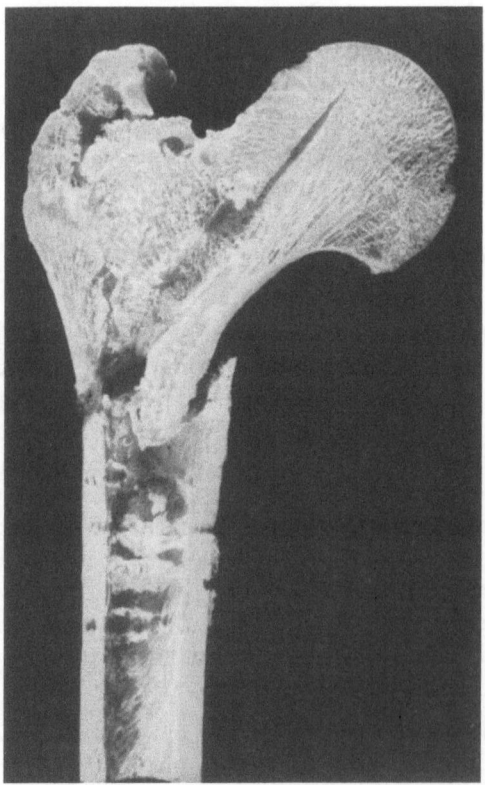

Fig. 235. Preparation to show the desired position with a spur of the calcar femorale engaging the shaft. If the shaft lies more laterally the fracture remains unstable in spite of nailing. With correct reduction, as in this case, the spur is impacted in the shaft and the angle of the femoral neck is maintained at 120—130°

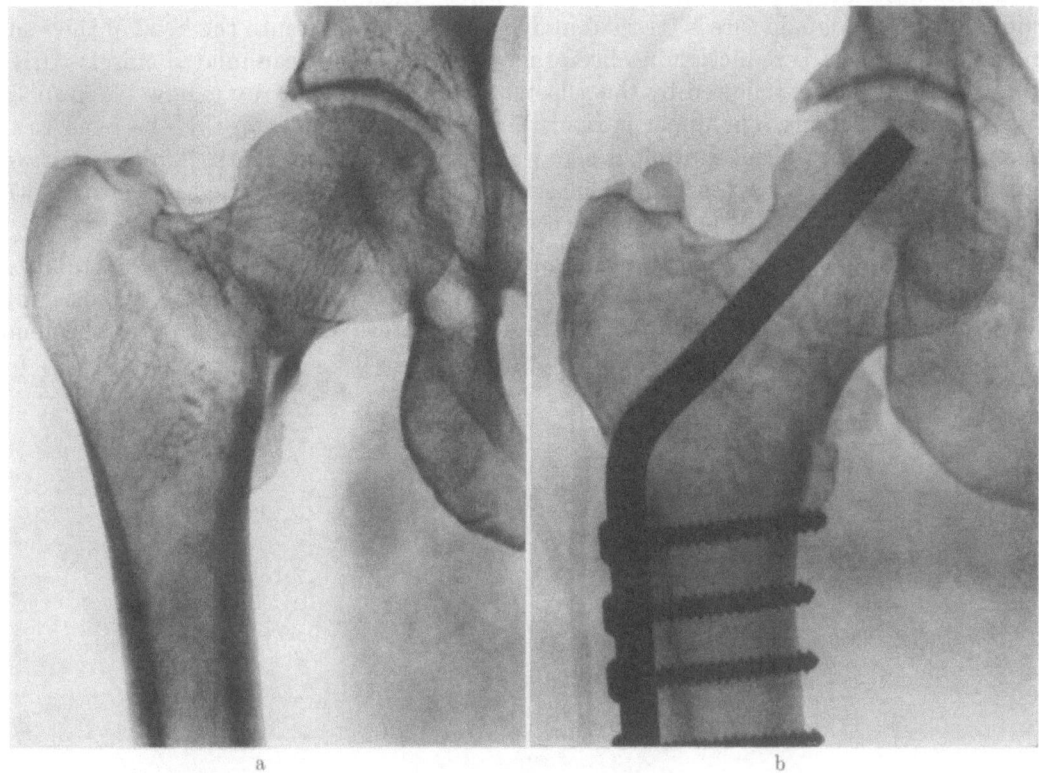

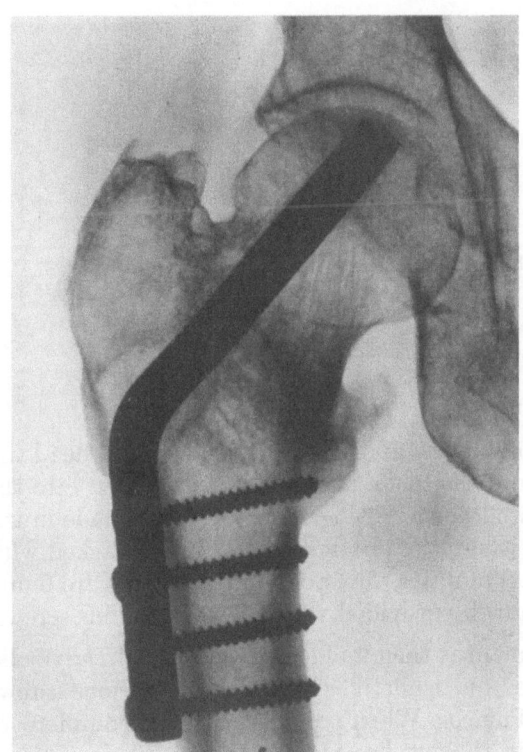

Fig. 236a—c. Pertrochanteric fracture held with only one nail, which was placed too high. a Before operation. b After internal fixation. c 1 year later.

The shaft was not medial, the spur was not impacted in the shaft, collapse of the fragments occurred with danger of the tip of the nail penetrating to the hip joint

To begin with, both main fragments are brought into alignment and the trochanter is fixed with a Steinman pin or thick Kirschner wires. Then, with the help of the triple drill guide, a Kirschner guide wire is inserted above the femoral neck into the head of the femur and an x-ray taken. If reduction has been successful the special cannulated chisel is driven in as described above, followed by the selected blade-plate. An x-ray is now taken in a. p. and lateral projections. The upper part of the shaft of the bone can then be fixed to the femoral neck with an 8 cm. cancellous screw and washer, and to the trochanter itself with one or two malleolar screws or cancellous screws. The plate is then fixed to the shaft with three or four screws and, if possible, one screw reaches the lesser trochanter.

If the bone is very porotic or the fracture so comminuted that it cannot be stabilized, it is advisable to fill the upper part of the medullary canal with acrylic, e. g. Palacos, after the femoral neck has been hollowed out and the plate fixed to the shaft of the femur (MÜLLER).

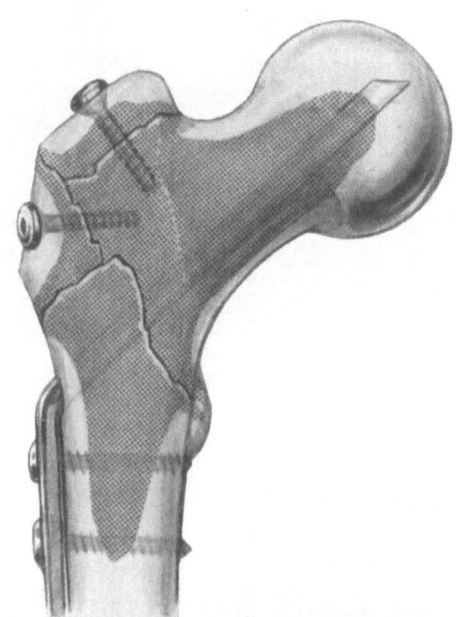

Fig. 237. Diagram to show a pertrochanteric fracture stabilised with the methylmetacrylate preparation "Palacos"

Technique

After exposure of the fracture the femoral neck and part of the femoral head are hollowed out. Reduction is then performed and the blade of the plate is inserted into the hollowed out femoral neck. The plate is screwed down. The space around the blade in the femoral neck and the upper end of the shaft where the proximal screw lies is packed with a first filling of acrylic cement. After about ten minutes the two main fragments are found to be stable. All secondary fragments must now be provided with short cancellous screws.

A second, smaller layer of fresh acrylic cement is then molded in over the already-solid first layer of polymerized methylmetacrylate, and while it is still soft the various screws in the smaller fragments are driven into the Palacos. When polymerization is complete all screws are found to have a solid anchorage in the acrylic (Fig. 237).

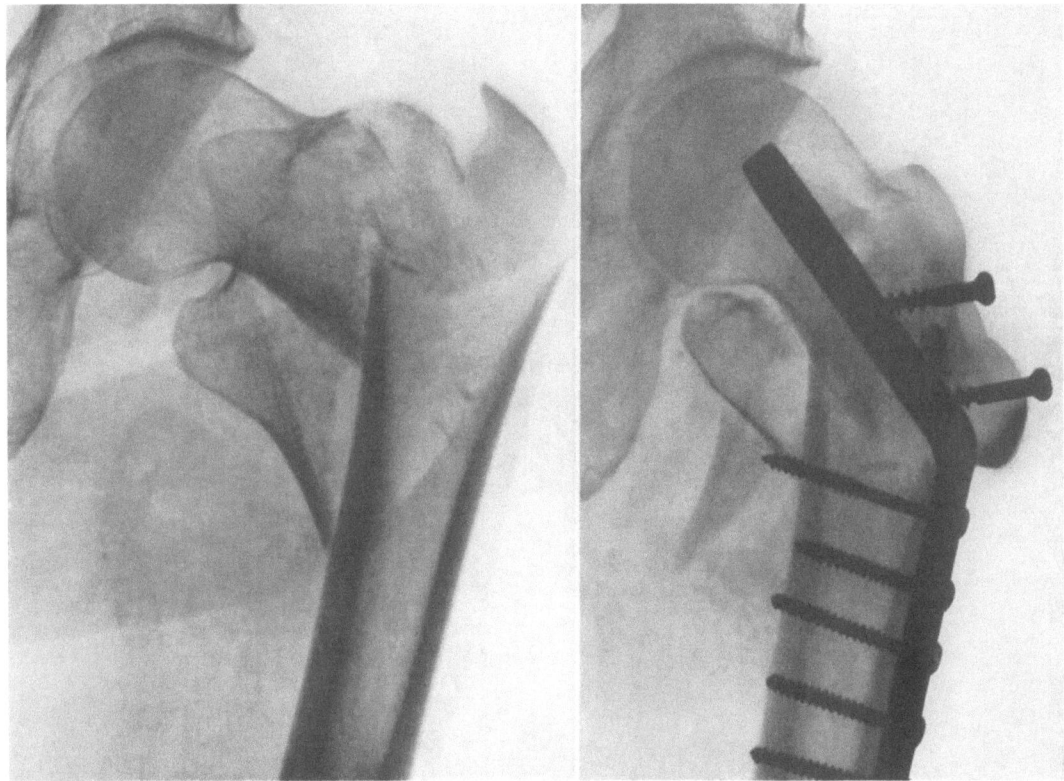

Fig. 238. Pertrochanteric fracture in a man of 74 with severe polyarthritis. Fixation of the main fragments with Palacos, blade-plate and screws. The patient was able to get out of bed on the 10th day

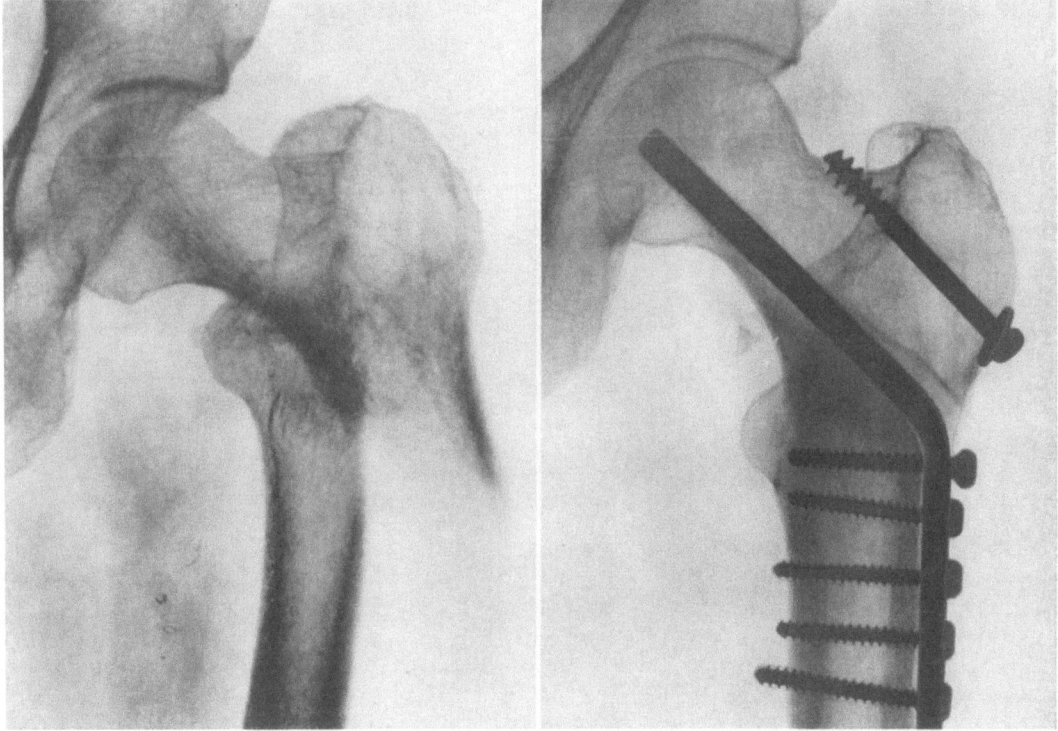

Fig. 239. Pertrochanteric and subtrochanteric fracture treated with a long blade-plate

Supplement

I. Internal Fixation of Compound Fractures

Even today the treatment of compound fractures is regarded as one of the least happy chapters in bone surgery.

For instance, ZOLLINGER (1951) reports in statistical records of the Swiss Accident Insurance Association (SUVA) that, in 1945, 60 compound leg fractures were reported to the Swiss Accident Insurance Companies. The mean period of treatment was 394 days and the average period of disability was 376 days. Compensation payments were made in 66% of all cases. Amputation was necessary in five cases, of which 2 were for late complications; 3 deaths following various operations were reported. But are today's results any better? We rather doubt it as almost every week infected pseudarthroses following compound fractures are admitted to our hospitals.

Primary or delayed internal fixation of compound fractures, as conservative treatment, produces good results only if certain *basic principles* are followed. Strict adherence to certain basic principles is more important than the pure technique of bone treatment. In evaluating the success of fracture treatment, the final functional result is a predominant factor. The occurrence of osteitis in a compound fracture represents the greatest danger and may lead to early failure in treatment. *Also in compound fractures, however, the goal of our efforts is to obtain the best possible functional end-result.*

Every compound fracture presents two problems: The wound treatment and the management of the fracture.

a) Wound Treatment

Careful bacteriological studies undertaken at the Mayo Clinic prove that in over 90% of infected compound fractures the bacteria recovered did not enter the wound at the time of the accident, but were hospital strains resistant to antibiotics.

For this reason we try to prevent the danger of added infection by avoiding any contact with the wound from the time the patient is first admitted. Any bandage applied before admission is removed only in the operating theatre by the surgeon himself; any undressed wound is immediately covered with sterile gauze and temporary bandages. The ambulance driver, orderly, nurse or houseman should never be allowed to inspect the wound, as more than 50% of the hospital staff are carriers of virulant bacteria.

It may be useful to remind the reader of a few well accepted facts. A soiled wound is not infected during the first few hours after its infliction; it is, at the worst, invaded by bacteria of varying pathogenicity. The bacteria which enter a wound can multiply only in favourable surroundings and this requires a latent period of between six and ten hours. POLICARD (1930) showed that liquefaction of devitalised tissue by leucocytic enzymes with a reduction of the large albumen molecules is required to allow bacterial multiplication. Therefore, if we excise the devitalised tissue as early as possible, we create the best conditions for undisturbed wound healing.

The *immediate débridement and excision of wound edges* are (since FRIEDRICH, 1898) the only forms of wound cleaning in which destroyed tissue is removed. As a rule, open soft tissue wounds are *extended in the long axis* of the limb and *fascial layers are split trans-versely*. Injured muscle which does not contract when pinched is excised, *nerves* and *arteries* are inspected and *foreign material* removed. To obtain a good view of fracture lines, the fragments may be angulated apart and possibly cleaned by brushing. Bone splinters that are quite free must be removed and may be washed and placed in a solution of penicillin. We usually re-insert them at the end of the operation because they are incorporated when bone reconstruction begins.

The operation may be lengthy, but must be performed carefully and good hemostasis achieved.

All antiseptics must be avoided, since, in the attempt to kill bacteria the local resistance of the host may also be destroyed. We do, however, use large quantities of physiological fluid and we prefer Ringer's solution to normal saline, as the former is more physiological, less toxic, and does not damage muscle. When devitalised tissue has been removed, there is always the question of *obtaining skin cover*. Substantial loss and necrosis of skin are usually followed by secondary infection which may extend to the bone. We must therefore *provide living tissue to cover the bone and also prevent any secondary necrosis*.

GOSSET (1959) emphasises two mechanisms that may lead to *skin necrosis*. First there is skin contusion without loss of dermis and without subcutaneous bleeding; secondly, contusion of the skin with loss of dermis and hematoma formation due to shearing effects. In the first group only the outer layer of skin is affected, leaving the deeper layers to provide protection for the bone. Here excision is unnecessary, but careful observation is required. As soon as the superficial necrotic layer separates, a split skin graft may be adequate.

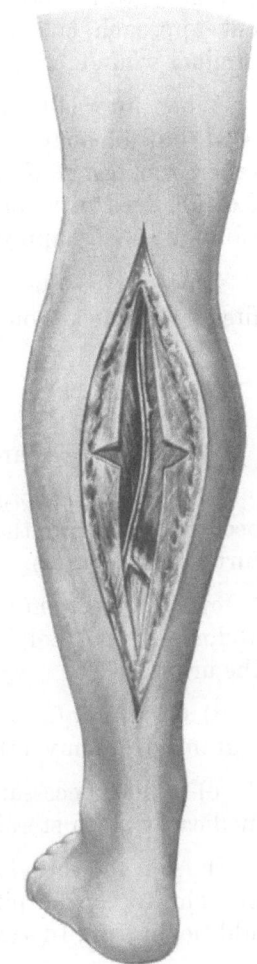

The second group occurs with more severe injuries. Here thorough excision of all contused or devitalised tissue is the best defense against secondary deep necrosis and should be followed by accurate skin closure without tension and with postoperative suction drainage.

As we have had some late necrosis in *primary flap grafts* and *other early pedicle procedures*, we no longer perform such operations as emergencies. We recommend, however, following PICOT, GOSSET (1959), and MERLE D'AUBIGNÉ (1959), that in all cases where skin cannot be closed without tension, a large relieving incision should be made on the opposite side, dividing skin and fascia (Fig. 240). This often allows primary skin closure, but if it is impossible we cover the wound with vaseline gauze, to be followed, as is the practice of MICHON and VILAIN (1959), by delayed pedicle grafts ten to fourteen days later.

b) Fracture Treatment

Almost all orthopaedic surgeons agree that *strict immobili-zation of the fractured bone is the first requirement*. The question, however, is whether this immobilization should be established by extension, plaster of paris cast, or internal fixation ? Widely varying views are held, and even today well known accident

Fig. 240. Tension relieving incision in the skin and fascia in the calf (after PICOT)

surgeons regard primary internal fixation of compound fractures as malpractice. Others are less emphatic and are willing *to perform internal fixation two to four weeks after the primary operation*, but only if the wound has healed by first intention. This solution has been recommended by KÜNTSCHER and others and seems sensible. Nevertheless, we feel that there is a grave danger of flare up of a latent infection after this procedure. Also the possible occurrence of thrombosis or embolism after immobilization for two weeks should not be underestimated.

The advocates of internal fixation cannot deny that the resistance of the tissues is greatly reduced in the region of the implanted material. In addition, internal fixation with wires, screws, plates or nails lessens the blood supply and the vitality of the bone and thus increases the danger of sequestra forming. The absolute stabilization of fragments by a rigid fixation on the other hand minimizes tissue necrosis, restores the original contour of the bone, limits postoperative immobilization to a few days, gives freedom from pain, shortens the period of treatment and saves time and money. In addition, the cosmetic and functional results are incomparably better than those achieved by conservative treatment.

It is therefore very tempting to complete the operation with internal fixation in every compound fracture. *Internal fixation of compound fractures, however, allows no imperfection.* Operation has to be performed during the first eight hours, all dead tissue must be carefully excised and the *metal implant* must never be covered by tissue of doubtful vitality. Internal fixation should not be regarded as the second part of the operation, but as a separate operation. After fresh exposure and towelling of the operation site, instruments are changed, gowns and gloves are changed and the skin is prepared anew. If possible, a different approach is employed for the internal fixation procedure at a distance from the original wound.

When internally fixing compound fractures, *a minimum of foreign material* should be used, but adequate rigidity must be obtained to allow early mobilization. Care must be taken, too, *that all the metal is covered by living tissue*. In general, the techniques for internal fixation used with compound fractures correspond with those used for simple ones. In the tibia we usually apply a single compression plate on the lateral side (Fig. 241).

Procedures to be adopted for the internal fixation of fresh compound fractures in the first ten hours are outlined in the following:

1. On Admission

a) *Open wounds* are immediately covered with a sterile dressing.

b) A careful *history* is taken and recorded, including how, when and where the accident occurred (the time that has elapsed since the accident, and the type of wound determine further procedures).

c) *General examination.* Determine whether there are other injuries, especially of the abdomen, spine, pelvis, neck of femur, forearm, shoulder or of vessels and nerves. Examine the urine.

d) Give an *infusion of saline and dextrose* with antibiotics (penicillin 20 mega units and 1 gram Streptomycin) if there is no contraindication.

e) Where necessary, *treat shock* with plasma or with whole blood transfusions. For medication with steroids, arterenol, etc. see chapter on Shock (Page 248).

f) An *x-ray examination* is made with the patient still on the splint in which he was brought to the hospital. These films should be taken without causing the patient any additional pain. In severe accident cases x-rays of the pelvis and skull are always required.

g) The patient is undressed and prepared for operation.

h) In the *operating theatre* the wound is inspected after the patient has been anaesthetized. Only then is the first-aid dressing removed and the wound inspected, this under strict aseptic conditions by the surgeon. Gloves and masks are worn for this examination. A color photograph may be taken at this point to record local findings.

2. Preparation for Operation

Anaesthesia has been induced and in appropriate cases a pneumatic tourniquet applied. The wound is covered with a sterile pad and the skin washed with benzine and ether. A local disinfectant such as "Merfen" may be used and the area shaved with a sterile safety or open razor. The wound is now treated with a suitable antiseptic by the surgeon, avoiding touching any protruding bone fragments. The wound is irrigated with Ringer's solution and a thorough mechanical cleaning carried out. After the wound edges have been disinfected again and a pneumatic tourniquet applied in Trendelenburg position, an adhesive is painted on and a layer of plastic sheeting applied.

3. Operation

a) Wound Treatment

Irrigation is continued and suction used to wash out all pockets in the wound, using large quantities of Ringer's solution.

With stab wounds and internally caused wound and cuts, only limited excision of the wound edge is needed. Any protruding bone fragments may be rinsed with ether and then with Ringer's solution. The bone is then managed as in a closed fracture.

In contused cases a sparing excision of the wound edges is carried out and the wound is enlarged by incisions in the long axis of the limb, so as to get good exposure.

The wound is carefully examined layer by layer, with detailed removal of all dead tissue and longitudinal or transverse incisions made in the fascia. Foreign bodies are removed by irrigation with Ringer's solution and by suction. Loose bone splinters are removed, washed with ether and Ringer's solution and placed in a penicillin solution containing 100000 units per 10 ml. The limb is angulated at the level of the fracture so that the bone ends may be inspected and, if necessary, cleaned up. Sometimes in cancellous areas the bone may need to be freshened with an osteotome.

Torn ligaments and nerves are repaired with the finest catgut only, then after the removal of the tourniquet, vessels are ligated using a minimum of suture material.

b) Treatment of the Fracture

Except when there are very dirty bone splinters that cannot be cleaned up, which occurs rarely, *a primary rigid internal fixation is desirable.*

Internal fixation should be regarded as a separate operation after the wound has been treated; new instruments, gowns and gloves are used. After the tourniquet has been removed, the skin is prepared anew and covered with an adhesive and plastic sheeting.

Ideally the incision is made as far as possible from the primary wound, but in some cases extension of the original wound may be more adequate.

As with closed fractures, internal fixation is achieved using *screws, compression plates, Küntscher nails, etc.*

The use of a compression plate is often indicated in compound fractures of the tibia, as the periosteal circulation is usually so doubtful in these fractures that the intramedullary blood supply should be preserved as far as possible. All metal implants should, how-ever, be covered by well vascularized tissue, which in the lower leg is best guaranteed on the lateral side of the tibia.

Internal fixation is only rigid when no fracture interval remains and we therefore replace *every* bone fragment. Completely loose fragments, however, are only re-inserted into existing defects after they have been washed with ether and Ringer's solution and have been placed in a penicillin solution for more than five minutes (Fig. 241).

c) Primary Wound Closure

This is desirable and a large posterior tension relieving incision in the middle of the calf (PICOT) is often effective in allowing the skin to be sutured without tension (Fig. 240).

It is especially important to avoid tension when there has been contusion of the sub-cutaneous tissue, but if closure without tension is impossible the wound is covered with a non-adhesive bandage for fourteen days (Biogauze, for instance), after which a flap graft may be brought in. Primary grafts are not always successful. Cross-leg flaps are often needed when there is much soft tissue loss. The wound is drained with two or three Redon drains. Only when the wound is severely soiled should a local continuous infusion of anti-biotics, as in osteitis, be instituted.

4. Postoperative Treatment

Compression is applied with foam rubber and elastic bandages. A single back slab or double gutter plaster splint is applied to the foot in contrast to the treatment of closed fractures.

The leg is kept well elevated (over 40 cms.).

Antibiotics. Penicillin is given for five days by intravenous drip at the rate of 20 to 40 mega units a day and 1 gram Streptomycin a day, after which local examination will indicate whether further antibiotics are needed. If a patient is still febrile after three or four days, we start giving Chloramphenicol.

In general, active movements of muscles and joints are begun three days after the anti-biotics have been discontinued.

5. Tetanus Prophylaxis

There is considerable doubt about ATS in the prophylaxis against tetanus, and when a wound is thought to be prone to this infection it is recommended that penicillin be given in full doses for at least 5 days, as all strains of Clostridia have proved up to date to be sensitive to this antibiotic. At the same time active immunization using Tetanus Toxoid should be begun since this drug is both safe and effective, and when the third dose has been given the patient will be safe from tetanus for five years. This will be long enough to cover any further operative procedures for this injury, besides protecting the patient against tetanus developing from further traumata. We have abandoned the use of ATS without ill effects, but we realize that there is not yet complete agreement about the inefficiency of this drug.

Summary

The danger of infection is the chief consideration in the management of compound fractures. The prevention of secondary infection by resistant strains of hospital organisms

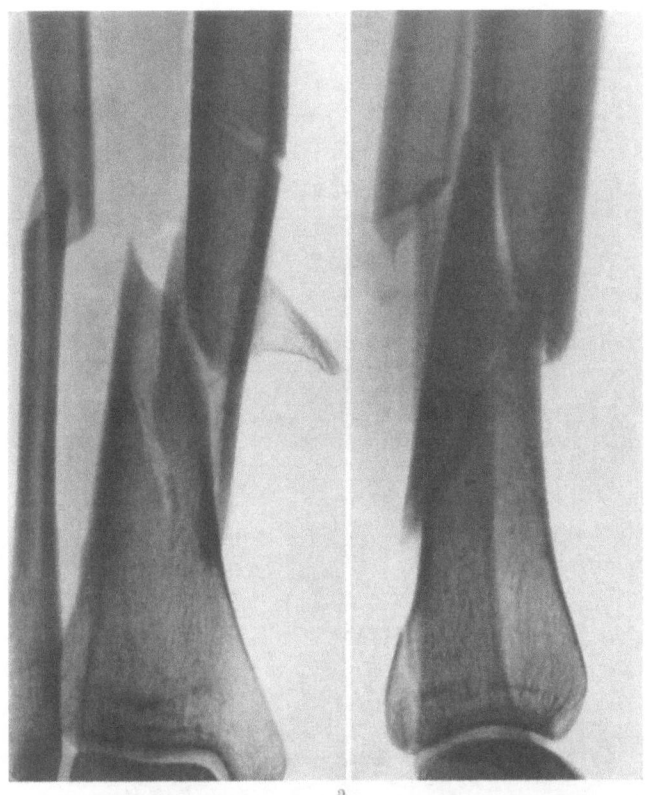

Fig. 241 a—c. a Compound fracture of the tibia with a fourth fragment projecting from the wound. b The avascular fragment was attached to the tap by a hole drilled in its middle and before the plate was tightened it was fitted precisely in its place. Internal fixation with a plate and 2 independent screws. c At 4 months the fracture was stable without osteoporosis. Even the small fragment had become completely incorporated into the bone
Separate fragments, wherever possible, are replaced exactly and compressed

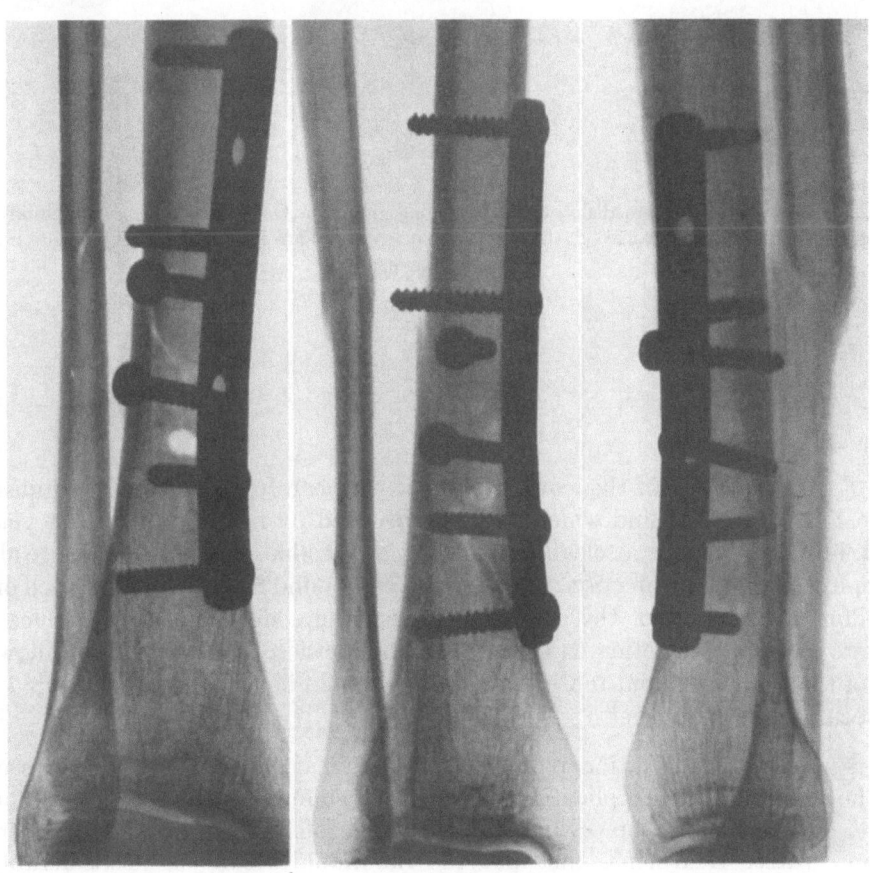

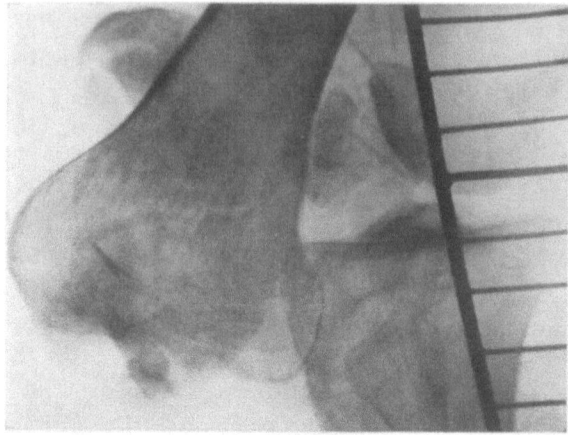

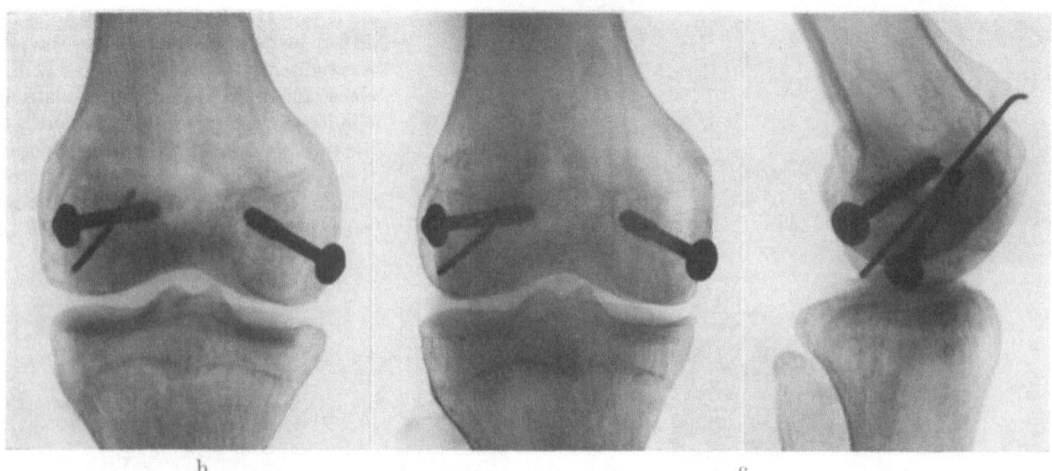

Fig. 242a—c. Compound fracture dislocation of the knee joint. a On admission. b After internal fixation with two screws and a Kirschner wire. c At 8 months. The condyles are stable, the knee joint has regained 110° of flexion

is vital. Early inspection of the wound together with careful excision of devitalised tissue, can transform a dirty wound which has been invaded by bacteria but is not yet actually infected, into one which is as clean and healthy as possible. These measures are always the best prophylaxis against infection. Converting a compound fracture into a closed one should not be done irrespective of the cost, since skin closure under tension produces necrosis and severe secondary infection. If a long relieving incision (PICOT) does not allow primary closure of the wound without tension, the defect should be left open and covered by grafts at between one and two weeks.

Emergency internal fixation performed under ideal conditions does not seem to increase the danger of the complications to which all compound fractures are prone. On the contrary, our experience shows that postoperative infection occurs less frequently than after conservative treatment, and that the functional results are considerably better.

II. Principles of Antibiotic Therapy and the Treatment of Infection Following Internal Fixation

1. Surgical Principles when Infection Follows Internal Fixation

Every operation is accompanied by some invasion of the wound by bacteria. Prevention of infection, however, depends not only upon the number of bacteria that enter the wound but as much on the blood supply of the surrounding tissues, the avoidance of dead spaces and the amount of foreign material used. It is well known that intact skin can tolerate an intra-dermal deposit of several million bacteria without the formation of an abscess, whereas the addition of a small foreign object favours abscess formation with a much smaller number of bacteria. This of course applies equally to the metal implants used in internal fixation, so that extra care is required in the treatment of the soft tissues.

What happens to metal implants in cases of frank bone and wound infection, when there is obvious purulent discharge from the wound? Two possibilities must be considered.

a) The Fixation Remains Secure

The implants must be left in place; though infection never heals completely while a foreign body remains in situ, bone healing nevertheless does in fact take place. Continuous administration of antibiotics and sometimes local chemotherapy by way of irrigating drains, especially with medullary nails, helps to gain time while bone union occurs (for details on the institution of irrigation drainage see page 236). If the objective of internal fixation i.e. bony union, has been achieved, the foreign material can be removed, the wound closed up primarily and irrigation drainage instituted for a few days. As a rule, primary wound healing follows.

b) The Internal Fixation is no Longer Rigid

If the implant is no longer fulfilling its purpose of providing rigidity, it should be removed as soon as possible. Situations of this nature may be difficult to master. As a general rule it is advisable to stimulate the formation of a periosteal bridge of callus by inserting a cancellous autograft if the fracture is unstable and infected. In fractures of the lower leg, the cancellous bone is placed on the interosseous membrane between the tibia and fibula.

Sometimes this cancellous graft can be inserted directly into the cavity remaining after all infected tissue has been excised and sequestra and bone of doubtful vitality resected widely enough until viable and vascular bone is reached. In other cases the condition of the soft tissues may demand an approach through an area of undoubted vitality even at a distance from the original wound.

2. Treatment of Infection with Antibiotics

a) General

The therapeutic efficacy of antibiotics is increasingly limited by the resistance of the bacteria. Successful management of an infection must therefore depend upon various chemotherapeutic agents.

Bacteria are regarded as resistant when they do not respond *in vitro* to the usual antibiotic concentrations. That is to say that resistance is not an absolute concept, but merely mirrors the reaction of bacteria towards antibiotics under standard conditions. Bacteria that are unaffected by a given quantity may respond to an increased dose. If it is assumed that an antibiotic has an antimetabolic effect, the improved response to a higher dose can be explained by the disturbance of the reaction equilibrium. One must never forget, however, that the defense mechanisms of the host are of decisive importance. With poor resistance — whatever that may mean — an antibiotic combination that seemed to be favourable *in vitro* may fail *in vivo*.

It is clear that the antibiogram, as it is routinely made out in bacteriological laboratories, cannot simply be applied to clinical conditions, though it does provide valuable clues. In some cases it is worth making a quantitative estimation with serial dilutions.

Resistance *in vitro* depends on the antibiotic on the one hand and on the micro-organism on the other. In theory the administration of any antibiotic may lead to the appearance of resistant strains. This tendency is marked with penicillin, but has to date never been observed with ristocetin. Staphylococci have proved to be the most adaptable and thus the most therapy resistant bacteria. The development of resistance probably corresponds directly to the selection of individuals with primary resistance from a bacterial population. The possibility of gene mutation, however, cannot be entirely disregarded.

The incidence of cross resistance is important. Bacteria which have become resistant to carbomycin or oleandomycin, for example, under certain circumstances can also show the same resistance to erythromycin. Cross resistance has also been observed with kanamycin and neomycin.

Antibiotic resistant strains of bacteria present grave problems in hospital practice. Here, rooms, utensils and to a considerable extent personnel as well, are often contaminated by such bacteria. It is clear that hospital infections can only be successfully combatted if a general effort is made to curb the development of resistance. This is best accomplished by a clear "policy on antibiotics", especially if outside doctors who refer cases to the hospital observe the same rules as the hospital itself. The following factors must be considered in implementing this policy:

1. Any unnecessary contact between antibiotic and germ must be avoided. As a rule, only confirmed bacterial infections should be treated with antibiotics. Antibiotics are ineffective and should not be used in the treatment of certain chronic bacterial infections and where the infection is present in necrotic tissue.

2. Only a few antibiotics should be used routinely, in order to hold the remainder in reserve. To this effect, it is best to begin treatment always with the same antibiotic and to change it if there is no clinical response after three days, or if intolerance develops.

3. Changing to a different antibiotic is less often necessary if the first one is given in maximal dosage.

4. The common method of counteracting resistance and at the same time of enhancing therapeutic effect, is to combine two different antibiotics. To do this, however, each antibiotic must be given in a dosage that would be effective if one were given in isolation. The combination of penicillin and streptomycin has proved effective, as has that of tetracycline with oleandomycin apparently. The latter is not entirely unobjectionable since it also produces a cross resistance with erythromycin, an antibiotic that is still very effective against staphylococci.

Some antibiotics show a certain mutual antagonism. Thus, for instance, penicillin in combination with a bacteriostatic agent such as tetracycline, has a diminished antibacterial effect. This phenomenon is explained by the fact that penicillin can only affect the metabolism of multiplying bacteria. Tetracycline in its bacteriostatic action, however, prevents the bacteria from reaching the multiplication phase. The respective antibacterial effects of individual antibiotics will be characterized in brief:

Bactericidal and bacteriostatic antibiotics:

Penicillin, streptomycin, bacitracin, thyrotricin.

Predominantly bacteriostatic antibiotics:

Tetracycline, chloramphenicol, erythromycin, oleandomycin, spiramycin, carbomycin.

Erythromycin and the tetracyclines in high dosage (approximately 6 gamma/ml.) have a bactericidal effect as well. This is especially true of erythromycin.

Purely bactericidal antibiotics:

Vancomycin, ristocetin, kanamycin, polymixin, neomycin.

A *side effect* of broad spectrum antibiotics is nausea. Chloramphenicol is also said to have an inhibiting effect on bone marrow. To our knowledge, however, this has not been observed in the more recent preparations. Tetracyclines, especially in cachectic patients, can increase the number of pathogens by killing off the saprophytes. Toxic side effects are often so severe that some antibiotics can only be applied locally. Used carefully, though, almost all antibiotics can be given parenterally.

The following have *neurotoxic* properties, especially on the auditory pathways: neomycin, kanamycin and streptomycin preparations. Of the latter, streptomycin itself damages the vestibular mechanism and dehydrostreptomycin the acoustic.

Thyrotricin, a mixture of 20% thyrocidin and 80% gramicidin, is hemolytic and cannot therefore be used parenterally.

Penicillin has the fewest toxic effects and it can be given in doses of 40 million units or more daily, which amounts to about 25 grams. Given intravenously, no reservoirs are formed so that the blood levels are genuinely controllable.

b) Principles in the Use of Antibiotics

It is most important to insist that the standard of asepsis of an operating suite is such that antibiotic medication in so-called clean operations is not only superfluous, but should be positively forbidden. During surgery, however, the wound may be irrigated with Ringer's solution containing neomycin and bacitracin (we use nebacetin 1 ampoule per 1000 ml.) about every thirty minutes. In our practice it is only in cases of internal fixation where the operation lasts more than two hours, that prophylactic antibiotic cover is given and this amounts to less than 3% of all cases.

The use of antibiotics is therefore restricted to cases of manifest infection and is only begun when local redness is seen, accompanied by a febrile reaction. When a decision is reached to use antibiotics a strict regime must be followed. There are few bacteria even today that are resistant to penicillin in high dosage, so that our first choice is to combine penicillin and streptomycin. In such a case we give 40 million units of penicillin and 1 gram of streptomycin daily by the intravenous route. This has the advantage that any sensitivity reaction can be quickly spotted and the drip stopped. As there is no reservoir of the drug in the body, any effects due to the penicillin subside at once. After using this method in several hundred patients, no untoward incidents have occurred.

In this, as in any other mode of antibiotic therapy, we observe the rule that, if there has been no clinical response after three days, the situation must be reviewed and the antibiotic changed. Next in order we use a tetracycline unless sensitivity tests suggest an alternative. Two grams of tetracycline are given daily and if the response is achieved, this is continued, but if not we change to chloramphenicol in doses of 2 grams daily. In this way, chloramphenicol has been kept as a reserve weapon in our hospital. If this too is ineffective, erythromycin is given in doses of 2 grams daily in addition to the chloramphenicol. If this routine has been followed through to the end, other bacteriological investigation may lead us to turn to rarer antibiotics, but this is only necessary in a very occasional case. Antibiotic doses can be summarized as follows:

Penicillin — between 20 and 60 mega units per day.

Streptomycin — 1 to 2 grams. Care must be exercised when the total dose has reached 60 grams.

Erythromycin, chloramphenicol, tetracycline — 2 to 3 grams using the same dosage with oral and parenteral administration.

Polymixin can be administered intra-muscularly in doses of 1.5 to 2.5 mg. per kilogram body weight. It is well tolerated by mouth also.

Neomycin is given orally, for disinfection of the gut in preparation for surgery, in a dose of 3 to 10 grams; intramuscularly it may be given in doses of 10 to 15 mg. per kilogram body weight, for a maximum of 10 days. As there are many better tolerated preparations there is usually no indication for its parenteral use.

Ristocetin — 2 to 3 grams intravenously.

Kanamycin — 2 grams up to a total of not more than 40 grams parenterally.

Vancomycin — 50 to 100 mg. 3 or 4 times daily intravenously for not longer than 7 days.

Oleandomycin — 1 to 2 grams intravenously, intramuscularly or orally.

Carbomycin — 2 to 4 grams by mouth.

In general, a continuous drip infusion should be used in emergencies, which is always applicable in fracture cases where antibiotics are required, as there is either an open wound or an obvious infection. This is the quickest way of achieving a uniform blood and tissue concentration.

c) Local Application of Antibiotics

When infection supervenes after internal fixation, local application of antibiotics has proved to be most reliable, especially when a drug to which the organism is shown to be sensitive, is given by continuous drip. The details of this technique, called "antibacterial irrigation drainage" (WILLENEGGER and ROTH, 1962) have been described elsewhere. The effectiveness of this system is due to its bacteriostatic effect on the infected surface combined with mechanical cleaning, both of which are important. The continuous removal of the products of inflammation and of necrotic particles enhances bacteriostasis and allows the tissue defences to eliminate the remaining bacteria.

The best indication for antibacterial irrigation drainage is when infection complicates medullary nailing, whether the infection is recent, or of longstanding. If the infection is not well localized, systemic chemotherapy should precede the instillation of an antibiotic locally, but when the general condition has improved, the point of entry of the medullary nail is exposed if the nail is still firm. This incision is made just large enough to accommodate two plastic drains, one of which is passed down to the distal end of the nail along its lumen. In the tibia for instance one drain is brought out medial and the other lateral to the patellar tendon, taking care not to penetrate the knee joint. The incision at the proximal end can be left open or loosely closed, depending on the severity of the infection. The proximal drain is used for infusing the antibiotic while the other is connected to a suction apparatus. If the infection is severe or of long standing or accompanied by periosteal abscesses or fistulae, it is better not to use the closed irrigation system but to infuse the antibiotic fluid through both drains, draining it out through any existing fistula or sinuses (open antibacterial irrigation drainage). When the medullary nail has become loose and is serving no useful purpose, it is removed and irrigation of the medullary canal is performed.

Continuous irrigation in this way quickly controls the infection in the bone and soft tissues. Where bone retains or renews contact with soft tissue, revascularization is always possible, even when there has been severe osteitis, especially in cancellous bone. Bone fragments without soft tissue contact remain necrotic and must be removed as sequestra. As soon as the stage of innocuous surface infection has been reached, irrigation for mechanical cleaning may be continued with normal saline alone and in many cases this need only be done intermittently, during the night or once a day. Meanwhile, suction drainage with a vacuum bottle is adequate. When this stage is reached the patient may be allowed to walk about if the medullary nail is still firm. When x-ray shows evidence of consolidation the nail is removed, antibiotic irrigation is renewed and soon replaced by saline. Suction drainage is instituted thereafter with progressively shortened drains. Under certain circumstances a long continued artificial fistula should be maintained, which in most cases will prevent subsequent flare-ups besides allowing egress for any remaining sequestra that were not apparent on x-ray.

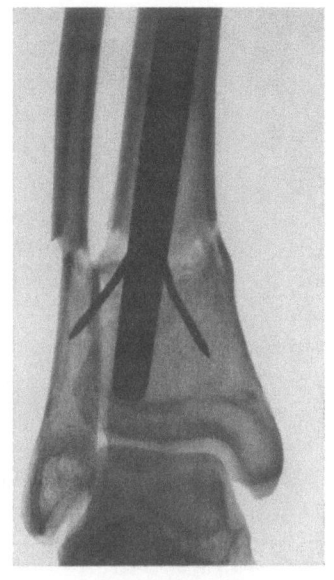

Fig. 243 illustrates this type of irrigation drainage in a case of infected medullary nailing, where osteomyelitis has already developed. It should be noted that the bone that was the site of osteitis became fully revascularized and ossification occurred in the cavity resulting from the removal of two metal splinters.

a Postoperative x-ray: Severe wound infection, abscess formation at the site of insertion of the nail and over the fracture, sinus down to the wound. Bacteria: hemolytic staphylococcus aureus, sensitive to chloramphenicol.

1st stage of treatment of the infection (b—e)

b 4 weeks after internal fixation, removal of the anti-rotational wires

c General chemotherapy for 8 days, irrigation drainage with entry and exit drains in the lumen of the medullary canal

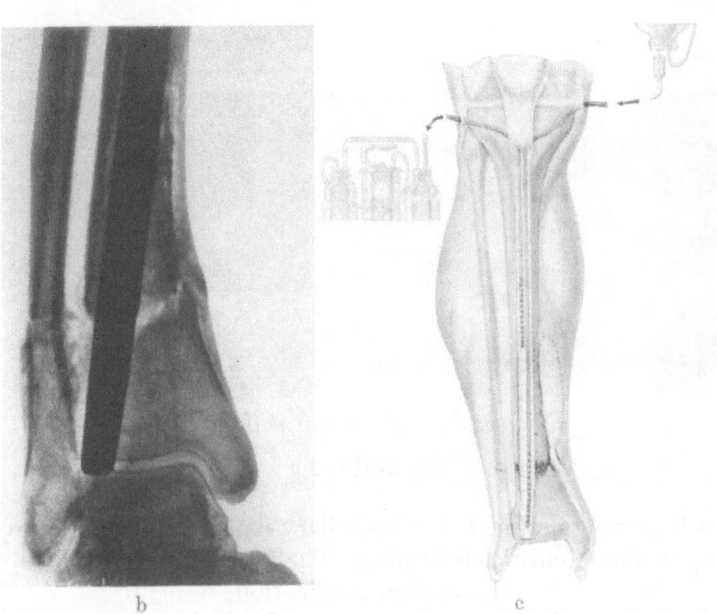

Fig. 243a—o. Antibacterial irrigation drainage to the site of an infected medullary nail (see text)

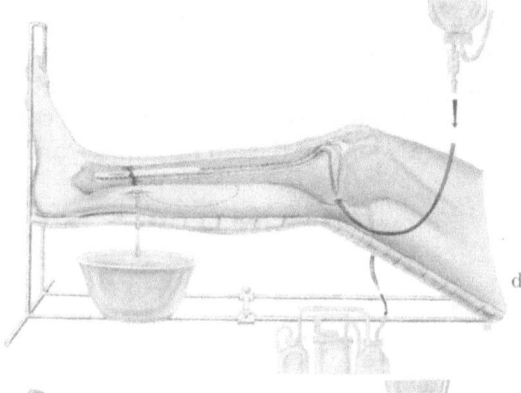

d and e Some of the irrigation fluid is evacuated as in open drainage through the enlarged surgical wound. Osteomyelitis three weeks after institution of irrigation drainage, or 7 weeks after internal fixation.

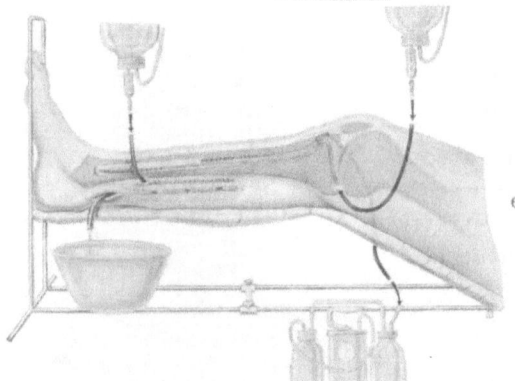

Method used: continuous drip with a $^1/_4\,^0/_{00}$ chloramphenicol for $4^1/_2$ weeks, alternating with physiological saline solution for 1 week and saline alone for 2 weeks until the nail is removed.

Fig. 243 d and e

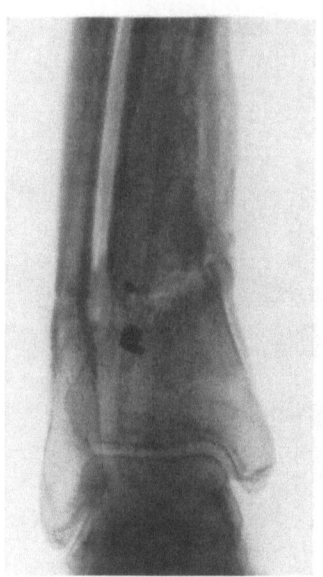

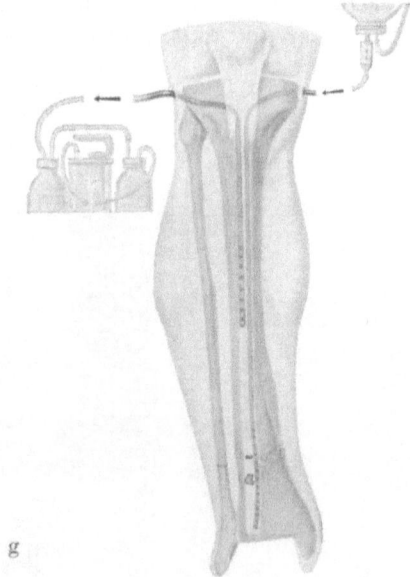

2nd phase of treatment (f, g)

Fig. 243 f and g

f $7^1/_2$ weeks after beginning drainage, the medullary nail is removed: 2 broken off pieces of the reamer are for the moment left in place. The fracture is clinically stable and x-ray shows clear ossification.

g In place of the nail, medullary drainage is established, irrigation with $^1/_4\,^0/_{00}$ chloramphenicol for 2 weeks and saline for another three weeks.

3rd phase of treatment (h, i)   *4th phase of treatment (k, l)*

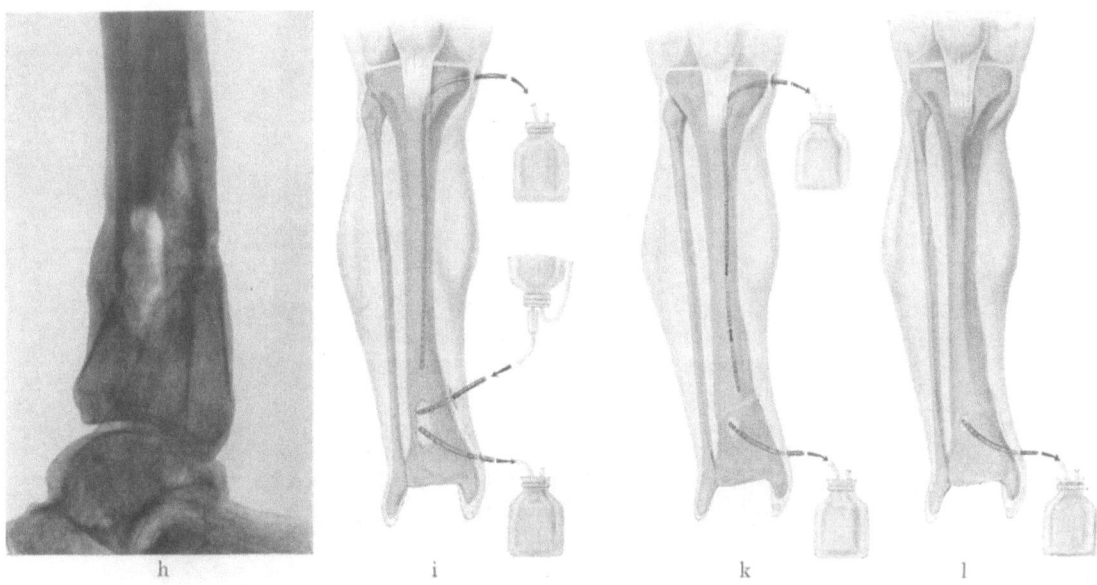

Fig. 243 h—l

h 5 weeks after removal of the nail or $12^1/_2$ weeks after the beginning of drainage, the two metal fragments are removed after suitable fenestration.

i Again, irrigation drainage is established for 3 weeks with $^1/_4 \,^0/_{00}$ chloramphenicol followed by saline alone for $4^1/_2$ weeks.

k and l 20 weeks after the beginning of the local treatment, the irrigation is replaced by suction drainage, the tube being shortened successively over $3^1/_2$ weeks. Total hospital treatment lastet 24 weeks.

5th phase of treatment (m, n)

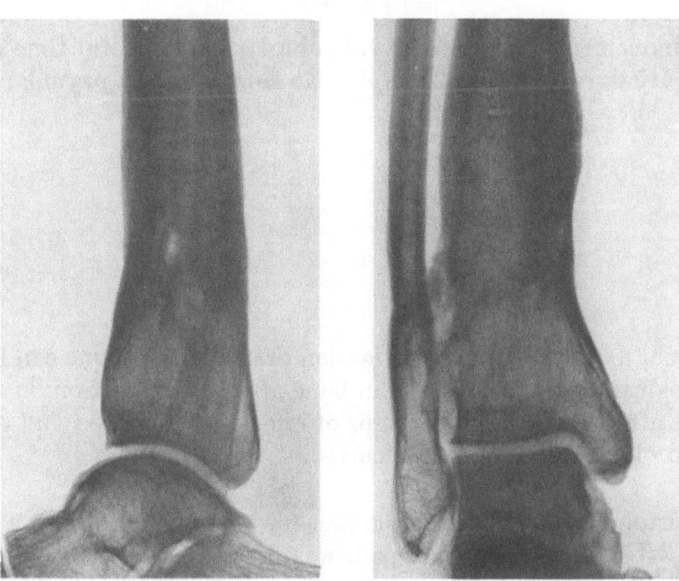

Fig. 243 m and n

A small medial fistula down to the bone is kept open with gauze for a long period, subsequently two small sequestra are discharged.

m and n After two years there is bony union without any flare up.

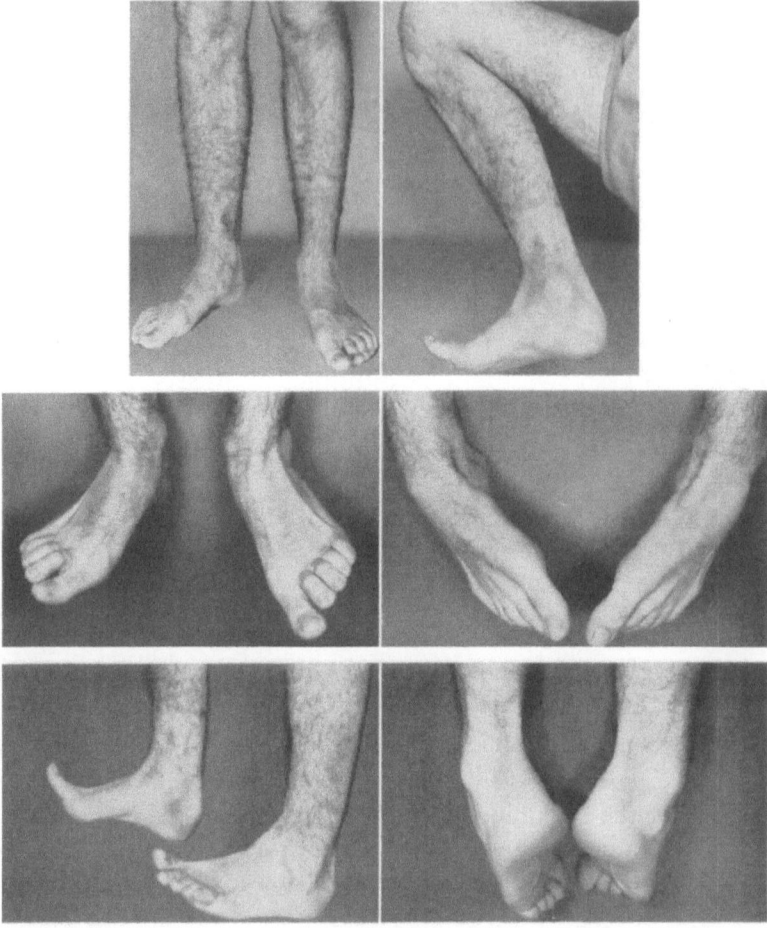

Fig. 243 o

Fig. 243 o. Full movement at the ankle and subtalar joints. Total time away from work 212 days, or about 30 weeks. No compensation payable.

In other internal fixations the same irrigation drainage technique can be used. Fig. 244 shows the radiological course of infection in bone after screw fixation, in which treatment began a few days after the first clinical signs of infection. Here, too, full revascularization and consolidation of the infected bone occurred.

Uneventful postoperative course for the first few days. After 8 days a plaster cast was applied. 5 weeks after internal fixation pain was first experienced in the wound and the patient was pyrexial.

6 weeks after internal fixation the plaster cast was removed: a discharge from the purulent hematoma appeared between the sutures: the organisms proved to be hemolytic streptococci and B. coli, both responding to chloramphenicol.

First phase of treatment of the infection

The surgical wound was re-opened and the infected hematoma evacuated. The heads of two screws were exposed on the medial surface of the tibia but the bone was covered. Closed irrigation drainage was introduced to the site of infection and continuous installation of $^1/_4{}^0/_{00}$ chloramphenicol was given for 2 weeks; thereafter suction drainage. Skin flaps were closed primarily with wire sutures (a). Satisfactory progress.

(a) x-ray 3 weeks after insertion of the drainage, i.e. 9 weeks after internal fixation. The patient became pyrexial again which, with further distal inflammatory swelling and a more obvious fracture line on the x-ray, was suggestive of osteomyelitis. Irrigation within the bone was therefore instituted.

2nd phase of treatment

Removal of two screws: introduction of two drainage tubes into the medullary canal, one passed through the hole of the removed screw, the other through an oblique hole drilled in the subcutaneous border of the tibia proximal to the fracture. Continuous instillation of $^1/_4{}^0/_{00}$ chloramphenicol for 20 days: subsequent suction drainage. Without interferring with the irrigation drainage, the remaining two screws were removed through separate stab incisions two weeks after the irrigation had been begun.

(b) x-ray 7 weeks after instituting drainage which was 13 weeks after internal fixation: progressive ossification of the fracture and re-ossification of the infected bone. Clinically the fracture was stable and neighbouring joints had full movement. The whole treatment of the infection took place without additional plaster casts.

(c) x-ray at 3 years and 8 months after internal fixation. Full bony union and restoration of function. No compensation was payable.

One big advantage of this form of therapy is that it avoids the need for any external support, so that active exercises can be begun a few days after institution of local drainage. Most of the cases treated in this way so far have resulted in full restoration of joint and muscle function.

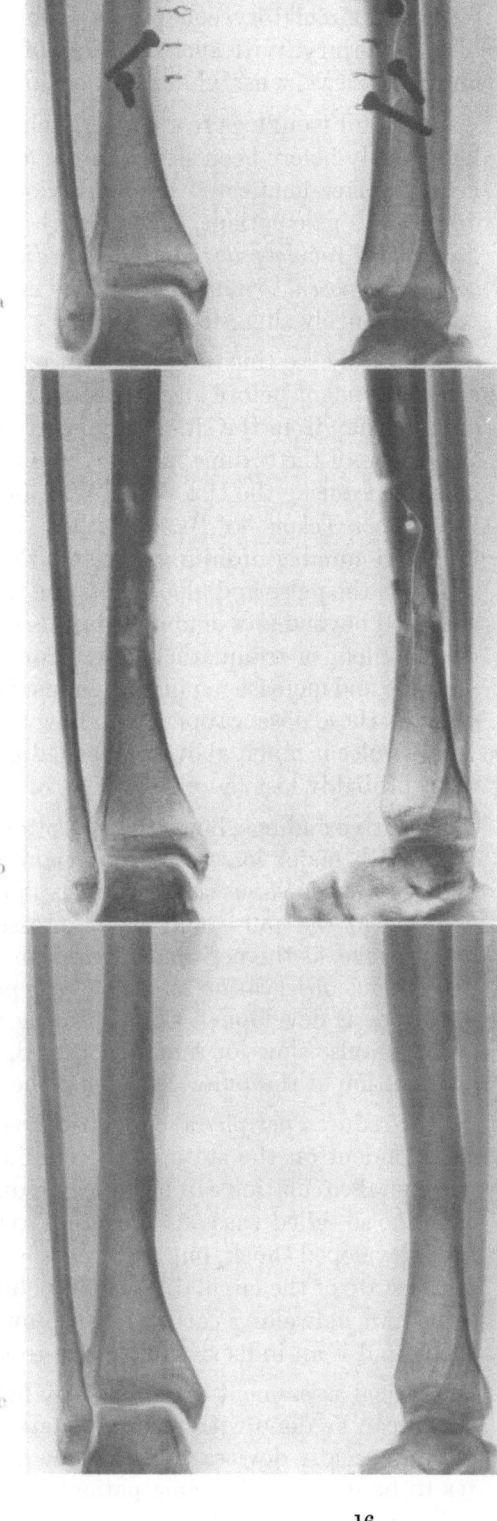

Fig. 244a—c. Wound infection after screw fixation (see text)

III. The Problem of Shock in Accident Surgery

1. Diagnosis of Shock

The clinician is inclined to make an intuitive diagnosis of shock and many doctors refer to any distressed patient, especially after injury, as being "in shock". This term therefore includes conditions with widely differing causes, ranging from the common fainting attack to severe circulatory collapse as occurs in myocardial infarction, peritonitis or a major bleeding injury. With such a variety of meanings, this term must necessarily remain vague and is not a very useful description for treatment.

In 1870 FISCHER gave a masterly clinical description of an accident victim in shock who had shortly before been struck in the abdomen by the shaft of a cart. This description has held its place unaffected by the various theories of shock that have come and gone. He described a pale patient, covered with perspiration, with cyanotic lips, *cool extremities, cool nose and a racing pulse, hardly recordible blood pressure, nausea, thirst and with an almost completely absent urinary output*. The man was clearly conscious but his reactions appeared to be strangely sluggish.

We rarely see this full picture in peace time, as patients have usually been given some early treatment before all the responses to trauma have developed. In war time or after a long journey from the site of injury, observation and/or treatment usually begin later and the effects of the trauma may develop fully. Patients in this condition have been carefully examined during the last World War and during the Korean War. Much credit must go to the "Shock Teams" of BEECHER et al. (1942) and GRANT and REEVE (1951) for examining in a large number of injured patients the relationship of simple circulatory disturbance, as shown in the pulse and blood pressure, to the actual blood volume. Their observations have classified beyond any doubt the primary significance of loss of blood or blood volume in the development of traumatic shock. From this sprang the recognition that the fall in blood pressure and increase in pulse rate must be carefully observed and that in the great mayority of cases these observations can allow an estimation of the volume of blood lost. Patients whose pulse is much above a hundred and whose blood pressure is below a hundred, have most probably lost more than 30% of their blood volume.

Negative findings, however, as is often the case in medicine, are of much less significance. Even with major losses of blood, pain can maintain the blood pressure at an artificially high level while vagus stimulation can produce a deceptively slow pulse. In our experience, changes in the pulse and blood pressure appear especially late with intra-abdominal hemorrhage, as the peritoneal irritation at the onset counteracts the fall in blood pressure. Continuous observation in such a case provides variable clues to the manner in which the syndrome is developing. Compensating mechanisms can only keep the blood pressure up and the pulse slow for a limited period, however, and soon the fall in blood pressure and acceleration of the pulse will reveal the true danger of the condition.

The reduced peripheral circulation, as shown by the cool extremities and slight cyanosis, is dependent on the state of the cardio-vascular system and the blood volume, but the peripheral circulation can be greatly reduced even without significant loss of blood volume, as in the so-called vasovagal reaction to trauma. Cool extremities are indeed a clear sign in fully developed shock, but a diagnosis must not be made on this alone. The best indication of the state of the circulating blood volume is obtained by measuring the hourly output of urine. An indwelling catheter has proved a useful means of estimating the state of the shock and is an indispensable guide to the progress of treatment.

Clinical assessment can be greatly helped by direct measurement of the blood volume, which can be done with reasonable speed with the help of radioactive isotopes. Recently semi-automatic devices have become available that allow repeated blood volume estimates to be made in the same patient at short intervals. We have experienced good results using the Volemetron (WILLIAMS and FINE, 1961; ALLGÖWER and STUDER, 1962; SIEGRIST et al., 1962; GRUBER and ALLGÖWER, 1964). Direct blood volume estimates are especially useful in patients who have already received blood and electrolytes, as the clinical signs are no longer as trustworthy as in an untreated case.

From what has been said four dependable signs that allow a firm diagnosis of shock to be made are: *arterial blood pressure, pulse rate, condition of the peripheral circulation and urinary output.* The development of the condition can be assessed by observing changes in these four signs. Based on these criteria the following reactions to trauma can be recognized:

a) Impending Shock

Cold, normotensive tachycardia (cold extremities and nose, pulse 100 to 120, blood pressure over 100, urinary output diminished to 20 ml. per hour). Such patients have generally lost not more than 30% of their blood volume. Transfusion is indicated, but there is no mortal danger, though careful observation is needed as the blood pressure may be kept deceptively high because of pain.

Cold, hypotensive bradycardia (cold extremities and nose, pulse below 100, blood pressure also below 100, urinary output generally normal if there is adequate filtration pressure). These signs usually indicate the so-called vasovagal reaction which is a condition related to "fainting". Owing to the stimulation of the vagus there is vasodilatation in the muscles. The cerebral circulation becomes inadequate and "collapse" results. This condition is often due to psychogenic factors, especially traumatic experiences and pain, and is quite transient.

b) Established Shock

Cold, hypotensive tachycardia (cold extremities and nose, pulse above 110, blood pressure below 100, urinary output below 20 ml. per hour). Here there is grave danger if the blood pressure falls below 70 and the pulse rises above 140. With this picture it may be assumed that about 50% of the blood volume has been lost.

This classification is based on simple clinical criteria, and avoids the introduction of unsupported clinical opinions into the terminology describing the pathogenesis of shock. The object of these definitions is to give information in terms of changes in blood pressure, pulse, skin colour and urinary output that are more informative than the laconic statement that the patient is "in shock" or, even worse, that he is in this or that condition of shock.

After operation some patients exhibit a special circulatory reaction which is not particularly significant, but should alert the staff to watch for the development of cold, hypotensive tachycardia. This is the condition called *warm hypotensive tachycardia* with a blood pressure below 100, a pulse above 100, but warm extremities.

2. Pathogenesis of Posttraumatic Circulatory Disturbances

It is beyond the scope of this book to discuss the pathogenesis of shock in general and we will limit ourselves to describing the causative factors that lead to shock after fractures and other injuries. Fractures always involve a relatively significant loss of blood as shown by CLARKE's (1957) valuable quantitative data. GANZONI (1959) has been able to confirm these figures from a large series of lower leg fractures. A blood loss of between 100 and 500 ml. in fractures of the lower leg and 500 to 3000 ml. in the femur must be expected. The blood loss may be widely distributed in the tissues so that estimating its quantity by direct inspection of local swelling is difficult. In modern traffic accidents, there are very often several fractures in one patient. If the blood loss from different lesions is added up in the case of multiple injury it may well be found that the patient has suffered a loss of between 20 and 50% of his blood volume. Observations of the blood pressure and pulse rate provide a good basis for estimating the volume of blood loss, but much more exact measurements can be obtained nowadays using radioisotopes (ALLGÖWER and STUDER, 1962). From this it becomes clear that every injured patient who is in a condition of established shock, must from the outset be regarded as having a severely depleted blood volume.

Having emphasized the significance of blood loss and in consequence the importance of blood replacement, it must be stated that the loss of circulating red cells is not always explained simply by extravasation of blood. Observations on these lines were published by SEAMAN and PONDER as early as 1943. They found that simply removing blood did not produce anemia as readily as the loss of the same quantity of blood due to an operation. GELIN (1956) deserves the credit for confirming this phenomenon and for establishing its relationship to another important source of circulatory disturbance after trauma, the pseudo-agglutination of red cells in small vessels known as "sludging", as had been found by KNISELY in 1942. Developing THORSEN's work (1950), GELIN was able to show that the same degree of anemia could be due to very different causes, in some of which there was no actual loss of red cells. The degree of anemia was related to the amount of sludging and the prevention of sludging would prevent the anemia.

Sludging is the direct result of the reduced suspension stability of the blood. Intra-vascular aggregation of red cells, which is easily observed in the conjunctiva in man and animals, is present three to eight hours after injury. The rise in the sedimentation rate occurs much later. The increased aggregation of red cells, however, persists as long as the raised sedimentation rate continues. Sludging appears to be a relatively unspecific reaction as it occurs after fractures, burns, contusions etc. to the same extent. It can also be due to the infusion of substances with large molecules like high molecular weight dextran, when the same decrease in circulating red cells occurs. THORSEN's observations confirmed by GELIN, are most valuable, showing that low molecular weight dextran (Rheomacrodex) effectively counteracts the tendency to sludging and thereby clearly improves the micro-circulation. Furthermore, low molecular weight dextran is able to restore to normal the number of circulating red cells which had been reduced by sludging. This is equally true with burns, contusions, fractures and experimentally-induced sludging caused by high molecular weight dextran.

There is a synergistic relationship between the extravascular loss of blood and the intravascular sludging. The decreased suspension stability of the blood, because of the resulting red cell stasis in the capillaries, reduces the oxygen carrying power. Both factors together reduce the microcirculation in the tissues, which in turn is particularly harmful in areas where vasoconstriction has occurred to compensate for the reduced circulating blood volume, especially in the abdominal viscera. In order to preserve life the body attempts to supply most of the available blood to the heart and the central nervous system, but this mechanism of centralization operates within narrow limits.

The microcirculation of the intestine and liver are clearly of special importance and impaired microcirculation of the gut disturbs permeability in two directions. On the one hand the capillary wall, which has suffered damage from anoxia, allows blood protein to enter the intestine, on the other, the metabolites from inside can enter the blood stream.

With a normal circulation the liver detoxicates small amounts of intestinal metabolites. In health, the equilibrium between the intestinal tract and the liver is well maintained, but an intestine damaged by anoxia makes far greater demands on the liver in this respect, which the liver can only meet if it is functioning optimally. The microcirculation of the liver, however, is just as badly disturbed as that of the intestine and it can no longer perform the necessary detoxication. Thus, a vicious circle is begun. The failure of the liver's detoxicating action in shock is not only related to toxins originating in the intestine but to all toxins, including those produced by bacteria. It is not commonly realized that very dirty wounds have a significant bacterial population within even a few hours, which produce equivalent quantities of toxin. An amount of toxin that would have little effect on a healthy body can be very deleterious to one that has been severely damaged.

Formerly much attention has been given to the effects on the kidney of the *"crush syndrome"*, i.e., posttraumatic renal insufficiency. It has been found that this is caused by two factors.

a) The diversion of the major part of the circulating blood volume to the vital centres greatly diminishes the renal blood flow, which in health amounts to about one-fifth of the cardiac output and which, in this condition, may be reduced to as little as one fiftieth. The kidney cannot tolerate this amount of hypoxia for more than two hours, after which irreversible damage is caused. In wartime such renal damage was often seen because the wounded only received full blood replacement after some delay. In peace time this syndrome is very rare, as proper blood replacement usually is available within a two hour limit. In this syndrome prophylaxis is especially successful, whereas therapy usually fails when the kidney has been damaged.

b) When muscle or blood pigments also reach the kidney, spasm of the vessels may be induced, resulting in further renal damage which would not have happened in a kidney with a normal blood supply.

In the kidney with reversible damage, the course runs from a relatively long lasting polyuric phase to an eventual state of substantial recovery. The polyuric phase needs the most careful replacement therapy which can only be successfully performed with daily control of the body weight. The basic rule is to replace the amount of water lost on the preceding day, plus 1000 ml. of glucose in water. The fluids given must contain the electrolytes secreted on the previous day.

The decreased suspension stability of the blood following trauma involves almost certainly not only the red cells, but the platelets and the chylomicrons too. This decreased suspension stability and the disturbance of the micro-circulation, however, cannot by themselves explain the incidence of *fat embolism* as BERGENTZ (1963) assumed in his development of GELIN's work. In our case histories of nearly 2000 surgically treated fractures, we have had no case of fat embolism in 1500 fractures resulting from sport accidents, whereas four severe cases and a number of minor ones were found in 500 traffic accidents. Damage to significant parts of the whole body seems to be a prerequisite for the development of severe fat embolism.

A number of authors consider the transport of fat from the fractured bone to be insufficient to explain the incidence of fat embolism. They point out that the pressure of the medullary canal falls to a very low level immediately after the fracture is sustained (REHM, 1957) and that thus the entry of fat into a vein is difficult to explain. It is also doubtful whether the femur contains sufficient fat to account quantitatively for a massive fat embolism (LEHMANN and MOORE, 1927). SEVITT's recently published (1962) monograph on the problem of fat embolism gives a very good survey of the theories on the pathogenesis of fat embolism. He draws particular attention to the interesting experiments of YOUNG and GRIFFITHS (1950) who did find an explanation for the entry of fat into the venous circulation of the injured bone.

"A thin-walled collapsible tube is placed horizontally in a container partly filled with fluid. One end of the tube is connected with a fluid reservoir, the height of which can be varied, and the other end is used for the outflow. If the pressure in the collapsible tube is higher at the proximal end and lower at the outlet, fluid will leave the tube, but if the outside pressure is then raised, the distal end of the tube collapses until the pressure from the proximal end is greater than that outside the tube, when it opens up again. Thus a cycle of collapse and distension is repeated rhythmically and it was found that if holes were made in the compressible tube, this rhythmic emptying resulted in fluid from outside being drawn into the tube and expelled from the distal end. When small beads were suspended in the outside fluid, they found their way, as a result of this pumping action, into the lumen and were expelled distally along it. The same may happen with the fat from the medullary canal, when there is a shift in the differential pressure that allows the extra-vascular pressure to rise even slightly and momentarily above that within the vessel".

After a critical survey of current literature, SEVITT reaches the conclusion that minor degrees of fat embolism can be triggered by various mechanisms (burns, severe infections, etc.). Severe fat embolism, however, is without exception associated with massive and generalized concussion of the skeleton. SEVITT therefore is of the opinion that in severe fat embolism there is always a massive transfer of fat from the injured bone especially, and that the mechanism described by YOUNG and GRIFFITHS explains the mode of transport.

The observation that fat embolism occurs rarely in sporting injuries but commonly in traffic accidents, is difficult to explain. The method of transfer described by YOUNG and GRIFFITHS should be present equally in both types of injury. It would seem possible therefore that the abnormal conditions in injured veins cannot be present in a fractured bone only and the classical experiment to induce fat embolism by bone concussion without fracture (RIPPERT, 1894, and FRITSCHE, 1910) points the same way. Undoubtedly the alteration in microcirculation and the decreased suspension stability may play a role in triggering the vicious circle that increases the anoxic damage to important tissues.

It has been shown that the vascular system of the lung tolerates a massive infiltration of fat without adverse results. The clinical signs of fat embolism originate only when fat has lodged in the larger vessels, expecially in the brain and parenchymatous organs. Later, however, there is usually significant change in the lungs. So far it has not been clarified whether this is a direct reaction to the toxic breakdown products of fat in the lung and in the bronchial capillaries, or whether it is the result of damage to the respiratory centre.

Up to date there is no specific treatment for clinically obvious fat embolism. The best prophylaxis may be regular full replacement of the blood volume and when possible the maintenance of a good microcirculation. The operative treatment of fresh fractures does not increase the risk of fat embolism statistically (see SEVITT, 1962). It seems rather that successful fixation has a certain prophylactic effect against further transport of fat emboli when injured extremities are moved.

The most severe successfully treated case of cerebral fat embolism with concurrent extensive lung involvement that we have seen was a case with fractures of both lower legs due to a traffic accident. The fractures had been internally fixed immediately after the accident and the very difficult nursing care needed (including postural drainage and percussion etc., for the chest) could hardly have been carried out with two unstable lower legs.

Today the prognosis in severe fat embolism has undoubtedly improved since we are better able to control the secondary effects. The disturbances of respiration are treated by immediate tracheostomy and intermittent positive pressure respiration, as well as by frequent bronchial toilet. When there is cerebral irritability and hyperpyrexia, chlorpromazine and its newer derivatives may be used. During the stage of unconsciousness or severe central nervous depression, blood gas analysis is desirable. Electrolytes are accurately measured, both in their serum values and their urinary excretion and are replaced in step with their elimination.

As a "specific" therapy, unsaturated fatty acids in the form of the phospholipids (Lipostabil) were mentioned recently (see HOSSLI and GATTIKER, 1960). It is recommended that for twenty-four hours, 1 to 1.5 grams of this be given intravenously. It appeared to have a favourable effect in two of the four cases of severe fat embolism we observed since the patient's recovery of consciousness seemed to coincide with the administration of the drug, but no conclusions can be drawn from so few cases and we mention this merely as a suggestion for further experimental use.

A complete remission will occur after even the most severe cerebral fat embolism, which justifies the use of all therapeutic means to prevent the patient dying from disturbances of ventilation and excretion during the critical days.

3. Treatment of Shock

No time should be lost in treating shock. The first two hours of increasing shock may be decisive as to whether or not the patient will suffer organic damage to his kidney or liver, or to his power of resistance against infection and toxins. A simple immediate fluid replacement combined with energetic chemotherapy can save patients who will not be savable a few hours later in spite of the most intensive treatment.

Replacement therapy in hypovolemia. The primary importance of a low blood volume in posttraumatic shock demands commensurate blood replacement. A therapeutic motto coined by GORDH "give the heart blood and the blood oxygen" can be supplemented by "give it soon and quickly".

The method used to replace the blood volume hardly needs further discussion. The traumatized patient will, in almost every case, require whole blood, in quantities estimated either by the described clinical criteria or with the help of blood volume determination. The equipment for the latter is only available in a few hospitals at present, so that clinical judgement will have to be used in most places. Blood pressure should not be used as the sole indication as it may be increased by compensating mechanisms before the loss has been replaced. A shut-down of the renal blood supply combined with maintenance of good blood flow to the vital organs, can be accompanied by a relatively high blood pressure. The accurate recording of the hourly urinary excretion is therefore most important, as it gives information about the activity in an organ which is very early affected by hypoxia, and can give an index of the degree of vasoconstriction occurring which seems to be directly proportional to the reduction in the blood volume.

It is not wise to try and force an adults "normal urinary output" of 50 ml. per hour as the body may become overloaded during the period of traumatic oliguria. The output of urine should, however, be at least 30 ml. per hour and optimally 40 ml. The exact amount can only be determined with the use of an indwelling catheter. Besides the urinary output, other physical signs of shock provide valuable information about its progress and the success of treatment. An increase in the blood pressure with a fall in the pulse rate, together with a rise in the temperature of the extremities and face are good signs. Nausea, vomiting, restlessness and thirst indicate inadequate replacement. Under-transfusion and over-transfusion can be avoided in most cases with the help of two measurements which we regard as important.

1. A minimum urinary output of 30 ml. per hour.

2. A venous pressure of not more than 15 cm. of water. Both of these are very simple measurements which can be done immediately even under very primitive conditions.

Although electrolyte solutions have little place in the restoration of blood volume, the mineral balance must be attended to during therapy for shock. In any severe accident case, alterations in electrolytes and acid base balance may give rise to disturbances and the time factor is important. The later treatment begins, the more important is the administration of electrolytes in addition to simple volume replacement in order to counter any development of acidosis. During each hour of waiting, about 200 ml. of electrolyte solution is transferred from the tissues into the blood vessels until the blood volume has been restored. We use Ringer's lactate solution, then infuse according to the rule of thumb, 200 ml. for every hour that has elapsed between the accident and the beginning of treatment.

In all cases where, despite adequate replacement of blood loss, the patient's microcirculation remains unsatisfactory, infusion of 500 to 1500 ml. of Rheomacrodex (low molecular weight dextran) is recommended. Rheomacrodex is probably the only available drug today capable of interrupting the vicious circle of inadequate micro-circulation and cellular aggregation in the postcapillary venules. A prophylactic infusion of Rheomacrodex (500 to 1500 ml. in 24 hours) seems indicated in all cases of cold hypotensive tachycardia. Operation is only allowed when the peripheral circulation is fully restored to normal, blood volume is checked or at least a normal hourly urinary output is obtained. Apart from all of the measures taken to restore blood volume in a freshly injured patient, we value immediate operative stabilization as an adjunct in the prophylaxis against fat embolism, particularly in multiple fractures.

Control of pain. Drugs to relieve pain should always be administered intravenously in shock and a dose of 50 mg. of pethidine has proved effective (BEECHER). Pain is relieved and side effects are rare.

Phenothiazine and hypothermia. The time when phenothiazine was so strongly advocated in treating shock, has passed. It may have occasional use in special conditions and then only in the hands of one with extensive experience in this field. It is vital that fluid replacement never lags behind the dilatation of the blood vessels that the drug may induce, as the body's regulating mechanisms are largely put out of action by it.

Chemotherapy. Chemotherapy is indicated irrespective of the type of injury as a lowered resistance to infection and increased sensitivity to toxins are present in the patient with shock. Over the last few years we have convinced ourselves of the values of large doses of penicillin given intravenously to every patient suffering from shock or with a compound wound. Between 10 and 40 mega units of penicillin and 1 gram of streptomycin are given intravenously on admission. The other uses of antibiotics are discussed in detail in the section on infections and antibiotics.

Hormones. There is no place for the routine administration of hormones. In animal experiments some types of shock were improved by the administration of aldosterone combined with hypertensin, but the exact applications to clinical practise are uncertain. As in the dog with severe endotoxin shock, this combination has proved useful, we can deduce that it is possible that in cases of blood loss accompanied by severe infection, steroids and hypertensin could by used as long as they are combined with intensive antibiotic treatment.

Drugs acting on the circulation. The use of this type of drug in shock is commonly discussed. When the body's compensatory mechanisms are conserving a reduced blood volume for the supply of the vital centres, it is unphysiological to use a drug with a constrictive action on the peripheral circulation, thereby increasing the danger produced by hypoxia. A sympathomimetic drug should never be used in preference to adequate blood volume replacement. From experimental evidence we know that noradrenaline with a reduced adrenal function can induce shock (LEVINE, 1953). It is always advisable therefore to combine noradrenaline or a similar substance, with prednisolone to prevent complications. If there is acidosis the effect of noradrenaline is diminished, though this can be corrected by giving sodium lactate or bicarbonate to restore the pH (WEIL, 1960).

To summarize, it may be said that steroids and drugs acting on the circulation should only be very rarely used in shock due to reduced blood volume. Where vasovagal reactions are predominant, sympathomimetics may be used though the diagnosis must be very accurate. Shock due to loss of red cell volume can begin with a vasovagal attack and the administration of a sympathomimetic drug makes the later assessment of the condition more difficult. In many cases today in which neurogenic factors are blamed for dysfunctions as may happen during anaesthesia, there may nevertheless be a genuine lack of blood volume. We all know how difficult it is to estimate the loss of blood during an operation.

Drugs acting on the heart. Recent experimental work has shown that the circulatory failure occurring in shock may have myocardial causes also, particularly when the critical two hour limit before treatment is begun, has been exceeded. Whenever signs of cardiac decompensation appear, especially when the pulse rate remains above 120, it is therefore advisable, to administer digitalis. We use digitoxin intravenously, up to 1 mg. or lanatosid C up to 1.6 mg., and later 0.1 or 0.2 mg. as booster doses.

4. Indications for Surgery in Patients with Shock

Surgeons in the last century, such as GUTRI (1850) or H. FISCHER (1870) used to warn against surgery in patients with shock. This opinion may still be held with justice but unlike surgeons in the last century we can now treat shock itself and with energetic treatment it should be possible to render patients fit for surgery within two hours.

If possible, anaesthesia should be delayed in shocked patients until the blood pressure has risen above 100 and the pulse rate started to fall. If a large blood volume deficit is suspected one should be prepared while inducing anaesthesia to infuse larger amounts of blood under pressure. One should never be taken unawares by a further fall of blood pressure in such a patient and this may be best controlled by having two drips running simultaneously. Blood should be given under pressure as soon as the first signs of hypotension develop, when the level of anaesthesia is deepened.

Again and again there are cases when, because of persistent blood loss that will endanger the patient's life, surgery must be undertaken with the patient still in shock. In such cases, a very large quantity of blood must be held in reserve while anaesthesia is induced. Intraarterial transfusion is never actually necessary and in view of the possible complications we think it is actually contra-indicated. The same goal can be reached more rapidly and less dangerously if blood is given under pressure into two or more veins.

The victims of shock have usually suffered a certain loss of blood volume, but by the beginning of treatment the continued loss is usually arrested. Replacement then is the only treatment required, and this is a most important measure in the preparation for surgery and to avoid disturbance of the microcirculation. We believe that little is gained by delaying surgery for a long time in shocked patients and that much may be lost by doing so. JAHNKE and SEELEY (1953), during the Korean War, for example, performed half their vascular surgery immediately after combatting severe degrees of shock. Their injured patients had lost between 30 and 60% of their blood volume, but early surgery proved to be detrimental in no single case although many of these operations must have been of long duration.

We are still far from understanding the etiology and pathogenesis of severe shock in all its details. Fortunately, however, some guides can be established for surgery as follows:

1. In the stage of cold hypotensive tachycardia surgery should not be performed if possible.

2. Two to three hours of appropriate treatment are generally sufficient to enable the patient to undergo surgery. Thereafter he is able to withstand surgery, even of long duration.

The indications for surgery can therefore be based on consideration for the later full restoration of function of the injured part. The early internal fixation of broken bones with adequate prophylaxis against shock appears to have an additional value in the prevention of fat embolism.

Literature

ABEL, A.: Eine technische Neuerung zur blutigen Knochenbruchfeststellung mit einer in sich verschiebbaren Knochenplatte. Chirurg 23, 446 (1952).

ACKERMANN, W.: Ein kombiniertes Einschlag- und Ziehgerät für Marknägel. Chirurg 16, 93 (1944).

Acta orthop. belg. 24, Suppl. III (1958): Le traitement des traumatismes récents de la main. Journées Orthopédiques et Chirurgicales de Bruxelles, 8—14 mai 1958. Bruxelles: Editions Acta med. belg.

ADAMS, J. C.: Outline of fractures. London: Livingston Ltd. 1957.

ADERHOLD, K.: Mediale Bohrdrahtwanderung nach Schenkelhalsdrahtung. Zbl. Chir. 78, 2003 (1953).

AHNEFELD, F. W., u. M. ALLGÖWER: Der Schock. Entstehung, Verlauf und Therapie. Dtsch. med. Wschr. 87, 425 (1962).

AICHNER, H., u. G. RUPP: Die gedeckte Markdrahtung frischer, unstabiler, geschlossener Schaftbrüche des Vorderarmes. Chir. Praxis 1, 55 (1960).

ALBRECHT, K. F.: Seltene Komplikation nach Nagelung einer Schenkelhalspseudarthrose. Chirurg 27, 228 (1956).

ALLGÖWER, M.: Verschraubung von Tibiafrakturen. Helv. chir. Acta 28, 214 (1961).

— Indikation und Technik der Osteosynthese. Bericht über die Unfallchirurg. Tagg., Mainz 1962, S. 161.

— Toxic factors in shock. In: Shock, p. 240. Berlin-Göttingen-Heidelberg: Springer 1962.

— C. BURRI, P. VON GRAFFENRIED, U. F. GRUBER, U. HEIM, J. MENG, G. SEGMÜLLER, J. SIEGRIST u. E. STUDER: Quantitative Untersuchungen der Wirkung entzündungshemmender Substanzen bei Unterschenkelfrakturen. Schweiz. med. Wschr. 93, 565—567 (1963).

—, u. A. ROSIN: Das periossäre Gewebe des normalen und frakturierten Knochens in der Gewebekultur. Bull. schweiz. Akad. med. Wiss. 9, 181 (1953).

—, u. E. STUDER: Methodik und Ergebnisse einer Schnellbestimmung des Blutvolumens mit Jod^{131} in der Klinik. Arch. klin. Chir. 301, 122 (1962).

— M. E. MÜLLER, R. SCHENK u. H. WILLENEGGER: Biomechanische Prinzipien bei der Metallverwendung am Knochen. Arch. klin. Chir. 305, 1 (1963).

ANDREESEN, R.: Mangelhafte Knochenneubildung bei Innenknöchelbrüchen (Pseudarthrosen), ihre Verhütung und Behandlung. Zbl. Chir. 65, 2213 (1938).

— Schienbeinkopfbrüche und ihre Behandlung. Vorträge aus der praktischen Chirurgie, H. 41. Stuttgart: Ferdinand Enke 1955.

ARDEN, G. P.: Radioactive isotopes in fractures of the neck of the femur. J. Bone Jt. Surg. 42 B, 21 (1960).

ARENS, W.: Zur Behandlung schwerer offener Unterschenkelbrüche. Mschr. Unfallheilk. 60, 276 (1957).

ASHHURST, A., and R. BROMER: Classification and mechanism of fractures of the leg bones involving the ankle. Arch. Surg. 4, 51 (1922).

AXHAUSEN, W.: Die Hüftarthrosis nach Schenkelhalsnagelung. Wiederherstellungschir. u. Traum. 1, 162 (1953).

BALBI, E.: Spätresultate der Operation der habituellen Schulterluxation nach CLAIRMONT-EHRLICH an der Chirurgischen Universitätsklinik Zürich. Thesis Zürich 1946.

BANDI, W., u. M. ALLGÖWER: Zur Therapie der Osteochondritis dissecans. Helv. chir. Acta 26, 552 (1959).

—, u. G. SOMMER: Erfahrungen mit der Falzcerclage nach LEEMANN. Helv. chir. Acta 26, 95 (1959).

BARACCHINO, G.: Osteosynthese mit Metallschrauben bei Frakturen des hinteren Pfannenrandes des Hüftgelenks. Arch. Putti Chir. Organi Mov. 1, 99 (1951). Ref. Zbl. Chir. 77, 2347 (1952).

BARNETT, C. H., and I. N. NAPIER: The axis of rotation of the ankle joint in man. Its influence upon the form of the talus and the mobility of the fibula. J. Anat. (Lond.) 86, 1 (1952).

BASSETT, C. A. L.: Current Concepts of Bone Formation. J. Bone Jt. Surg. 44 A, 1217 (1962).

—, D. K. CREIGHTON, and F. E. STINCHFIELD: Contributions of endosteum, cortex, and soft tissues to osteogenesis. Surg. Gynec. Obstet. 112, 145 (1961).

BASSLEER, R., et. C. DESAIVE: Effets de faibles doses de béryllium sur la croissance et l'ossification d'ébauches osseuses d'embryons de poulet, cultivées en „roller tubes", C. R. Soc. Biol. (Paris) 154, 458 (1960).

BATEMAN, J. E.: Trauma to nerves in limbs. Philadelphia and London: W. B. Saunders Company 1962.

BAUD, B.: Coxa vara als Komplikation von fächerförmigen Drahtfixationen pertrochanterer Femurfrakturen. Chirurg 26, 468 (1955).

BAUER, K. H.: Frakturen und Luxationen. Berlin: Springer 1927

BAUERMEISTER, A.: Experimentelle Grundlagen für den Aufbau einer neuen Knochenbank. Mschr. Unfallheilk., Beiheft 58, 1958).

BAUMANN, E.: Die Fraktur als Notfall und ihre dringliche Versorgung. Helv. med. Acta 2, 191 (1935).

— Zur Behandlung der Knochenbrüche am Ellbogengelenk. Ber. VIII. Intern. Kongr. Unfallmed. u.Berufskr., 26.—30. 9. 1938, Frankfurt a. M.

— Ursache und Prophylaxe der Pseudarthrose des inneren Knöchels. Z. Unfallmed. Berufskr. 48, 3 (1955).

— Wirkliche und vermeintliche Wachstumsstörungen nach kindlichen Ellbogenbrüchen. Helv. chir. Acta 26, 577 (1959).

— Zur Behandlung der Knochenbrüche am Ellbogengelenk. Arch. klin. Chir. 295, 300 (1960).

— Zur Behandlung der Brüche des distalen Humerusendes beim Kind. Chir. Praxis 4, 317 (1960).

BAUMANN, W.: Zur Indikation der pertrochanteren Schenkelhalsnagelung. Zbl. Chir. **83**, 229 (1958).

BAUMGARTL, F., H. GREMMEL u. K. H. WILLMANN: Die Durchblutung von frakturierten Unterschenkeln während der Heilung an Hand von arteriographischen Untersuchungen. Zbl. Chir. **83**, 1386 (1958).

BAUR, E.: Zur Therapie der geschlossenen Unterschenkelschaftfrakturen. Schweiz. Unfallversicherungsanstalt, Mitt. **39** (1959).

BAYNE, L. G., H. MORRIS, and J. WICKSTROM: Evaluation of intramedullary fixation of the tibia with Lottes nail. Sth. med. J. (Bgham. Ala.) **53**, 1429 (1960).

BECHTOL, C. O., A. B. FERGUSON, and P. G. LAING: Metals and engineering in bone and joint surgery. Baltimore: Williams & Wilkins Co. 1959.

BECK, W.: Chirurgische Behandlung der Knöchelbrüche. Mschr. Unfallheilk. **42**, 241 (1951).

BEECHER, H. K., J. D. MacCARRELL, and E. J. EVANS: Barbiturates in traumatic and hemorrhagic shock. Ann. Surg. **116**, 658 (1942).

BELENGER, M., E. VANDERELST et R. MINEZ: Les séquelles des fractures malléolaires chez les accidentés du travail. Acta orthop. belg. **16**, 404 (1950).

BERENTEY, G.: Chirurgische Behandlung der pertrochanteren Brüche. Zbl. Chir. **81**, 1122 (1956).

— S. SOMOGYI u. G. PEER: Behandlung der Pseudarthrose des medialen Knöchels. Zbl. Chir. **81**, 832 (1956).

BERENYI, P. vide FORGON, M., u. P. BERENYI.

BERGENTZ, S.-E.: Studies on the genesis of posttraumatic fat embolism. Acta chir. scand., Suppl. **282** (1961).

BERGERMANN, H.: Die Behandlung geschlossener und offener Frakturen durch perkutane Fixierung unter Anwendung von Gewindedrähten mit Spannhaltevorrichtung. Bruns' Beitr. klin. Chir. **192**, 374 (1956).

BERGMANN, E.: Ulnarisspätlähmung nach Ellbogenbrüchen. Mschr. Psychiat. Neurol. **117**, 203 (1949).

BERNHART, G.: Erfahrungen mit der Marknagelung nach KÜNTSCHER bei Oberschenkelfrakturen am Kantonspital St. Gallen 1942—1945. Thesis Zürich 1947.

BESSLER, W., et M. MÜLLER: Le diagnostic précoce de la nécrose de la tête fémorale. Ann. Radiol. **4**, 21 (1961).

— — Autoradiographische Studien bei Femurkopfnekrose. Arch. orthop. Unfall-Chir. **53**, 320 (1961).

BISTRÖM, O.: Surgical treatment of non-union and delayed union of long bones. Acta orthop. scand. **24**, 160 (1955).

BLANGUERNON, S.: L'enclouage centro-médullaire des os longs, selon KÜNTSCHER. Son application au Kantonsspital de Winterthur. Rev. Chir. (Paris) **66**, 42 (1947).

BLANKE, K.: Die Spanplastik nach PHEMISTER. Theoretische Grundlagen, Indikationen, Technik und Ergebnisse. Hefte Unfallheilk. **53** (1956).

BLIESENER, R.: Über die durch die Bardenheuersche Extensionsmethode an den Brüchen der unteren Gliedmaßen erhaltenen funktionellen Ergebnisse. Langenbecks Arch. klin. Chir. **55**, 277 (1897).

BLOCH, H. R.: Die Druckplatten-Osteosynthese der Vorderarmschaftfrakturen. Helv. chir. Acta **30**, 98 (1963).

BLOCK, W.: Die percutane Drahtfixierung des Ellbogenbruchs. Mschr. Unfallheilk. **55**, 289 (1952).

— Die percutane Drahtfixierung bei Frakturen, Luxationen, Resektionen. Arch. orthop. Unfall-Chir. **46**, 619 (1954).

BLOUNT, W. P.: Fractures in children. Baltimore: Williams & Wilkins Co. 1955.

BLÜMEL, P.: Die Behandlung der pertrochanteren und infratrochanteren Oberschenkelbrüche mit der nichtsperrenden Laschenschraube. Brun's Beitr. klin. Chir. **191**, 85 (1955).

BLUM, H.: Beitrag zur operativen Behandlung der Unterschenkelfrakturen. Thesis Zürich 1956.

BOCCANERA, L., e. A. SLAVAGNI: Considerazioni sulla terapia delle gravi fratture comminute del gomito. Chir. Organi Mov. **50**, V (1961). Ref. Minerva ortop. **13**, 417 (1962).

BÖHLER, J.: Bankspanverpflanzung bei frischen Schaftbrüchen der langen Röhrenknochen. Chirurg **26**, 76 (1955).

— Gekreuzte Bohrdrähte, ein einfaches Prinzip der Osteosynthese. Arch. orthop. Unfall-Chir. **47**, 242 (1955).

— Operative Behandlung des Bruches des medialen Knöchels und des großen hinteren Schienbeinkeiles. Verh. dtsch. orthop. Ges., Beiheft Z. Orthop. **88**, 138 (1957).

BÖHLER, L.: Technik der Knochenbruchbehandlung, 12.—13. Aufl. Wien: W. Maudrich 1957.

— Neues zur Behandlung der Fersenbeinbrüche. Arch. klin. Chir. **287**, 698 (1957).

— Bericht über die bei 3308 Unterschenkelbrüchen in den Jahren 1926—1950 im Wiener Unfallkrankenhaus erzielten Behandlungsergebnisse unter Benützung des Hollerithverfahrens. Hefte Unfallheilk. **54** (1957).

BÖHLER, L. jr.: Kritik der operativen Behandlung von Knöchelbrüchen. Verh. dtsch. orthop. Ges., Beiheft Z. Orthop. **88**, 350 (1957).

— Behandlung der suprakondylären Oberarmbrüche bei Kindern und Jugendlichen. Mschr. Unfallheilk. **64**, 1 (1961).

— E. TROJAN u. H. JAHNA: Behandlungsergebnisse von 734 frischen einfachen Brüchen des Kahnbeinkörpers der Hand. Wiederherstellungschir. u. Traum. **2**, 86 (1954).

— jr.: Kritik der operativen Behandlung von Knöchelbrüchen. Verh. dtsch. orthop. Ges., Beiheft Z. Orthop. **88**, 350 (1957).

BOLIN, H.: The fibula and its relationship to the tibia and talus in injuries of the ankle due to forced extensal rotation. Acta radiol. (Stockh.) **56**, 439 (1961).

BONET, H.: Fracture de l'extrémité inférieure des deux os de l'avant-bras avec complications graves et inattendues. Acta orthop. belg. **21**, 217 (1955).

BONNIN, G. J.: Injuries of the ankle. London: William Heinemann, Medical Books Ltd. 1950.

BOTHE, R. T., L. E. BEATON, and H. A. DAVENPORT: Reaction of bone to multiple metallic implants. Surg. Gynec. Obstet. **71**, 598 (1940).

—, and H. A. DAVENPORT: Reaction of bone to metals; lack of correlation with electrical potentials. Surg. Gynec. Obstet. **74**, 231 (1942).

BOYD, H. B., and L. D. ANDERSON: Management of unstable trochanteric fractures. Surg. Gynec. Obstet. **112**, 633 (1961).

—, and R. B. KNIGHT: Fractures of the astragalus. Sth. med. J. (Bgham, Ala.) **35**, 160 (1942).

—, and ST. W. LIPINSKI: Nonunion of trochanteric and subtrochanteric fractures. Surg. Gynec. Obstet. **104**, 463 (1957).

— D. B. ZILVERSMIT, and R. A. CALANDRUCCIO: The use of radioactive phosphorus (P^{32}) to determine the viability of the head of the femur. J. Bone Jt. Surg. **37**A, 260 (1955).

BRAUN, W.: Über vollständige Verrenkungen und Verrenkungsbrüche im oberen Sprunggelenk. Zbl. Chir. **85**, 1256 (1960).

BRAUNSTEIN, P. W., and P. A. WADE: Treatment of unstable fractures of the ankle. Ann. Surg. **149**, 217 (1959).

BRAV, E. A.: Further evaluation of the use of intramedullary nailing in the treatment of gunshot fractures of the extremities. J. Bone Jt. Surg. **39**A, 513 (1957).

—, and V. H. JEFFRESS: Modified intramedullary nailing in recent gunshot fractures of the femoral shaft. J. Bone Jt. Surg. **35**A, 141 (1953).

BREITENFELDER, H.: Der lange Drehbruch des äußeren Knöchels. Spätschäden und ihre Verhütung. Verh. dtsch. orthop. Ges. ,Beiheft Z. Orthop. **88**, 333 (1957).

— Komplikationen während und nach der Nagelung der Epiphyseolysis capitis femoris und ihre Verhütung. Zbl. Chir. **85**, 2041 (1960).

BREMNER, A.-E., et C. K. WARRICK: Les fractures du calcanéum. Acta orthop. belg. **17**, 217 (1951).

BROCHER, J. E. W.: Die Wirbelsäulenleiden und ihre Differentialdiagnose, zweite erweiterte Aufl. Stuttgart: Georg Thieme 1959.

BRUCK, H., u. H. MOSER: Über die Cerclage bei Unterschenkelbrüchen. Arch. orthop. Unfall-Chir. **46**, 536 (1954).

BRÜCKNER, H.: Die perkutane Kirschner-Drahtfixation in der Fraktur- und Luxationsbehandlung. Zbl. Chir. **87**, 85 (1962).

BRÜTSCH, H., u. W. J. PIROZYNSKI: Zur Behandlung der pertrochanteren Frakturen. Helv. chir. Acta **15**, 209 (1948).

BRUNNER, W.: Unsere Erfahrungen mit der Marknagelung nach KÜNTSCHER. Z. Unfallmed. Berufskr. **40**, 103 (1947).

BRUSSATIS, F.: Technische Probleme der Osteosynthese. Verh. Dtsch. Orthop. Ges. 49. Kongr. Zürich 27. bis 30. 9. 1961. Stuttgart: Ferdinand Enke 1962.

—, u. M. E. MÜLLER: Metallbeschaffenheit und Korrosionserscheinungen an Platten und Schrauben. Arch. klin. Chir. **305**, 15 (1963).

BUCHBORN, E.: Handbuch für innere Medizin, 4. Aufl. Bd. IX. Berlin-Göttingen-Heidelberg: Springer 1952.

BUCK-GRAMCKO, D.: Zur metallischen Osteosynthese im Bereiche des oberen Sprunggelenkes. Arch. orthop. Unfall-Chir. **47**, 211 (1955).

BÜHLMANN, E.: Über die Behandlung der Navicularepseudarthrose mit Verschraubung. Z. Unfallmed. Berufskr. **41**, 253 (1948).

BÜRKLE DE LA CAMP, H.: Operative Knochenbruchbehandlung. Tagungsber. des Berufsgenossenschaftstags 1949 in München.

— Wandlungen und Fortschritte in der Lehre von den Knochenbrüchen. Arch. klin. Chir. **76**, 163 (1953).

— Auswirkungen der Fortschritte der Chirurgie auf die Unfallchirurgie. Hefte Unfallheilk. **45**, 1 (1953).

— Die Knochenregeneration bei der Transplantation kältekonservierten homoioplastischen Knochens. Ber. 16. Tgg. Internat. Ges. Chirurgie in Lissabon 1963. Bruxelles: Médical et Scient. 1954.

— Allgemeinchirurgische Grundsätze für operative Eingriffe. In: Chir. Operationslehre, Bd. 1. Wien: Urban & Schwarzenberg 1955.

— Grundzüge der operativen Technik und der plastischen Chirurgie. In: Chir. Operationslehre, Bd. 1. Wien: Urban & Schwarzenberg 1955.

— Gedanken zur Pseudarthrosenbehandlung. In: Festschrift „Leistungen und Ergebnisse der neuzeitlichen Chirurgie". Stuttgart: Georg Thieme 1958.

— Klinischer Erfahrungsbericht über chronische Folgen traumatischer Einwirkungen an den Stützgeweben. Verh. Dtsch. Ges. Pathologie, 43. Tgg. Stuttgart 1959. Stuttgart: Gustav Fischer.

— Die Druckosteosynthese und ihre Beziehungen zur Kallusentwicklung. Medizinische **37**, 1671 (1959).

— Knochentransplantationen. Kongreßber. d. XVIII. Tagg. der Soc. Internat. de Chirurgie in München 1959. Brüssel: Médical et Scient. 1960.

— Die einfachste Frakturenbehandlung einschließlich Extension. Arch. klin. Chir. **296**, 271 (1960).

— Betrachtungen über die Knochenverpflanzung. Med. Welt **3**, 139 (1960).

— Fehler und Gefahren bei der operativen Behandlung frischer Frakturen. Dtsch. Z. Chir. **298**, 87 (1961).

— Zum Thema: Eitrige Osteomyelitis und Unfall. Zbl. Chir. **86**, 1202 (1961).

— Plastiken und Transplantationen. In: Lehrbuch der Chirurgie, 3. Aufl. Stuttgart: Georg Thieme 1962.

BUHR, A. J., and A. M. COOKE: Fracture patterns. Lancet **1959**I, 531.

BURKHARDT, V., u. F. WEISS: Zur Behandlung von Frakturen mit Piacryl- und Igamid-B-Stiften. Zbl. Chir. 85, 1319 (1960).

BURMAN, M.: Primary torsional fracture of the radius of ulna. J. Bone Jt Surg. 35 A, 665 (1953).

BURRI, C.: Die Tibiapseudarthrose. Die Möglichkeit der Druckdosierung am Gerät nach KEY. Thesis Bern 1959.

BUXTORF, P.: Die Behandlung der Humerusfrakturen mittels Vertikalextension. Helv. med. Acta 4, 289 (1937).

CADEN, J. G.: Internal fixation of fractures of the forearm. J. Bone Jt Surg. 43 A, 1115 (1961).

CAMPBELL, C.: Operative orthopedics, vol. I, fifth edit. Saint Louis: C. V. Mosby Comp. 1964.

CARR, C. R., and D. TURNIPSEED: Experiences with intramedullary fixation of compound femoral fractures in war wounds. J. Bone Jt Surg. 35 A, 153 (1953).

CAUCHOIX, J.: Sur le traitement des pseudarthroses de la diphyse fémorale. Acta orthop. belg. 18, 1 (1952).

CAVE, E. F.: Carpus with reference to fractured navicular bone. Arch. Surg. 40, 54 (1940).

— Retroulnar dislocation of capitate with fracture or subluxation of naviculare bone. J. Bone Jt Surg. 23, 830 (1941).

— Medullary nails in pathological conditions of the femur. Amer. Ac. Orthop. Surg. Instr. C. Lect. VIII, 46 (1951).

— Injuries to the wrist joint. Amer. Ac. Orthop. Surg. Instr. C. Lect. VII, 1 (1953).

— Fractures and other injuries. Chicago: The Year Book Publishers Inc. 1958.

— Fractures of the femoral neck. Amer. Ac. Orthop. Surg. Instr. C. Lect. XVII, 79 (1960). St. Louis: G. V. Mosby Comp. 1960.

— J. T. NICHOLSON, F. E. WEST, W. R. MACAUSLAND JR., C. R. SULLIVAN, P. R. LIPSCOMB, R. G. EVANS, C. A. COBB, and J. W. HILLMAN: Symposium on fractures about the knee. Amer. Ac. Orthop. Surg. Instr. C. Lect. XVIII, 73 (1961). St. Louis: C. V. Mosby Comp. 1961.

CHANDLER, S. B., and P. H. KREUSHER: A study of the blood supply of the ligamentum teres and its relation to the circulation of the head of the femur. J. Bone Jt. Surg. 14, 834 (1932).

CHAPUT: Pronostic des fractures bimalléolaires. Bull. Soc. Chir. (Paris) 32, 927 (1906).

— Les fractures malléolaires du cou-de-pied et les accidents du travail. Paris: Masson & Cie. 1907.

— De la réduction des fractures malléolaires compliquées de luxation du pied. Bull. Soc. Chir. (Paris) 38, 656 (1913).

CHARNLEY, J.: Compression arthrodesis. Including central dislocation as a principle in hip surgery. Edinburgh: E. & S. Livingston Ltd. 1953.

— N. J. BLOCKEY, and D. W. PURSER: The treatment of displaced fractures of the neck of the femur by compression. J. Bone Jt Surg. 39 B, 45 (1957).

CLARKE, A. R.: Recent advances in haemorrhage and shock. Brit. med. J. 1957 II, 721.

CLARKE, E. G. C., and J. HICKMAN: Investigation into correlation between electrical potentials of metals and their behaviour in biological fluids. J. Bone Jt Surg. 35 B, 467 (1953).

CLAWSON, D. K.: Intertrochanteric fracture of the hip. Amer. J. Surg. 93, 580 (1957).

CLERMONT: Sur la disjonction tibio-péronière et les fractures du cou-de pied. Rev. Chir. (Paris) 47, 143 (1913).

CLEVELAND, M., D. M. BOSWORTH, and F. R. THOMPSON: Intertrochanteric fractures of the femur. J. Bone Jt Surg. 29, 1049 (1947).

— D. M. BOSWORTH, F. R. THOMPSON, H. J. WILSON JR., and T. ISHIZUKA: A ten-year analysis of intratrochanteric fractures of the femur. J. Bone Jt Surg. 41 A, 1399 (1959).

—, and G. FIELDING: A continuing end result study of intracapsular fractures of the neck of the femur. J. Bone Jt Surg. 36 A, 1020 (1954).

— and J. W. FIELDING: Intracapsular fracture of the neck of the femur. Amer. Ac. Orthop. Surg. Instr. C. Lect. XII, 35 (1955). Ann. Arbor: J. W. Edwards 1955.

COHEN, J.: Corrosion testing of orthopaedic implants. J. Bone Jt Surg. 44 A, 307 (1962).

COMPERE, E. L.: Treatment of osteomyelitis and infected wounds by closed irrigation with a detergent antibiotic solution. Acta orthop. scand. 32, 324 (1962).

CONSTENSOUX, G.: A propos d'un cas de paralysie tardive du nerf cubital survenue vingt-cinq ans après une fracture du coude. Rev. neruol. 1, 363 (1918).

CORDREY, L. J., and M. FERRER-TORELLS: Management of fractures of the greater multangular. J. Bone Jt Surg. 42 A, 1111 (1960).

CORNIOLEY, C.: Dans quelles conditions faut-il opérer les fractures graves du cou-de-pied (Genre Dupuytren)? Lyon chir. 26, 305 (1929).

CORRODI, E.: Die Ergebnisse der Behandlung frischer Unterschenkelfrakturen Erwachsener mittels Zugschraubenosteosynthese. I. Nachkontrolle einer geschlossenen Serie von 113 Fällen (Nov. 1957 bis Mai 1959). Thesis Basel 1962.

COWIE, R. S.: Fractures of the forearm treated by open reduction and plating. Brit. J. Surg. 44, 263 (1956).

COZZOLINO, A.: Risultati a distanze delle fratture dell'olecrano trattate cruememente. Arch. Ortop. (Milano) 72, 1594 (1959).

CREYSSEL, J., G. DE MOURGUES, J. GOUNAT et A. BOUCHET: Le fixateur externe d'HOFFMANN dans les fractures ouvertes de jambes. Lyon chir. 51, 241 (1956).

DAHLGREN, S.: Venography in fractures of the femoral neck. Acta chir. scand. 117, 494 (1959).

DANIS, R.: Théorie et pratique de l'ostéosynthèse. Paris: Masson & Cie. 1947.

— Le vrai but et les dangers de l'ostéosynthèse. Lyon chir. 51, 740 (1956).

Debeyre, J., et P. Doliveux: Arthroplasties de la hanche. Etude critique à propos de 200 cas opérés. Paris: Editions Médicales Flammarion 1954.

Debrunner, A. M.: Ergebnisse der Unterschenkelbruchbehandlung am Bürgerspital Solothurn 1954—1958. Thesis Zürich 1961.

Decoulx, P., et. J. P. Razemon: La pression interfragmentaire dans l'ostéosynthèse. Lyon chir. 51, 211 (1956).

Delaney, M. W., and D. M. Street: Fracture of femoral shaft with fracture of neck of same femur. Treatment with medullary nail for shaft and Knowles pins for neck. J. int. Coll. Surg. 19, 303 (1953).

Delaunoy, A.: Quelques cas d'ostéosynthèse métallique chez le noir africain. Acta orthop. belg. 21, 139 (1955).

Demark, G. E. van, and R. E. van Demark: Hip nailing in patients of eighty years or older. Amer. J. Surg. 85, 664 (1953).

Desenfans, G.: Notes à propos de la fracture de Monteggia chez l'adulte. Acta orthop. belg. 16, 520 (1950).

—·, et H. Evrard: Le traitement chirurgical des fractures du cou-de-pied. Acta orthop. belg. 18, 303 (1952).

Detzel, H.: Traumatische Hüftluxation mit Femurfraktur — eine seltene Unfallfolge. Mschr. Unfallheilk. 56, 1 (1953).

Dickson, J. A.: The "unsolved" fracture. A protest against defeatism. J. Bone Jt Surg. 35A, 805 (1953).

Dienberg, F. J.: Ermüdungsbruch der linken Ulna bei einem 24jährigen Mann und die sich daraus ergebenden Probleme. Arch. orthop. Unfall-Chir. 49, 15 (1957).

Diener, A., Dörr u. K. O. Herrmann: Untersuchungen und Ergebnisse der physikalischen und physiologischen Gesetzmäßigkeiten bei der Anwendung von Kunststoff in der Knochenchirurgie. Zbl. Chir. 81, 2376 (1956).

Dietl, H.: Über die Sprengung der Knöchelgabel, ihre Erkennung und Behandlung. Zbl. Chir. 81, 2154 (1956).

Dohn, K.: Luxatio acromio-clavicularis supraspinata. Acta orthop. scand. 25, 183 (1956).

Dowling, J. J., and J. R. Sawyer: Comminuted Colles' fractures. J. Bone Jt Surg. 43A, 657 (1962).

Drapanas, Th., J. McDonald, and H. W. Hale jr.: A rational approach to classification and treatment of the surgical neck of the humerus. Amer. J. Surg. 99, 617 (1960).

Drescher, C.: Über Nagelungen am Schenkelhals. Zbl. Chir. 83, 959 (1958).

Dressler, W.: Ein Beitrag zum Krankheitsbild der arthrogenen Ulnarislähmung (Ulnaris-Spätlähmung). Chirurg 29, 487 (1958).

Droste, W. v.: Die sog. zentrale Hüftgelenkluxation (Pfannengrundbruch) und ihre Behandlung. Arch. orthop. Unfall-Chir. 45, 1 (1952).

Düben, W.: Konservative oder operative Behandlung veralteter Kahnbeinbrüche und -pseudarthrosen. Arch. klin. Chir. 295, 309 (1960).

Duesberg, R., u. W. Schröder: Pathophysiologie und Klinik des Kollapszustandes. Leipzig: S. Hirzel 1944.

—·, u. H. Spitzbarth: Klinik und Therapie der Kollapszustände. Stuttgart: Friedr.-Karl Schattauer 1963.

Dupuis, P. V.: Etude des diverses variétés des fractures en écuelle du plateau tibial externe et leur traitement. Acta orthop. belg. 21, 113 (1955).

Dupuy de Frenelle et F. A. Maloine: Techniques des opérations et pansements plaies de guerre. Paris: 1916.

Dupuytren, G.: Leçons orales de clinique chirurgicale 2e édit., vol. 1, p. 378. Paris: Germer-Baillière 1839.

Dziadek, J.: Extraartikuläre Nagelung des Schenkelhalsbruches ohne Hilfsapparate. Zbl. Chir. 83, 1847 (1958).

Earle: Simple, succeeded by compound dislocation forwards, of the inferior extremity of the tibia. Lancet 1828/29II, 346.

Eckmann, L.: Tetanus. Prophylaxe und Therapie. Basel u. Stuttgart: Benno Schwabe 1960.

Edwards, P.: Internal fracture fixation with Rush's pin. Experiences of a series of 116 cases. Acta chir. scand. 117, 480 (1959).

Eggeling, W., R. Panzner u. K. Hübner: Behandlungsergebnisse konservativ und operativ behandelter Unterschenkelschaftbrüche in der Chirurgischen Universitätsklinik Halle/Saale in den letzten 10 Jahren. Bruns' Beitr. klin. Chir. 199, 289 (1959).

Eggers, G. W. N.: The contact splint. Rep. Biol. Med. 4, 42 (1946).

— Internal contact splint. J. Bone Jt Surg. 30A, 40 (1948).

— W. H. Ainsworth, T. O. Shindler, and Ch. M. Pomerat: Clinical significance of the contact-compression factor in bone surgery. Arch. Surg. 62, 467 (1951).

— Th. O. Shindler, and Ch. M. Pomerat: The influence of the contact-compression factor on osteogenesis in surgical fractures. J. Bone Jt Surg. 31A, 693 (1949).

Ehalt, W.: Erfahrungen mit der Marknagelung nach Küntscher. Zbl. Chir. 69, 1849 (1942).

— Nagelung pertrochanterer Oberschenkelbrüche. Z. Orthop. 80, 3 (1950).

— Erfahrungen bei der Marknagelung offener Unterschenkelbrüche. Arch. orthop. Unfall-Chir. 44, 500 (1951).

Eiermann, H.: Das teleologische Prinzip in der Lehre von der Frakturheilung. Dtsch. med. Wschr. 85, 384, 395 (1960).

Emneus, H., u. U. Stenram: Reaction of tissues to alloys used in osteosynthesis. Acta orthop. scand. 29, 315 (1960).

Ender, J.: Behandlung der intraartikulären Schenkelhalsbrüche und ihre Folgen mit Ergebnissen der Nachuntersuchung. Arch. orthop. Unfall-Chir. 45, 237 (1952).

— H. Krotschek u. R. Simon-Weidner: Die Chirurgie der Handverletzungen. Wien: Springer 1956.

Endler, F.: Die medikamentöse Lokalbehandlung der Osteomyelitis und ihre Ergebnisse. Wien. med. Wschr. 107, 653 (1957).

ENZLER, A.: Spätresultate der Operationen nach EDEN und EDEN-BRUN bei habitueller Schulterluxation. Thesis Zürich 1946.

ERIKSSON, E., O. SAHLIN and U. SANDAHL: Late results of conservative and surgical treatment of fractures of the olecranon. Acta chir. scand. **113**, 153 (1957).

ERLER, F.: Zur Arthrodese des hinteren unteren Sprunggelenks, insbesondere nach früherem Fersenbeinbruch. Chirurg **27**, 512 (1956).

EVANS, D. L.: Fatigue fractures of the ulna. J. Bone Jt Surg. **37**B, 618 (1955).

EVANS, E. M.: Fractures of the radius and ulna. J. Bone Jt Surg. **33**B, 548 (1951).

— Trochanteric fractures. A review of 110 cases treated by nail-plate fixation. J. Bone Jt Surg. **33**B, 192 (1951).

EVANS, F. G.: Stress and strain in bones. Their relation to fractures and osteogenesis. Springfield: Ch. C. Thomas 1957.

FACKERT, S.: Zur operativen Behandlung von Knöchelbrüchen und -pseudarthrosen. Arch. orthop. Unfall-Chir. **46**, 513 (1954).

FASEL, A.: Wiederholte Oberschenkelbrüche bei einem Jugendlichen und Unfallbegutachtung. Mschr. Unfallheilk. **63**, 270 (1960).

FAYSSE, R., et A. LAPRAS: Résultats du traitement des fractures de l'extrémité supérieure du radius. Lyon chir. **57**, 101 (1961).

FEHR, A.: Die Drahtnaht des geschlossenen Unterschenkelspiralbruches. Erfahrungen mit der grundsätzlichen und frühen Operation. Helv. chir. Acta **12**, 233 (1945).

FEHR, A. M.: Die Behandlung der Pseudarthrose und ihre Ergebnisse. Helv. chir. Acta **20**, 355 (1963).

—, u. W. RIEBEN: Weitere Erfahrungen mit Phemisterplastik. Helv. chir. Acta **21**, 411 (1954).

FELSENREICH, F.: Untersuchungen über die Pathologie des sog. Volkmannschen Dreieckes neben Richtlinien moderner Behandlung schwerer Luxationsfrakturen des oberen Sprunggelenkes. Arch. orthop. Unfall-Chir. **29**, 491 (1931).

— Die percutane Nagelung des sog. Volkmannschen Dreiecks. Arch. klin. Chir. **169**, 712 (1932).

— Schlottergelenke nach Malleolarfrakturen. Arch. orthop. Unfall-Chir. **37**, 149 (1936/37).

— Die Klinik der „posttraumatischen Arthritis" und verwandter Zustände. Wien. med. Wschr. 87, 1140, 1163 (1937).

FERGUSON, A. B., Y. AKAHOSHI, P. G. LAING and E. S. HODGE: Trace metal ion concentration in the liver, kidney, spleen and lung of normal rabbits. J. Bone Jt Surg. **44**A, 317, 313 (1962).

—, P. G. LAING and E. S. HODGE: The ionization of metal implants in living tissues. J. Bone Jt Surg. **42**A, 77 (1960).

FICK, K. F.: Ergebnisse von 921 mittels Marknagelung nach KÜNTSCHER versorgten Unterschenkelbrüchen. Arch. klin. Chir. **287**, 713 (1957).

FINK, C. G., and J. S. SMATKO: Bone fixation and the corrosion resistance of stainless steels to the fluids of the human body. J. electrochem. Soc. **94**, 271 (1948).

FINK, R.: Die Marknagelung nach KÜNTSCHER bei multiplen Frakturen. Z. Unfallmed. Berufskr. **49**, 162 (1956).

FISCHER, H. G.: Nagelverbiegung nach Küntscher-Nagelung, zugleich ein Beitrag zur Pseudarthrosebehandlung. Zbl. Chir. **81**, 1133 (1956).

FISCHER-WASELS, J., u. H. B. SCHÜNEMANN: Zur Frage der Marknagelung. Arch. orthop. Unfall-Chir. **46**, 207 (1953).

FLEMING, A.: Penicillin. London 1950.

FLEMING, J. L.: The pugh nail in the treatment of hip fractures. Surg. Clin. N. Amer. **39**, 1507 (1959).

FLOREY, M. E., and H. W. FLOREY: General and local administration of penicillin. Lancet **1943**I, 387.

FORD, L. T., J. O. LOTTES and J. A. KEY: Experimental study of the effect of pressure on the healing of bone grafts. Arch. Surg. **62**, 475 (1951).

FORGON, M.: Percutane Drahtfixation der suprakondylären Oberarmbrüche der Kinder. Arch. orthop. Unfall-Chir. **46**, 338 (1954).

— Über percutane Schenkelhalsnagelung (Vereinfachung der Technik). Zbl. Chir. **81**, 109 (1956).

— Über percutane Hülsendruckosteosynthese. Chirurg **28**, 67 (1957).

—, u. P. BERENYI: Die Versorgung des typischen Speichenbruches mit Drahtfixation durch die Elle. Arch. orthop. Unfall-Chir. **47**, 70 (1955).

— — Technisches zur orthopädischen Unfallchirurgie von Malleolarfrakturen und -pseudarthrosen. Arch. orthop. Unfall-Chir. **50**, 182 (1958).

FORSSMANN, W.: Die Versorgung von Knochenbrüchen aus der Sicht des mittleren Krankenhauses. Ther. Umsch. **19**, 2 (1962).

FRANK, E., u. F. KISSLER: Gedeckte Markdrahtung beim Querbruch des Unterschenkels und isolierten Schienbeinbruch. Chirurg **31**, 206 (1960).

FREDENHAGEN, H.: Die Stufenbildung im oberen Sprunggelenk. Z. Unfallmed. Berufskr. **50**, 204 (1957).

FRIEDENBERG, Z. B., and G. FRENCH: The effect of known compression forces on fracture healing. Surg. Gynec. Obstet. **94**, 743 (1952).

FRIEDMAN, PH.: The Phemister method in the treatment of pseudarthrosis. Thesis Bern 1958.

FRIEDRICH, P. L.: Die aseptische Versorgung frischer Wunden unter Mitteilung von Tierversuchen über die Auskeimungszeit von Infektionserregern in frischen Wunden. Langenbeck's Arch. klin. Chir. **57**, 288 (1898).

FRIES, L., u. H. WILLENEGGER: Spätresultate nach gebolzten Tibiakopfbrüchen. Z. Unfallmed. Berufskr. **53**, 242 (1959).

FRITSCHE, E.: Experimentelle Untersuchungen zur Frage der Fettembolie mit spezieller Berücksichtigung prophylaktischer und therapeutischer Vorschläge. Dtsch. Z. Chir. **107**, 456 (1910).

FUCHS, G., u. H. KÄMMERER: Indikation zur konservativen Behandlung des Innenknöchelbruches und zur operativen Versorgung mit dem Rush-Pin. Chirurg **31**, 254 (1960).

FÜRMAIER, A.: Zur Diagnose und Therapie der Bandverletzungen und Gabelsprengungen am oberen Sprung-gelenk. Arch. orthop. Unfall-Chir. **44**, 541 (1951).

GALLAGHER, J. T. F.: Ankle fractures, transarticular pin fixation in fracture dislocations. Amer. J. Surg. **79**, 573 (1950).

GANDOLFI, M., e. S. ZANOLI: La frattura isolata dell'eminenza capitata. Arch. Ortop. (Milano) **72**, 1485—1493 (1959).

GANZONI, R.: Messungen bei Frakturhämatomen. Helv. chir. Acta **26**, 35 (1959).

GASSER, H.: Personal communication.

GATELLIER, J.: The juxtoretroperoneal route in the operative treatment of fracture of the malleolus with posterior marginal fragment. Surgey **52**, 67 (1931).

GAY, J. R., and J. G. LOVE: Diagnosis and treatment of tardy paralysis of ulnar nerve. Based on a study of 100 cases. J. Bone Jt Surg. **29**, 1087 (1947).

GEISER, M.: Kritische Bemerkungen zur Frage der Cerclage von Torsions- und Schrägfrakturen des Schaft-knochens, insbesondere der Tibia. Schweiz. med. Wschr. **88**, 137 (1958).

GELBKE, H.: Tierversuche zur Frage der Frakturcallus- und Pseudarthrosenentstehung. (Eine Analyse der Experimente und Schlüsse OBERDALHOFFs.) Arch. klin. Chir. **277**, 306 (1953).

— Die „dynamische Osteosynthese" nach RUSH, eine wertvolle Vervollständigung der Küntscher-Nagelung. Chirurg **26**, 529 (1955).

— Inwiefern ist die intramedulläre Frakturfixation nach RUSH etwas Neuartiges und Wertvolles in der Unfall-chirurgie. Hefte Unfallheilk. **55**, 237 (1956).

—, u. H. DZIEKAN: Spätergebnisse genagelter Schenkelhalsfrakturen. Zbl. Chir. **77**, 316 (1952).

GELIN, L. E.: Studies in anemia of injury. Acta chir. scand., Suppl. 210 (1956).

GIANNESTRAS, N. J.: Primary bone graft with pinning of intracapsular fractures of the femur. Amer. J. Surg. **93**, 588 (1957).

GIESEKING, H.: Die Nagelung als Behandlungsmaßnahme beim frischen und alten Kahnbeinbruch. Z. Orthop. **80**, 597 (1950/51).

GISSANE, W.: A dangerous type of fracture of the foot. J. Bone Jt Surg. **33**B, 535 (1951).

GLÖCKNER, U.: Vereinfachte Schenkelhalsnagelung. Zbl. Chir. **78**, 700 (1953).

GÖTHMAN, L.: Arterial changes in experimental fractures of the monkey's tibia treated with intramedullary nailing. A microangiographic study. Acta chir. scand. **121**, 56 (1961).

GOLDMAN, M. A., R. K. JOHNSON, and N. M. GROSSBERG: New approach to chronic osteomyelitis. Ortho-pedics, April 1960.

GOSSET, J.: A propos du traitement des fractures ouvertes des jambes. Actualités Chir. orthop. et rép. p. 12. Paris: Expansions Sci. 1959.

GRAF, R., u. H. WERNER: Die Phlebographie des Schenkelkopfes bei der frischen medialen Schenkelhalsfraktur. Fortschr. Röntgenstr. **92**, 331 (1960).

GRAFFENRIED, P. VON, u. M. ALLGÖWER: Frakturen und Fettembolie. Z. Unfallmed. Berufskr. **57**, (1964), in Press.

GRANT, R. T., and E. B. REEVE: Observations on the general effects of injury in man (with special reference to wound shock). Spec. Rep. Ser. med. Res. Counc. (Lond.) No. 277 (1951).

GRAU, E.: Behandlung der Luxationsfrakturen des oberen Sprungggelenkes mit Längssprengung aus der Tibia (sog. Volkmann-Dreieck) mit Extension und percutaner Fixation durch einen Kirschner-Draht. Mschr. Unfallheilk. **58**, 345 (1955).

GREIFENSTEINER, H.: Die operative Behandlung der Unterschenkelpseudarthrose und Unterschenkelbrüche mit verzögerter Kallusbildung unter besonderer Berücksichtigung der Kompressions-Osteosynthese. Bruns' Beitr. klin. Chir. **187**, 219 (1953).

GREISSINGER, H., u. H. KEISSLER: Zur Behandlung des medialen Schenkelhalsbruches mit dem Laschennagel. Chirurg **31**, 176 (1960).

GRENSHAW, A. H., and F. D. WILSON: The surgical treatment of fractures of the patella. Sth. med. J. (Bgham, Ala.) **47**, 716 (1954).

GRUBER, U. F., and M. ALLGÖWER: The use of the Volemetron for blood volume measurements. Bull. Soc. int. Chir. **23**, 218 (1964).

—, u. J. SIEGRIST: Der Volumeneffekt verschiedener Plasmaersatzstoffe. Arch. klin. Chir. **301**, 128 (1962).

GRUSS, D.: Spätresultate nach operativ behandelter habitueller Schulterluxation. Thesis Basel 1952.

GURLT, E.: Handbuch der Lehre von den Knochenbrüchen. Berlin 1862.

HACHEZ-LEBLANC, M.: Le vissage direct des fractures trimalléolaires basses par torsion avec diastasis tibio-astragalien. Acta orthop. belg. **16**, 307 (1950).

HACKETHAL, K. H.: Küntscher- oder Rush-Nagelung? Arch. klin. Chir. **287**, 703 (1957).

— Die Bündelnagelung. Wien: Springer 1961.

HÄBLER, C.: Die Leistungsfähigkeit der verschiedenen Osteosynthese-Methoden bei frischen geschlossenen Brüchen. Chirurg **22**, 433 (1952).

HÄUPTLI, O.: Unsere Erfahrungen mit der Cerclage der Unterschenkelfrakturen. Z. Unfallmed. Berufskr. **49**, 147 (1956).

HAFNER, R. H. V.: Trochanteric fractures of the femur. A review of eighty cases with a description of the "low-nail" method of internal fixation. J. Bone Jt. Surg. **33**B, 513 (1951).

HAINZL, H.: Zur Knochenbolzung der Kahnbeinpseudarthrose. Zbl. Chir. **82**, 1708 (1957).

HALSTENBACH, H.: Über die Behandlung der Frakturen des proximalen Femurendes (unter Ausschluß der intrakapsulären Schenkelhalsfraktur). Thesis Bern 1959.

HAMPTON, O. P., and W. T. FITTS JR.: Open reduction of common fractures. New York: Grune & Stratton 1959.

—, and E. P. HOLT: The present status of intramedullary nailing of fractures of the tibia. Amer. J. Surg. **93**, 597 (1957).

HAUCK, G. J.: Die individuelle Behandlung des Drehbruchs. Chirurg **27**, 16 (1956).

HEDENBERG, I., and R. POMPEIUS: Shaft fractures of the lower leg. Comparing the early results of open and closed treatment in 120 cases. Acta chir. scand. **118**, 339 (1959/60).

HEDSTRÖM, Ö.: End results in the treatment of Monteggia fractures. Acta orthop. scand. **32**, 46 (1962).

HEINZEL, J.: Behandlungsergebnisse der kindlichen Oberschenkelfrakturen der letzten 10 Jahre. Arch. klin. Chir. **295**, 309 (1960).

HEISE, E.: Zur Behandlung der Pseudarthrose nach KÜNTSCHER. Mschr. Unfallheilk. **63**, 88 (1960).

HELFERICH, HRCH.: Atlas und Grundriß der traumatischen Frakturen und Luxationen. 10. neubearb. und vermehrte Aufl. München: J. F. Lehmann 1922.

HELLNER, H.: Die haematogene Osteomyelitis und ihre Behandlung. Vorträge aus der praktischen Chirurgie. Stuttgart: Ferdinand Enke 1954.

HENKE, G.: Vergleichende Ergebnisse der konservativen und operativen Knöchelbruchbehandlung unter Berücksichtigung der Einteilung nach NIELS LAUGE-HANSEN. Diss. Basel 1962.

HENSCHEN, C.: Behandlung der medialen Schenkelhalsbrüche durch femoro-pelvine Auffädelungsverschraubung. Med. Welt **7**, 474 (1933).

HENSELL, V.: Die arthrogene Ulnarislähmung. Zbl. Chir. **78**, 1999 (1953).

HERRMANN, L.: Ein fixierender Kunststoffverband. Zbl. Chir. **83**, 1171 (1958).

HERZOG, H.: Die suprakondyläre Humerusfraktur. Thesis Zürich 1943.

HERZOG, K.: Die Nagelung von Oberarmbrüchen mit geradem, starrem Marknagel. Mschr. Unfallheilk. Beiheft, **42**, 224, 226 (1951).

— Verlängerungsosteotomie unter Verwendung des percutan gezielt verriegelten Marknagels. Hefte Unfallheilk. **42**, 221 (1951).

— Die geborgte Kraft als Behandlungsprinzip der Knochenbrüche. Hefte Unfallheilk. **43**, 203 (1952).

— Nagelung der Tibiaschaftbrüche mit einem starren Nagel. Dtsch. Z. Chir. **276**, 227 (1953).

— Technik und Ergebnisse von Nagelungen schwieriger Tibiabrüche und Pseudarthrosen. Arch. klin. Chir. **287**, 693 (1957).

— Die Technik der geschlossenen Marknagelung frischer Tibiafrakturen mit dem Rohrschlitznagel. Chirurg **29**, 501 (1958).

— Die Behandlung von Tibiabrüchen mit Rohrschlitznägeln. Zbl. Chir. **83**, 512 (1958).

— Über die Eignung dicker Marknägel (Rohrschlitznägel) zur Behandlung von Tibiapseudarthrosen unter Belassung des Pseudarthrosengewebes. Chirurg **31**, 21 (1960).

— Die Technik der geschlossenen Marknagelung des Oberschenkels mit dem Rohrschlitznagel. Chirurg **31**, 465 (1960).

HICKS, J. H.: Pathological effects from surgical metal, modern trends in surgical material. London: L. Gillis 1958.

— External splintage as a cause of movement in fractures. Lancet **1960** I, 667.

— Fractures of the forearm treated by rigid fixation. J. Bone Jt. Surg. **43**B, 680 (1961).

HILL, ST. A.: Practical points in elbow fractures. Sth. med. J. (Bgham, Ala.) **47**, 26 (1954).

HILTBRUNNER, A.: Erfahrungen mit 51 mit Falzcerclagen (Spanninstrument Leemann) behandelten Unterschenkeltorsionsfrakturen. Z. Unfallmed. Berufskr. **48**, 207 (1955).

HINDMARSCH, J., and L. UNANDER-SCHARIN: Osteosynthesis in pseudarthrosis of the humerus diaphysis. Acta orthop. scand. **32**, 121 (1962).

HIPPS, H. E.: Surgical repair of patellar fractures. Amer. J. Surg. **101**, 198 (1961).

HÖNEISEN, H.: Die Knöchelfrakturen des Jahres 1945. Thesis Zürich 1949.

HOFFA, A.: Lehrbuch der Frakturen und Luxationen. IV. Aufl. Stuttgart: Ferdinand Enke 1904.

HOFFMANN, R.: L'Osteotaxis. Paris: Editions Gead 1951.

— Enclouage médullaire et „ostéotaxis". Lyon chir. **50**, 309 (1955).

HOFMEISTER, F.: Die orthopädisch-chirurgische Behandlung der traumatisch bedingten Schenkelkopfnekrosen. Arch. orthop. Unfall-Chir. **49**, 556 (1958).

HOHL, M., and J. V. LUCK: Fractures of the tibial condyle. J. Bone Jt Surg. **38**A, 100 (1956).

HOHMANN, G.: Zur Behandlung der frischen und der veralteten schlecht verheilten Knöchelbrüche. Arch. orthop. Chir. **44**, 271 (1950).

— Fuß und Bein. München: J. F. Bergmann 1951.

HOLDER, E.: Die Doppelfrakturen einer Extremität. Arch. klin. Chir. **279**, 402 (1954).

HOSSLI, G., u. R. GATTIKER: Aufgaben des Anaesthesisten bei der Behandlung der Fettembolie. Anaesthesist **9**, 285—291 (1960).

HUGGLER, A.: Zuggurtung der Patella. Z. Unfallmed. Berufskr. **57** (1964), in Press.

HUGHSTON, J. C.: Fracture of the distal radial shaft. J. Bone Jt Surg. **39** A, 249 (1957).

HULLIGER, L.: Personal communication.

HULTH, A.: Fermoral head phlebography. A method of predicting viability. J. Bone Jt Surg. **40** B, 844 (1958).

HUNDEMER, W.: Beitrag zur extraartikulären Knochenbolzung der Kahnbeinpseudarthrose der Hand. Zbl. Chir. **77**, 274 (1952).

HUNT, J. R.: Tardy or late paralysis of the ulnar nerve. A form of chronic progressive neuritis developing many years after fracture dislocation of the elbow joint. J. Amer. med. Ass. **66**, 11 (1916).

ILLES, T.: Die Behandlung der Knochenbrüche mit perkutaner kortikaler Fixation. Zbl. Chir. **81**, 1089 (1956).

INGRAM, A. J., and B. BACHYNSKI: Fractures of the hip in children. Treatment and results. J. Bone Jt Surg. **35** A, 867 (1953).

ISLER, W.: Über die Indikation zur Osteotaxis nach HOFFMANN. Helv. chir. Acta **18**, 289 (1951).

JACKSON, R. A., and I. MACNAB: Fractures of the shaft of the tibia. Amer. J. Surg. **97**, 543 (1959).

JANIK, B.: Zur Behandlung der subcapitalen Oberarmbrüche und -pseudarthrosen durch Aufstülpung der Fragmente. Bruns' Beitr. klin. Chir. **190**, 196 (1955).

JANTZEN, P. M.: Zur Drahtumschlingung bei Unterschenkelbruch des Skiläufers. Münch. med. Wschr. **102**, 718 (1960).

JERGESEN, F.: Open reduction of fractures and dislocations of the ankle. Amer. J. Surg. **98**, 136 (1959).

JEWETT, E. L.: New approach for subtrochanteric and upper femoral shaft fractures using a dual flange nail plate. Amer. J. Surg. **81**, 186 (1951).

— Rigid internal fixation of intracapsular femoral neck fractures. Amer J. Surg. **91**, 621 (1956).

JINKINS, W. J., L. D. LOCKHART, and G. W. N. EGGERS: Fractures of the forearm in adults. Sth. med. J. (Bgham, Ala.) **53**, 669 (1960).

JOHNSON, W., R. C. HICKSON, B. E. MALSTROM, and E. G. BEHRENDTS: Fracture of the forearm. J. int. Coll. Surg. **11**, 175 (1951).

JONAS, J.: Bimalleolarfraktur mit Absprengung des hinteren Dreiecks. Thesis Zürich 1954.

JUDET, J.: Traitement des fractures du coup-de pied et des cals vicieux du cou-de-pied. Acta orthop. belg. **16**, 436 (1950).

— R. JUDET, J. LAGRANGE et J. DUNOYER: Résection — reconstruction de la hanche. Arthroplastie par prothèse acrylique. Paris: L'Expansion scientifique française, Editeur 1952.

— — — — A study of the arterial vascularisation of the femoral neck in the adult. J. Bone Jt Surg. **37** A, 663 (1955).

—, et J. LAGRANGE: Fractures des membres chez l'enfant. Paris: Librairie Maloine 1958.

JUNGE, H.: Stabile Osteosynthese bei der subtrochanteren Femurfraktur. Chirurg **28**, 120 (1957).

JUNGHANNS, H.: Die Brüche des knienahen Unterschenkelabschnittes (Schienbeinkopfbrüche). Arch. klin. Chir. **276**, 242 (1953).

KAPLAN, E. B.: Surgical approach to the lateral (peroneal) side of the knee joint. Surg. Gynec. Obstet. **104**, 346 (1957).

KAPLAN, I. W., and C. C. CRAIGHEAD: Two-plane fixation of fractures of the femoral shaft with Eggers' plates. Amer. J. Surg. **89**, 862 (1955).

KARITZKY, B.: Zur Marknagelung von Frakturen der langen Röhrenknochen. Zbl. Chir. **77**, 148 (1953).

KARLINGER, T., u. J. SAS: Die Rolle mechanischer Faktoren in der Kallusbildung (eine experimentelle Arbeit). I. Durch Marknagelung gewonnene Angaben. Bruns' Beitr. klin. Chir. **202**, 265 (1961).

KARNBAUM, S.: Zur Behandlung der pertrochanteren Oberschenkelfraktur. Chirurg **26**, 312 (1955).

KAUCKY, B.: Klinische Erfahrungen mit Knochenmarksnagelung von infizierten Brüchen. Rozhl. Chir. **35**, 363 (1956). Ref. Zbl. Chir. **82**, 932 (1957).

KEIL, H. R.: Ergebnisse der Behandlung offener und geschlossener Unterschenkelschaftbrüche. Zbl. Chir. **84**, 142 (1959).

KEIL, W.: Über ein Hilfsgerät zur Entfernung tiefsitzender oder gebrochener Schenkelhalsnägel. Zbl. Chir. **77**, 1407 (1952).

— „Re"fraktur eines kindlichen Oberschenkels nach Drahtumschlingung. Zbl. Chir. **83**, 1938 (1958).

KENNEDY, J. C., R. M. McFARLANE, and A. D. McLACHLIN: The Moe plate in intertrochanteric fractures of the femur. J. Bone Jt Surg. **39** B, 450 (1957).

KESSLER, G.: Beitrag zur Frage der operativen Behandlung geschlossener Unterschenkeltorsionsbrüche mit der Drahtringnaht. Thesis Basel 1952.

KEY, J. A.: Stainless steel and vitallium in internal fixation of bone. Comparison. Arch. Surg. **43**, 615 (1941).

—, and J. O. LOTTES: Complications and errors in technique in medullary fixation of the femur. Amer. Ac. Orthop. Surg. Instr. C. Lect. VIII, 27 (1951). Ann Arbor: J. W. Edwards.

—, and F. C. REYNOLDS: The treatment of infection after medullary nailing. Surgery **35**, 749 (1954).

KEYER, T. F.: Simple method of blind nailing for fractured neck of the femur. Amer. J. Surg. **80**, 571 (1950).

KING, T.: Recurrent dislocation of the elbow. J. Bone Jt Surg. **35** B, 50 (1953).

KIRSCH, J.: Die Stabilität des Küntscher-Nagels. Ein Beitrag zur Marknagelung. Mschr. Unfallheilk. **62**, 143 (1959).

KLEIGER, B.: The mechanism of ankle injuries. J. Bone Jt Surg. **38**A, 59 (1956).

KLEIN, A., R. J. JOPLIN, J. A. REIDY, and J. HANELIN: Slipped capital femoral epiphysis. Springfield: Ch. C. Thomas 1953.

KLÖSS, J.: Zur Osteosynthese der Ellbogengelenksbrüche. Vortrag Tagg. Mittelrhein. Chirurgen, Würzburg 1961.

—, u. S. WELLER: Möglichkeiten und Grenzen der Osteosynthese bei Ellbogengelenksfrakturen. Vortrag Mittelrhein. Chirurgen, Schaffhausen 1962.

KLOSE, H., u. B. JANIK: Spezielle Chirurgie (H. KLOSE). Frakturen und Luxationen (B. JANIK). Berlin: W. de Gruyter & Co. 1953.

KNESE, K.-H.: Knochenstruktur als Verbundbau. Zwanglose Abhandlungen aus dem Gebiet der normalen und pathologischen Anatomie, H. 4. Stuttgart: Georg Thieme 1958.

KNIGHT, R. A., and G. D. PURVIS: Fractures of both bones of the forearm in adults. J. Bone Jt Surg. **31**A, 755 (1949).

KNISELY, M. H.: Microscopic observations of intravascular agglutination of red cells and consequent sludging of blood in human diseases. Anat. Rec. **82**, 426 (1942).

KNOBLAUCH, H.: Beitrag zur operativen Behandlung der Tibiakopfgelenkbrüche. Mschr. Unfallheilk. **56**, 340 (1953).

KNÜPPER, H.: Die Fixation schwer einstellbarer Knochenbrüche durch schräge Drahtung. Zbl. Chir. **77**, 722 (1952).

KÖHNLEIN, E., u. S. WELLER: Über Frakturen im Bereich des Kniegelenks. Zbl. Chir. **86**, 849 (1961).

KÖNIG, F.: Moderne Behandlung der Frakturen der unteren Extremitäten. Z. ärztl. Landpraxis **3**, 330, 363 (1894).

— Über die Berechtigung frühzeitiger blutiger Eingriffe bei subcutanen Knochenbrüchen. Langenbecks Arch. klin. Chir. **76**, 23 (1905).

— Operative Chirurgie der Knochenbrüche. 1. Bd.: Operationen am frischen und verschleppten Knochenbruch. Berlin: Springer 1931.

KÖNIG, P.: Zur Therapie der subtrochanteren Oberschenkelbrüche. Arch. orthop. Unfall-Chir. **48**, 641 (1957).

KOLB, O.: Nachuntersuchungen an genagelten Schenkelhalsfrakturen. Chirurg **21**, 467 (1950).

KOSLOWSKI, L.: Frakturbehandlung mit dem Rush-Federstab. Möglichkeiten und Grenzen. Chirurg **29**, 108 (1958).

— Zur Technik der Schenkelhalsnagelung mit dem Drei-Lamellen-Nagel. Chirurg **31**, 306 (1960).

— Aktuelle Fragen der Knochenbruchbehandlung. Wehrmed. Mitt. **5**, 1 (1962).

—, u. H. RAUCH: Über Mehrfachbrüche an den unteren Gliedmaßen. Mschr. Unfallheilk. **62**, 263 (1959).

—, u. S. WELLER: Tücken der Marknagelung. Chirurg **33**, 460 (1962).

KOTHE, W.: Beitrag zur operativen Behandlung von Oberarmkopffrakturen. Zbl. Chir. **78**, 421 (1953).

KRISTENSEN, T. B.: Treatment of malleolar fractures according to Lauge-Hansen's method. Preliminary results. Acta chir. scand. **97**, 362 (1948/49).

— Fractures of the ankle. VI. Follow-up studies. Arch. Surg. **73**, 112 (1956).

KROMPECHER, S.: Die Knochenbildung. Jena: Gustav Fischer 1937.

KRULL, F.: Beitrag zur operativen Behandlung der Schienbeinkopfbrüche. Arch. orthop. Unfall-Chir. **46**, 114 (1953).

KUCHENREUTER, G.: Erfahrungen bei Verschraubung der Verrenkung im Acromio-claviculargelenk nach BOSWORTH. Chirurg **27**, 250 (1956).

KÜNTSCHER, G.: Einführung in die Marknagelung. J. int. Chir. **11**, 85 (1951).

— Die stabile Osteosynthese. Arch. klin. Chir. **270**, 444 (1951).

— Die Nagelung der Malleolarpseudarthrose. Mschr. Unfallheilk. **56**, 107 (1953).

— Die vollautomatische Schenkelhalsnagelung. Z. Orthop. **84**, 17 (1953).

— Zur Frage der Marknagelfrakturen (Bemerkungen zu der gleichnamigen Arbeit von J. FISCHER-WASELS und H. B. SCHÜNEMANN). Arch. orthop. Unfall-Chir. **46**, 429 (1954).

— Fünfzehn Jahre Marknagel. Arch. klin. Chir. **282**, 211 (1955).

— Zur Behandlung der schweren Verrenkungsbrüche des oberen Sprunggelenkes. Mschr. Unfallheilk. **59**, 295 (1956).

— Ein entscheidendes Experiment der Knochenchirurgie. Zbl. Chir. **81**, 817 (1956).

— Pseudarthrose nach „Marknagelung". Z. Orthop. **87**, 225 (1956).

— Die Marknagelung des Oberarms vom proximalen Ende aus. Chirurg **28**, 218 (1957).

— Die Trochanterimplantation mittels geradem Oberschenkelmarknagel. Z. Orthop. **89**, 406 (1957).

— Geschlossene Marknagelung des Unterschenkels. Chir. Praxis **1**, 73 (1957).

— Die Nagelung des Schenkelhalsbruches. Chir. Praxis **3**, 317 (1957).

— Stabile Osteosynthese gelenknaher Brüche. Zbl. Chir. **82**, 1641 (1957).

— Zur Technik der Drehosteotomie der langen Röhrenknochen. Mschr. Unfallheilk. **60**, 225 (1957).

— Das Callusproblem. Arch. orthop. Unfall-Chir. **49**, 1 (1957).

— Der Knochen als Entzündungsmodell. Z. ges. exp. Med. **130**, 279 (1938).

— Ein einfacher Distraktionsbügel für die Marknagelung. Chirurg **29**, 333 (1958).

— Die Technik des Aufweitens der Markhöhle. Chirurg **30**, 28 (1959).

Küntscher, G.: Marknagelung bei infolge alter Fraktur deformierten Knochen. Mschr. Unfallheilk. 63, 401 (1960).
— Zur Marknagelung des Trümmerbruchs. Chirurg 31, 503 (1960).
— Die Behandlung der Unterarmpseudarthrose. Chirurg 32, 37 (1961).
— Die Marknagelung. Berlin: W. Springer 1962.
Künzli, H. F.: Zur operativen Behandlung der Ellbogenfrakturen. Thesis Basel 1960.
Küppermann, W.: Osteosynthese mit konservierten Knochen. Mschr. Unfallheilk. 60, 74 (1957).
Kummer, A.: The treatment of pertrochanteric fractures. Arch. chir. neerl. 10, 250 (1958).
Labes, H.: Zur Spießung der Klavikular- und Unterarmfrakturen durch Kirschnerdraht. Zbl. Chir. 82, 1166 (1957).
Lacroix, P.: Sur la réparation des fractures. Les mécanismes locaux. Soc. int. Chir., 15ᵉ Congr., Lisbonne 1953, p. 553.
Laffitte, H., P. Suire et C. Assi: Le traitement des fractures diaphysaires de l'humérus et du fémur. Mém. Acad. Chir. 79, 509 (1953).
Laing, P. G., and J. M. O'Donnel: The engineering design of hip nails and the development of the H-beam nail. Surg. Gynec. Obstet. 112, 567 (1961).
Lambotte, A.: Notice sur l'emploi du fil de fer et de vis du même métal dans la suture osseuse. Presse méd. belge 44, 125 (1892).
— L'intervention opératoire dans les fractures. Paris: A. Maloine 1907.
— Le traitement des fractures. Paris: Masson & Cie. 1907.
— Chirurgie opératoire des fractures. Paris: Masson & Cie. 1913.
Lang, F.: Das distale Radio-Ulnargelenk. Seine Bedeutung in der Unfallmedizin. Mschr. Unfallheilk., Beih. 36 (1942).
Lange, M.: Die Behandlung der Trümmerbrüche im Bereich der großen Gelenke (Schulter-, Hüft- und Knie-gelenke). Z. Orthop. 84, 373 (1953).
Lange, P., u. G. Rosolleck: Zwei seltene Abrißfrakturen. Zbl. Chir. 83, 1000 (1958).
Lauge, N. (Lauge-Hansen): Fractures of the ankle. Analytic historic survey as the basis of new experimental, roentgenologic and clinical investigations. Arch. Surg. 56, 259 (1948).
Lauge-Hansen, N.: "Ligamentous" ankle fractures. Diagnosis and treatment. Acta chir. scand. 97, 544 (1948).
— Fractures of the ankle. II. Combined experimental-surgical and experimental-roentgenologic investiga-tions. Arch. Surg. 60, 957 (1950).
— Fractures of the ankle. IV. Clinical use of genetic roentgen diagnosis and genetic reduction. Arch. Surg. 64, 488 (1952).
— Fracture of the ankle. V. Pronation-dorsiflexion fracture. Arch. Surg. 67, 813 (1953).
— Fractures of the ankle. Amer. J. Roentgenol. 71, 456 (1954).
Laurent, L. E.: Pseudarthrosis of the internal malleolus. Ann. Chir. Gynaec. Fenn. 45, 49 (1956).
Lecutier, M. A., and A. H. Smith: Air embolism as a complication of medullary nailing. J. Bone Jt Surg. 39 B, 534 (1957).
Leemann, R.: Die Falz-Cerclage und der Falzspanner. Helv. chir. Acta 19, 119 (1952).
— Modifizierte Draht-Cerclage mit neuem Spanninstrument. Z. Unfallmed. Berufskr. 1, 52 (1952).
Leemann, R. A.: Die „Falzcerclage" als technische Verbesserung der Drahtumschlingung bei Brüchen des langen Röhrenknochens. Chirurg 28, 60 (1957).
Lehmann, E. M., and R. M. Moore: Fat embolism including experimental production without trauma. Surgery 14, 621 (1927).
Lehv, S. P.: A headless self-drilling screw. Amer. J. Surg. 80, 608 (1950).
—, and M. S. Beinfield: Clinical application of the Lehv headless screw. Amer. J. Surg. 81, 351 (1951).
Le Fort, J. A.: Note sur une variété non décrite de la fracture verticale de la malléole externe. Bull. gén. Thér. (Paris) 110, 193 (1886).
Lempert, H., u. G. Gurn: Ergebnisse der Marknagelung nach Küntscher (111 Nagelungen in 35 Kranken-häusern). Arch. orthop. Unfall-Chir. 45, 143 (1952).
Letournel, E.: Les fractures du cotyle, étude d'une série de 75 cas. J. Chir. (Paris) 82, 47 (1961).
Leveuf, J., et. P. Bertrand: Luxations et subluxations congénitales de la hanche. Leur traitement basé sur l'arthrographie. Paris: G. Doin & Cie. 1946.
Levine, R.: Metabolic requests in chronic stress situations. U. S. Gov. Print. Off. 1953, p. 46.
Lewis, D., and E. M. Miller: Peripheral nerve injuries associated with fractures. Ann. Surg. 76, 528 (1922).
Lewis, K. M.: Internal fixation with Smith-Petersen nail and extension bar in treatment of intertrochanteric fractures of femur. Amer. J. Surg. 80, 669 (1950).
Lichtenauer, F., and C. Benthien: Die Behandlung der Luxationsfrakturen des oberen Sprunggelenkes mit Längsabsprengung aus der Tibia (sog. Volkmannsches Dreieck) mit Extension und percutaner Fixation durch einen Kirschnerdraht. Mschr. Unfallheilk. 57, 338 (1954).
Lindahl, Ol.: Rigidity of immobilization of transverse fractures. Acta orthop. scand. 32, 237 (1962).
Lipscomb, P. R.: Vascular and neural complications in supracondylar fractures of the humerus in children. J. Bone Jt Surg. 37 A, 487 (1955).
Logroscino, D., e. E. de Marchi: Vascolarizzazione e trofo-patie delle ossa del carpo. Chir. Organi Mov. 23, 499 (1938).

LOTTES, J. O.: Treatment of fractures of the femur with a heavy large cored, three-flanged medullary nail. Surgery 29, 868 (1951).
— Intramedullary fixation for fractures of the shaft of the tibia. Sth. med. J. (Bgham, Ala.) 45, 407 (1952).
— L. J. HILL, and J. A. KEY: Closed reduction, plate fixation, and medullary nailing of fractures of both bones of the leg, a comparative end result study. J. Bone Jt Surg. 34 A, 861 (1952).
LÜDI, H., H. WILLENEGGER u. O. HASE: Behandlungsresultate von offenen Frakturen. Helv. chir. Acta 19, 269 (1952).
LÜTZELER, H.: Die Entstehungsursache der Pseudarthrose nach Bruch des Kahnbeins der Hand. Dtsch. Z. Chir. 235, 450 (1932).
LUTZEYER, W., u. U. GUSE: Behandlungsergebnisse von Ellbogengelenkfrakturen beim Jugendlichen unter besonderer Berücksichtigung der operativen Therapie und der Nachbehandlung. Arch. orthop. Unfall-Chir. 45, 629 (1953).
MAATZ, R.: Über die Formschlüssigkeit bei der Küntschernagelung. Zbl. Chir. 70, 1641 (1943).
— Die Wundmechanik in der Federosteosynthese. Z. Orthop. 80, 643 (1950/51).
— Pseudarthrosenbehandlung durch die Markfeder. Arch. klin. Chir. 270, 446 (1951).
— Die Behandlung der Tibiakopfbrüche mit der Spongiosafeder. Chirurg 27, 247 (1956).
— Osteosynthese an der Elle. Chirurg 28, 24 (1957).
MADSEN, E., and P. C. MADSEN: Primaer osteosynthese ved crusfracturer. Nord. Med. 60, 1835 (1958).
MAGNANT, M.: La dislocation radiocubitale inférieure au cours des fractures diaphysaires de l'avantbras avec luxation postérieure de la tête cubitale. Mém. Acad. Chir. 79, 441 (1953).
MAGNUSSON, R.: On the late results in non-operated cases of malleolar fractures. Acta chir. scand. 90, Suppl. 84 (1944).
— On the late results in non-operated cases of malleolar fractures. III. Fractures by supination together with a survey of the late results in non-operatively treated malleolar fractures. Acta chir. scand. 92, 259 (1945).
MAISONNEUVE, M. J. G.: Recherches sur la fracture du péroné. Arch. gén. Méd. 2ᵉ et N. sér. 7, 165 (1840).
MANCINI, G.: Die Osteosynthese der pertrochanteren Oberschenkelfraktur. Arch. Putti Chir. Organi Mov. 1, 18 (1951). Ref. Zbl. Chir. 77, 1806 (1952).
— Osteosynthese der pertrochanteren Oberschenkelfrakturen. Arch. Putti Chir. Organi Mov. 2, 53 (1952). Ref. Zbl. Chir. 78, 1119 (1953).
MANDRUZZATO, F. A.: Sur le traitement des fractures du calcanéum. Acta orthop. belg. 17, 220 (1951).
MAREK, F. M.: Treatment of fractures of shaft of tibia by intramedullary fixation with Lottes' nail. Amer. J. Surg. 91, 204 (1956).
— Axial fixation of forearm fractures. J. Bone Jt Surg. 43 A, 1099 (1961).
MARION, J., J. LAGRANGE, R. FAYSSE et P. RIGAULT: Les fractures de l'extrémité inférieure de l'humérus chez l'enfant. Rev. Chir. orthop. 48, 490 (1962).
MARNEFFE DE, D.: Indications du traitement orthopédique ou chirurgical dans les fractures malléolaires fermées. Revue de 81 observations. Acta chir. belg. 54, 411 (1955).
MARTIN, B.: Knochenveränderung nach Küntschernagelung. Zbl. Chir. 77, 76 (1952).
MARTIN DU PAN, R., S. WALTER et M. NEYROUD: A propos de 3 cas d'ostéomyélite aiguë. Rev. méd. Suisse rom. 81, 139 (1961).
MARWEGE, H.: Sollen Oberarmschaftbrüche genagelt werden? (Ein Beitrag zur Küntschernagelung von Oberarmschaftbrüchen.) Bruns' Beitr. klin. Chir. 189, 245 (1954).
—, u. G. TEICHERT: Weitere Erfahrungen mit der verbundenen Doppelschraube bei der Versorgung medialer Schenkelhalsbrüche. Chirurg 28, 505 (1957).
MASON, M. L.: Intracapsular fractures of the neck of the femur. A review of one hundred cases treated by internal fixation. Brit. J. Surg. 40, 482 (1952).
MATHE, E.: Unsere Erfahrungen mit den metallischen Osteosynthesen. Rozhl. Chir. 31, 180 (1952). Ref. Zbl. Chir. 78, 554 (1953).
MATTER, P., u. G. GUT: Ergebnisse der offenen Unterschenkelfrakturen im Churer Krankengut 1958—1962. Z. Unfallmed. Berufskr. 57 (1964), in Press.
MATTI, H.: Die Knochenbrüche und ihre Behandlung. 1. Aufl. Berlin: Springer 1918.
— Die Knochenbrüche und ihre Behandlung, second edition. Berlin: Springer 1931.
MATTNER, H. R.: Schenkelhalsfrakturen im Kindesalter. Arch. orthop. Unfall-Chir. 49, 473 (1958).
MATZEN, P. F.: Der Marknagel in der Pseudarthrosenbehandlung. Zbl. Chir. 78, 1624 (1953).
MAURER, G.: Zur Behandlung der Malleolarfrakturen mit Sprengung der Knöchelgabel. Dtsch. Z. Chir. 270, 460 (1951).
MAXFIELD, J. E., and F. J. MCDERMOTT: Experiences with the Palmer open reduction of fractures of the calcaneus. J. Bone Jt Surg. 37 A, 99 (1955).
MAYER, H.: Die operative Behandlung der Luxationsfrakturen des oberen Sprunggelenkes bei gleichzeitiger Sprengung des Ligamentum interosseum zwischen Tibia und Fibula. Chirurg. 27, 509 (1956).
MCADAM, J. W. J., J. P. DUGUID, and S. W. CHALLINOR: Systemic administration of penicillin. Lancet 1944 II, 336.
MCELVENNY, R. T.: An instrument to hold and to drive the stuck nail. Clin. Orthop. 5, 230 (1955).
— The treatment of nonunion of femoral neck fractures. Surg. Clin. N. Amer. 37, 251 (1957).
— The immediate treatment of intracapsular hip fracture. Clin Orthop. 10, 289 (1957).

McLaughlin, H. L.: Recurrent anterior dislocation of the shoulder. I. Morbid anatomy. Amer. J. Surg. **99** 628 (1960).

— Fracture of the carpal navicular (scaphoid) bone. J. Bone Jt Surg. **36** A, 765 (1954).

Menegaux, G., et. D. Odiette: L'ostéosynthèse au point de vue biologique. Influence de la nature du métal. Paris: Masson & Cie. 1936.

Merino, W.: Las seudarthrosis con perdida de substancia del antebrazo su tratamiento por los injertos oseos. J. int. Chir. **11**, 525 (1951).

Merle D'Aubigné, R.: Ununited fracture of the neck of femur. Proc. roy. Soc. Med. **53**, 437 (1959).

— Fractures ouvertes des jambes. Actualités Chir. orthop. et répat. p. 9. Paris: Exp. Sci. 1959.

—, et R. F. Mazas: Formes anatomiques et traitement des fractures de l'extrémité supérieure du tibia. Rev. Chir. orthop. **46**, 318 (1960).

Michon, J., et R. Vilain: Fractures ouvertes des diaphyses superficielles. Actualités Chir. orthop. et répar., p. 19. Paris: Exp. Sci. 1959.

Miles, J. E., G. A. Degenshein, and A. A. Kane: The double onlay bone graft in the treatment of delayed union and nonunion. Surg. Gynec. Obstet. **94**, 426 (1952).

Miller, D. S., and L. Markin: Simples method of bone grafting for nonunion of the tibia. Arch. Surg. **62**, 548 (1951).

Modny, M. T., and H. G. Kunz: Insertion, with a guide, of multiple nails in fractures of the femoral neck. Amer. J. Surg. **99**, 13 (1960).

Montmollin, B. de: Evolution du traitement des fractures. Rév. méd. Suisse rom. **82**, 457 (1962).

Moraes, F. de: La réduction des fractures de l'avant-bras par le levier démonte-pneu. Acta othop. belg. **16**, 5 (1950).

Morrison, G. M., and E. J. Coughlin jr.: Ski injuries. Amer. J. Surg. **80**, 630 (1950).

Moser, H. s. Bruck, H., u. H. Moser.

Müller, D. H.: Erfahrungen mit der Methode des Gewindebolzens in der Frakturbehandlung. Thesis Zürich 1946.

Müller, H., u. K. F. Pitzke: Ertl-Span und Umkehrspan. Ein Beitrag zur Spanplastik bei kallusverzögerter Unterschenkelfraktur und Pseudarthrose. Bruns' Beitr. klin. Chir. **202**, 399 (1961).

Müller, M. E.: Die Kompressionsosteosynthese unter besonderer Berücksichtigung der Kniearthrodese. Helv. chir. Acta **22**, 474 (1955).

— Zur Druckosteosynthese. Z. Unfallmed. Berufskr. **49**, 136 (1956).

— Zur Behandlung der Schenkelhalspseudarthrose. Z. Unfallmed. Berufskr. **50**, 125 (1957).

— Zur Reposition und Osteosynthese des Schenkelhalsadduktionsbruches. Helv. chir. Acta **24**, 237 (1957).

— Die hüftnahen Femurosteotomien. Stuttgart: Georg Thieme 1957.

— A propos des fractures trans-cervicales vraies du fémur. Lyon chir. **54**, 776 (1958).

— Traitement des retards de consolidation et des pseudarthroses par principes biomécaniques. Soc. int. Chir. orthop. et Traumatol., New York, 1960. Extrait du volume des rapports, p. 612, 1961.

— Zur operativen Behandlung der Kondylenbrüche im Kniebereich. Verh. Dtsch. orthop. Ges., Kongreß-band 49. Kongreß Zürich 1961. Stuttgart: Ferdinand Enke.

— Principes d'ostéosynthèse. Helv. chir. Acta **28**, 198 (1961).

— Die Verwendung von Kunstharzen in der Knochenchirurgie. Arch. orthop. Unfall-Chir. **54**, 513 (1962).

— L'ostéosynthèse précoce des fractures ouvertes. Z. Unfallmed. Berufskr. **55**, 240 (1962).

— A propos des fractures diaphysaires ouvertes. Acta othop. belg. **28**, 506 (1962).

— Internal fixation of fractures and for non-unions. Proc. roy. Soc. Med. **56**, 455 (1963).

— Kunstharze in der Knochenchirurgie. Helv. chir. Acta **30**, 121 (1963).

— Operative Behandlung der Malleolarfrakturen. Arch. klin. Chir **304**, 808 (1963).

—, u. M. Allgöwer: Zur Behandlung der Pseudarthrose. Helv. chir. Acta **25**, 253 (1958).

— — u. H. Willenegger: Die Gemeinschaftserhebung der Arbeitsgemeinschaft für Osteosynthesefragen. Arch. klin. Chir. **304, 808** (1963).

—, et. H. Vasey: A propos des fractures diaphysaires ouvertes. Acta orthop. belg. **28**, 506 (1962).

Müller, P.: Beitrag zur Frage der operativen Behandlung geschlossener Unterschenkelfrakturen. Thesis Bern 1959.

Müssbichler, H.: Arterial supply to the head of the femur. An arteriographic study in vivo of lesions attending fractures of the femoral neck. Acta radiol. (Stockh.) **46**, 533 (1956).

Mumenthaler, M.: Die Luxation des Nervus ulnaris am Ellenbogen. Darstellung von 60 eigenen Fällen mit klinischen Symptomen. Dtsch. Z. Nervenheilk. **178**, 163 (1958).

— Die Ulnarisparesen. Stuttgart: Georg Thieme 1961.

Murphy, J. B.: Cicatricial fixation of ulnar nerve from ancient cubitus valgus. Release and transference to new site. Surg. Clin. Mercy Hosp. **5**, 661 (1916).

Murray, R. A.: The one-bone forearm. A reconstructive procedure. J. Bone Jt Surg. **37** A, 366 (1955).

Navarre, M.: A propos des lésions du ligament latéral interne dans les fractures dites de la malléole externe. Acta orthop. belg. **28**, 138 (1962).

Neer, Ch. S., Th. H. Brown jr., and H. L. McLaughlin: Fracture of the neck of the humerus with dislocation of the head fragment. Amer. J. Surg. **85**, 252 (1953).

Neff, G.: Primäre Osteosynthese bei offenen Frakturen. Helv. med. Acta **11**, 515 (1944).

NEFF, G.: Zur operativen Behandlung der pertrochanteren Frakturen. Chirurg 21, 596 (1950).

NEUENFELDT, H. J.: Über die Behandlung und Spätresultate bei Tibiakopffrakturen. Thesis Hamburg 1939.

NICOLE, R.: Die Indikation beim Schenkelhalsbruch. Dtsch. Z. Chir. 251, H. 11 u. 12 (1939).

— Bilanz der heutigen Behandlung der Schenkelhalsfrakturen. Helv. med. Acta 6, 943 (1940).

— Metallschädigung bei Osteosynthesen. Helv. chir. Acta, Suppl. 3 (1947).

NIGST, H.: Die traumatische Neuritis des Nervus ulnaris. Eine Analyse von 73 operierten Fällen. Helv. chir. Acta 20, 37 (1953).

—, u. H. WILLENEGGER: La pénicilline en application locale dans les infections chirurgicales. Méd. Hyg. 11, 126 (1953).

NORDENSEN, N. G.: Sur la vascularisation de la tête du fémur par la voie du ligament rond fémoral. Lyon chir. 35, 178 (1938).

OBERHOLZER, J.: Beitrag zur Behandlung der Querfraktur des Vorderarmes in Schaftmitte. Helv. chir. Acta 13, 363 (1946).

OBLETZ, B. E., and B. M. HALBSTEIN: Non-union of fractures of carpal navicular. J. Bone Jt Surg. 20, 424 (1938).

OTT, W.: Zur Behandlung offener Trümmerfrakturen des Unterschenkels mit ausgesprochener Weichteilverletzung. Helv. chir. Acta 25, 213 (1958).

PALMER, I.: Fractures of the upper end of the tibia. J. Bone Jt Surg. 33 B, 160 (1951).

PAP, K., u. J. SZENTPETERY: Über die Bitorsionsdislokation der jugendlichen Epikondylenbrüche. Arch. orthop. Unfall-Chir. 49, 109 (1957).

PASCHOLD, K.: Über Patellarfrakturen und ihre Behandlungsergebnisse unter besonderer Berücksichtigung der Arthrosis deformans. Zbl. Chir. 83, 1532 (1958).

PAUWELS, F.: Der Schenkelhalsbruch, ein mechanisches Problem. Stuttgart: Ferdinand Enke 1935.

PEITSCH, H.: Erfahrungen mit der intramedullären Frakturfixation nach RUSH. Mschr. Unfallheilk. 62, 368 (1959).

— Ergebnisse der Marknagelung bei Schaftfrakturen der langen Röhrenknochen. Mschr. Unfallheilk. 63, 412 (1960).

PENROSE, J. H.: The Monteggia fracture with posterior dislocation of the radial head. J. Bone Jt Surg. 33 B, 65 (1951).

PEREGALLI, P. F.: Considerazioni sul trattamento delle fratture biossee d'avambraccio con infibulazione endomidollare. Arch. Ortop. (Milano) 65, 52 (1952).

PERKINS, G.: Fractures and dislocations. London: The Athlone Press 1958.

PETROKOV, V.: Die acromio-claviculare Luxation. Bruns' Beitr. klin. Chir. 199, 143 (1959).

PFAEHLER, E.: Zur Behandlung von Tibiakopfbrüchen aus dem Krankengut der Schweizerischen Unfallversicherungsanstalt der Jahre 1950—1954. Z. Unfallmed. Berufskr. 55, 325 (1962).

PHEMISTER, D. B.: The pathology of ununited fractures of the Neck of the femur with special reference to the head. J. Bone Jt Surg. 21, 681 (1939).

PHILIPPSEN, K. H.: Ein Beitrag zur Behandlung der Olecranonfrakturen. Arch. orthop. Unfall-Chir. 47, 649 (1955).

PLATZGUMMER, H.: Zur blutigen Behandlung irreponibler und veralteter Luxationsfrakturen des Schultergelenkes. Arch. orthop. Unfall-Chir. 45, 514 (1953).

POHL, E.: Nicht sperrende Schenkelhalsschrauben fourth edit. Mai 1956.

POHL, J.: Beitrag zur blutigen Behandlung der Fractura colli humeri und der Brüche des proximalen Humerusendes. Zbl. Chir. 77, 1056 (1952).

POILLEUX, M. F.: Traitement des fractures basses du tibia par enclouage percutanée à pénétration malléolaire. Mém. Acad. Chir. 79, 339 (1953).

POLICARD, A.: Aus: R. LERICHE et A. POLICARD, Physiologie phathologique chirurgicale. Paris: Masson & Cie. 1930.

POLTERA, R.: Die Erfahrungen bei operativ behandelten Schlüsselbeinbrüchen. Thesis Zürich 1959.

PORTIS, R. B., and H. A. MENDELSOHN: Conservative management of fractures of the ankle involving the medial malleolus. J. Amer. med. Ass. 151, 102 (1953).

PREISER, G.: Eine typische posttraumatische und zur Spontanfraktur führende Ostitis des Naviculare carpi. Fortschr. Röntgenstr. 15, 189 (1910).

PROSEK, G.: Kompressionsbehandlung von Schrägbrüchen durch Spanndrahtumschlingung. Chriurg 26, 368 (1955).

PUTTI, V.: Die operative Behandlung der Schenkelhalsbrüche. Stuttgart: Ferdinand Enke 1942.

QUÉNU, E.: Fracture de Maisonneuve (fracture dite par diastase). Bull. Soc. Chir. (Paris) 32, 943 (1906).

— Du diastasis de l'articulation tibio-péronière inférieure. Rev. Chir. (Paris) 27/36, 62 (1907).

— Etudes sur les fractures marginales postérieures du tibia. De leur rôle dans les luxations du pied en arrière. Bull. Soc. Chir. Paris 38, 1070 (1912).

— Etudes sur les fractures. Rev. Chir. (Paris) 32/45, 416 und 32/46, 257 (1912).

RACKER, CH. DE: La fracture isolée de la diaphyse radiale avec ou sans luxation du cubitus. Lyon chir. 50, 230 (1955).

RAMADIER, J. O., J. DUPARC, D. ROUGEMONT et F. DE FERRARI: Le traitement chirurgical des fractures trochanteriennes et juxta-trochanteriennes. Rev. Chir. orthop. 42, 759 (1956).

RASOVSKY, A.: Vorderarmbrüche durch intramedulläre Prothese mit Kirschnerdraht behandelt. Čas. Lék. čes. **94**, 480 (1955). Ref. Zbl. Chir. **81**, 80 (1956).

RAZEMON, J. P. s. DECOULX, P., et J. P. RAZEMON (1956).

REHBEIN, F.: Zur Behandlung des veralteten Kahnbeinbruches und der Kahnbeinpseudarthrose der Hand. Dtsch. Z. Chir. **260**, 356 (1948).

—, u. W. DÜBEN: Zur konservativen Behandlung des veralteten Kahnbeinbruches und der Kahnbeinpseudarthrose. Arch. orthop. Unfall-Chir. **45**, 67 (1952).

REHM, J.: Beobachtungen bei der Verwendung von V2A-Stahldrähten zur Markschienung von Unterarmfrakturen. Chirurg **26**, 390 (1955).

— Über die besonderen gefäßphysiologischen Bedingungen bei der Schenkelhalsfraktur und ihre Berücksichtigung bei der operativen Behandlung. Chirurg **27**, 303 (1956).

— Zur Behandlung schwerer Fersenbeinfrakturen mit primärer Bolzungsarthrodese im unteren Sprunggelenk. Zbl. Chir. **81**, 2194 (1956).

— Experimentelle Untersuchungen zur Entstehung der Fettembolie beim Knochenbruch. Dtsch. Z. Chir. **285**, 230 (1957).

—, u. H. J. SÜSSE: Transossale Venographie des Kopffragmentes bei Schenkelhalspseudarthrosen. Mschr. Unfallheilk. **58**, 137 (1955).

REHN, E.: Der Schock und verwandte Zustände des autonomen Systems. Stuttgart: Ferdinand Enke 1937.

REIMERS, C.: Die Verschraubung medialer Schenkelhalsbrüche. Dtsch. Z. Chir. **270**, 449 (1951).

— Die Brüche des fußnahen Unterschenkelabschnittes. Dtsch. Z. Chir. **276**, 260 (1953).

REME, H.: Bericht über 115 mit dem Rundnagel nach LEZIUS versorgte petrochantere Frakturen. Arch. klin. Chir. **287**, 709 (1957).

REMY, R.: Considérations sur l'enclouage médullaire dans les fractures des deux os de l'avant-bras chez l'enfant. Acta orthop. belg. **21**, 333 (1955).

RETTIG, H.: Frakturen im Kindesalter. München: J. F. Bergmann 1957.

RIBBERT, H.: Fettembolie, Korresp.-Bl. schweiz. Ärz. **24**, 457 (1894).

— Zur Fettembolie. Dtsch. med. Wschr. **26**, 419 (1900).

RICKLIN, E.: Erfahrungen mit der Nagelung der pertrochanteren Femurfrakturen nach MOSER-WINKELBAUER. Z. Unfallmed. Berufskr. **48**, 109 (1955).

RICKLIN, P.: Osteotaxis nach HOFFMANN zur Behandlung schlecht geheilter Frakturen. Z. Unfallmed. Berufskr. **50**, 52 (1957).

RIESS, J.: Die Indikationsstellung zur operativen Behandlung frischer Brüche des inneren Knöchels. Chirurg **26**, 103 (1955).

— Kahnbeinpseudarthrosen, operative Behandlung auf Spanverpflanzung und temporäre Verlängerung der Sehne des Musculus flexor carpi radialis. Chirurg **31**, 457 (1960).

RIEUNAU, G., et G. RAY: Enclouage du péroné dans les fractures supra-malléolaires. Lyon chir. **51**, 594 (1956).

RITCHEY, S. J., J. P. RICHARDSON, and M. S. THOMPSON: Rigid medullary fixation of forearm fractures. Sth. med. J. (Bgham, Ala.) **51**, 852 (1958).

ROBERTSON, R. C.: Intramedullary fixation of fractures of the forearm. Amer. J. Surg. **85**, 496 (1953).

RODECK, G.: Zur operativen Behandlung subtrochanterer Frakturen mit dem Küntscher-Nagel. Zbl. Chir. **81**, 613 (1956).

ROMBOLD, CH.: Depressed fractures of the tibial plateau. J. Bone Jt Surg. **42**A, 783 (1960).

ROSENFELD, W.: Die Fibula als Sperrknochen. Zbl. Chir. **82**, 68 (1957).

ROSTOCK, P.: Die Malleolarpseudarthrose. Arch. klin. Chir. **191**, 557 (1938).

ROTH, H.: Über Spätfolgen traumatischer Hüftgelenksluxationen. Thesis Zürich 1940.

— Knochenmarkveränderungen nach Marknagelung. Schweiz. med. Wschr. **75**, 7 (1945).

— Die Konservierung von Knochengewebe für Transplantationen. Wien: Springer 1952.

ROWE, J., and R. SUTHERLAND: Fracture fixation by transarticular pin. Amer. J. Surg. **74**, 24 (1947).

RÜCKERT, W.: Retrograde offene Marknagelung zur Vermeidung tödlicher Fettembolie. Z. Unfallmed. Berufskr. **49**, 209 (1956).

RUSH JR., H. L., W. T. FITTS JR., J. GIBBONS, and E. W. MONROE: Intramedullary nailing in the presence of infection. Surg. Gynec. Obstet. **94**, 727 (1952).

RUSSE, O.: Fracture of the carpal navicular. J. Bone Jt Surg. **42**A, 759 (1960).

— Nachuntersuchungsergebnisse von 22 Fällen operierter veralteter Brüche und Pseudarthrosen des Kahnbeins der Hand. Z. Orthop. **93**, 5 (1960).

SACHSE, H.: Vorschläge zu einer neuartigen Spanndrahtextension. Mschr. Unfallheilk. **53**, 176 (1950).

SAGE, F. P.: Medullary fixation of fractures of the forearm. J. Bone Jt Surg. **41**A, 1489, 1525 (1959).

SALEM, G.: Behandlung der Tibiapseudarthrosen mit dem Rohrschlitznagel. Chirurg **31**, 74 (1960).

SARTORA, A.: Le traitement des plaies de guerre. Paris: Berger-Levrault 1917.

SAVASTANO, A. A., L. A. SAGE, and V. ZECCHINO: Treatment of fresh fractures of neck of femur with intramedullary stem prostheses. Arch. Surg. **75**, 985 (1957).

SCAGLIETTI, O.: Anzeigestellung zur operativen Frakturbehandlung. Arch. Putti Chir. Organi Mov. **1**, 11 (1951). Ref. Zbl. Chir. **77**, 1806 (1952).

—, u. F. PERAZZINI: Die Kahnbeinpseudarthrosen. Wiederherstellungschir. u. Traum. **2**, 112 (1954).

SCALES, J. T., G. D. WINTER, and H. T. SHIRLEY: Corrosion of the orthopaedic implants. Screws, plates and femoral nail-plates. J. Bone Jt Surg. 41 B, 810 (1959).

SCHÄFER, R.: Zur Markschienung unstabiler Unterarmbrüche mit Kirschnerdrähten. Zbl. Chir. 82, 142 (1957).

SCHENK, R., u. H. WILLENEGGER: Zur Histologie der primären Knochenheilung. Arch. klin. Chir. 305 (1963). In Press.

SCHLEYER, H., v.: Zur Indikationsstellung der Marknagelung. Mschr. Unfallheilk. 53, 17 (1950).

SCHMIDT, E.: Über die Anwendung der Druckosteosynthese bei Kniescheibenbrüchen. Zbl. Chir. 84, 178 (1959).

SCHMORELL, H.: Zur Knochenbolzung bei Frakturen der langen Röhrenknochen mit Bolzen aus Amputationsknochen. Zbl. Chir. 77, 1751 (1952).

SCHNEIDER, R.: Die Marknagelung der Tibia. Helv. chir. Acta 28, 207 (1961).

SCHÖNBAUER, H. R.: Vermeidbare Behandlungsfolgen durch zu kurze Fixation von isolierten Brüchen des Ellenschaftes. Chir. Praxis 2, 183 (1960).

SCHÜRCH, O.: Über einen Drahtbinder. Zbl. Chir. 17, 1006 (1933).

— Wandlungen in der Frakturenbehandlung. Basel: Benno Schwabe & Co. 1944.

—, u. W. ACKERMANN: Über die Technik der Frakturbehandlung mit dem Gewindebolzen. Z. Unfallmed. Berufskr. 37 (1944).

SCHÜTZE, E.: Die Schenkelhalsfraktur "the unsolved fracture". Zbl. Chir. 81, 606 (1956).

SCHULTZ, H.: Laschenschraubung pertrochanterer Oberschenkel- und lateraler Schenkelhalsbrüche. Mschr. Unfallheilk. 56, 47 (1953).

SCHUMANN, G.: Über die operative Behandlung von Knochenbrüchen mit Gabelsprengung. Zbl. Chir. 80, 542 (1955).

SCHUMPELICK, W.: Die stabilere Osteosynthese des medialen Schenkelhalsbruches mit der verbundenen Doppelschraube. Chirurg 26, 131 (1955).

—, u. P. M. JANTZEN: Ergebnisse der Behandlung von Unterschenkelbrüchen mit der Drahtumschlingung. Bruns' Beitr. klin. Chir. 187, 129 (1953).

— — A new principle in the operative treatment of trochanteric fractures of the femur. J. Bone Jt Surg. 37 A, 693 (1955).

SCHWIER, V.: Osteosynthese von Unterschenkelbrüchen mit knöchernen Schrauben. Mschr. Unfallheilk. 61, 234 (1958).

— Zu den Problemen der Osteosynthese, der Knochenneubildung und der Knochenverpflanzung. Chirurg 31, 220 (1960).

SCUDERI, C.: Arthroplasty cup with center pin. Surg. Gynec. Obstet. 100, 631 (1955).

SEAMAN, B., and E. PONDER: Estimation and control of postoperative dehydration with aid of hemoglobin and plasma protein determinations. J. clin. Invest. 22, 673 (1943).

SEGMÜLLER, G., G. KESSLER u. E. CORRODI: Ergebnisse der Tibiaosteosynthese: Untersuchungen an 3 geschlossenen Serien von insgesamt 462 Fällen. Z. Unfallmed. Berufskr. 57, 252 (1964).

SEIFERT, E.: Eine technische Anregung zur blutigen Knochenbruchfeststellung nach LANE. Chirurg 22, 318 (1951).

SEIFFERT, K. E.: Die Behandlung der Finger- und Mittelhandfrakturen. Arch. klin. Chir. 295, 305 (1960).

SENFF, A.: Diskussionsbemerkung zu dem Hauptreferat von Prof. KÜNTSCHER-Schleswig über die Marknagelung auf der 60. Tagg. der Norwestdtsch. Chirurgenvereinig. in Hamburg am 10. 10. 1947.

— Die Gefahren der Fettembolie bei der Marknagelung nach KÜNTSCHER. Zbl. Chir. 76, 734 (1951).

SENGESSE, B.: Compression du cubital par un cal vicieux du coude. Résection de la gouttière épitrochléoolécranienne. Guérison. Ann. Policlin. Bordeaux 5, 641 (1898).

SEVITT, S.: Fat embolism. London: Butterworths 1962.

SEYFARTH, H.: Beitrag zur Anwendung von Metallen in der plastischen Chirurgie. Arch. orthop. Unfall-Chir. 47, 656 (1955).

SIEGRIST, J.: Blutvolumenmessungen bei Frakturpatienten. Z. Unfallmed. Berufskr. 57 (1964), in Press.

— F. W. AHNEFELD u. M. HALMAGYI: Indikationen und klinische Ergebnisse der Blutvolumenbestimmung mit radioaktivem Jod. Bericht. I. Europ. Kongr. Anaesthesiologie, Wien 1962.

SIGEL, A.: Zur Unterteilung und Behandlung der Verrenkungsbrüche des oberen Sprunggelenkes mit Abscherung eines hinteren Schienbeinbruchstückes (sog. Volkmannsches Dreieck). Arch. orthop. Unfall-Chir. 44, 341 (1951).

SIMON, H.: Die Extensionsfrakturen des unteren Humerusendes im Kindesalter und ihre Behandlungsergebnisse. Arch. orthop. Unfall-Chir. 49, 150 (1957).

SINKUS, R., u. E. SCHÜTZE: Zur Behandlung der pertrochanteren Oberschenkelfraktur. Zbl. Chir. 83, 1372 (1958).

SIPOS, I.: Luxationsfraktur des anatomischen Oberarmhalses durch Strom. Zbl. Chir. 81, 2304 (1956).

SJÖVALL, H.: Die Formen der Frakturen der langen Röhrenknochen. Zbl. Chir. 82, 1234 (1957).

SLEE, G. C.: Fractures of the tibial condyles. J. Bone Jt Surg. 37 B, 427 (1955).

SMITH, F. M.: Surgery of the elbow. Springfield: Thomas; Blackwell; Ryerson 1954.

SMITH, H., and F. P. SAGE: Medullary fixation of forearm fractures. J. Bone Jt Surg. 39 A, 91 (1957).

SMITH, J. E. M.: Internal fixation in the treatment of fractures of the shafts of the radius and ulna in adults. J. Bone Jt Surg. 41 B, 122 (1959).

SMITH-PETERSEN, M. N.: Treatment of fractures of the neck of the femur by internal fixation. Surg. Gynec. Obstet. 64, 287 (1937).

SOUZA CAMPOS BATALHA, E. DE: New method of intra-articular arthrodesis by transposition of local cancellous bone. Amer. J. Surg. **80**, 85 (1950).

SPEED, J. S.: Surgical treatment of condylar fractures of the humerus. Amer. Ac. Orthop. Surg. Instr. C. Lect. VII, 187 (1950). Ann Arbor: U. W. Edwards.

—, and H. B. BOYD: Treatment of fractures of the ulna with dislocation of the head of the radius (Monteggia fracture). J. Amer. med. Ass. **115**, 1699 (1940).

—, and R. A. KNIGHT: Malunion of Colles' fractures and its treatment. Amer. Ac. Orthop. Surg. Instr. C. Lect. II, 76 (1944). Ann Arbor: J. W. Edwards.

SPIGELMANN, L.: Positive pressure in the reduction of fractures of the tibial condyle. J. Bone Jt Surg. **35**A, 696 (1953).

STAPLES, O. S.: Arthrodesis of the elbow joint. J. Bone Jt Surg. **34**A, 207 (1952).

STEINMANN, F.: Lehrbuch der funktionellen Behandlung der Knochenbrüche und Gelenkverletzungen. Stuttgart: Ferdinand Enke 1919.

STOBER, W.: Zur Therapie der medialen Malleolarfraktur. Mschr. Unfallheilk. **60**, 115 (1957).

STONHAM, F. V.: Recurrent subluxation of the ankle joint. Med. J. Aust. **47**, 44 (1960).

STRAUMANN, F., S. STEINEMANN, O. POHLER u. H. WILLENEGGER: Neue experimentelle und klinische Ergebnisse über die Metallose. Arch. klin. Chir. **305**, 21 (1963).

STREICHER, H.-J.: Schenkelhalsfrakturen bei Kindern und Jugendlichen. Arch. klin. Chir. **287**, 716 (1957).

STREIFINGER, H.: Gerät zum Korrigieren (Ausrichten) einer mit Fehlwinkel liegenden Fraktur im Gipsverband. Chirurg **31**, 46 (1960).

STRELI, R.: Verwendung von Bohrdrähten zur Osteosynthese. Arch. klin. Chir. **287**, 722 (1957).

STRINGA, G.: Ergebnisse konservativer Behandlung der Schaftbrüche von Oberarm, Unterarm, Oberschenkel und Unterschenkel. Chir. Praxis **4**, 461 (1957).

STRUPPLER, V.: Verletzungen und Wiederherstellung der oberen Extremitäten. Die frischen Verletzungen. In: Neue dtsch. Chirurgie, Bd. 68. Stuttgart: Ferdinand Enke.

STULZ, E., J. FOLSCHWEILLER et J.-J. BADINA: Réflexions sur le traitement des fractures du calcanéum d'après 61 observations. Acta orthop. belg. **17**, 231 (1951).

STURZENEGGER, H.: Über die Behandlung der lateralen Malleolarfraktur mit Subluxation des Talus. Schweiz. med. Wschr. **84**, 1313 (1954).

TABANELLI, M.: Il metodo della triplice trazione con filo di Kirschner. Istituto Clin. Chir. Milano 1947.

TANNER, E. E.: Die Therapie der Fersenbeinbrüche unter Berücksichtigung der Spätresultate. Thesis Bern 1959.

TAYLOR, G. M., A. J. NEUFELD, and V. L. NICKEL: Complications and failures in the operative treatment of intertrochanteric fractures of the femur. J. Bone Jt Surg. **37**A, 306 (1955).

TERLEP, H.: Blutige Reposition und Erfolgsaussichten bei Brüchen am oberen Speichenende bei Kindern und Jugendlichen. Arch. orthop. Unfall-Chir. **49**, 507 (1958).

THOMSON, J. E. M.: The Küntscher nail in the treatment of fractures of the tibia and fibula. Surg. Gynec. Obstet. **94**, 189 (1952).

— D. A. WILLANDER, and E. S. MAXIM: Küntscher nailing of the forearm in problem cases. Amer. J. Surg. **85**, 486 (1953).

THORSÉN, G., and H. HINT: Agglutination, sedimentation and intravascular sludging of erythrocytes. Acta chir. scand., Suppl. **154** (1950).

TILLAUX, P.: Recherches cliniques et expérimentales sur les fractures malléolaires. Bull. Arch. méd. Paris, Sér. II 1, 817 (1872).

TRILLAT, A.: Fractures spiroides du tibia à plusieurs fragments. Lyon chir. **50**, 319 (1955).

TROJAN, E.: Die Behandlung der Knöchelbrüche mit Abscherung eines großen hinteren Schienbeinkeiles. Z. Orthop. **84**, 636 (1953).

— Arthrodesen nach Fersenbeinbrüchen. Chir. Praxis **5**, 61 (1961).

— Zur Diagnose des Kahnbeinbruches der Hand. Chir. Praxis **5**, 311 (1961).

—, et G. DE MOURGUES: Fractures et pseudarthroses du scaphoide carpien. Etude thérapeutique. Rev. Chir. orthop. **45**, 614—677 (1959).

TRUETA, J.: Appraisal of the vascular factor in healing of fractures of the femoral neck. J. Bone Jt Surg. **39**B, 3 (1957).

—, and M. H. M. HARRISON: The normal vascular anatomy of the femoral head in adult man. J. Bone Jt Surg. **35**B, 442 (1953).

TSCHERNAWSKIJ, W. A.: Die Taktik des Chirurgen in der operativen Behandlung von Diaphysenbrüchen. Zbl. Chir. **85**, 840 (1960).

TUCKER, F. R.: Arterial supply to the femoral head and its clinical importance. J. Bone Jt Surg. **31**B, 82 (1949).

VALLS, J.: Late treatment of post-traumatic aseptic necrosis of the hip in fractures and dislocations of the neck of the femur, with special reference to arthrodesis and arthroplasty. Wiederherstellungschir. u. Traum. **5**, 74 (1960).

VASLI, S.: Operative treatment of ankle fractures. Acta chir. scand, Suppl. **226**, 1 (1957).

VERBRUGGE, J.: Luxation postérieure de la hanche compliquée d'une fracture de la tête et de la diaphyse fémorales. Acta orthop. belg. **21**, 357 (1955).

VIERNSTEIN, K., u. P. M. JANTZEN: Die Verletzungen im Bereich des oberen Sprunggelenkes. Z. Orthop. **88**, 87 (1957).

VERNE, J.: Cellular sensitivity to drug action in short-term tissue cultures: in vitro correlations with sensitiviyt in vivo. Ann. N. Y. Acad. Sci. **58**, 1195 (1954).

VOIGT, H. E.: Doppelseitige, subtrochantere, luetische sogenannte Spontanfrakturen der Oberschenkel mit Bruch eines Marknagels. Arch. orthop. Unfall-Chir. **49**, 312 (1957).

VOLKERT, R.: Ergebnisse der Nagelung medialer Schenkelhalsfrakturen. Arch. orthop. Unfall-Chir. **45**, 86 (1952).

VOLKMANN, R.: Beitrage zur Chirurgie. Leipzig: Breitkopf & Härtel 1875.

VOM SAAL, F. H.: Intramedullary fixation in fractures of the hand and fingers. J. Bone Jt Surg. **35**A, 5 (1953).

VOORDE, C. VAN DE, et P. ALEXANDER: L'ostéosynthese de la clavicule. Opération justifiée. Acta orthop. belg. **17**, 174 (1951).

VOSS, O., u. K. W. HARTMANN: Die Nagelung des Oberarmkopfbruches. Zbl. Chir. **78**, 414 (1953).

WADE, P. A., R. D. CAMPBELL JR., and R. J. KERIN: Management of intertrochanteric fractures of the femur. Amer. J. Surg. **97**, 634 (1959).

—, and A. J. OKINAKA: The problem of the supracondylar fracture of the femur in the aged person. Amer. J. Surg. **97**, 499 (1959).

WAGNER, C. J.: Fractures of the head of the radius. Amer. J. Surg. **89**, 911 (1955).

WAGNER, H.: Neue Osteosyntheseschrauben und ihre Gewebsverträglichkeit. Verh. Dtsch. Orthop. Ges. 49. Kongr. 1961, 418 (1962).

— Die Einbettung von Metallschrauben im Knochen und die Heilungsvorgänge des Knochengewebes unter dem Einfluß der stabilen Osteosynthese. Arch. klin. Chir. **305**, 28 (1963).

WAGNER, J. H., and F. P. FERRARO: Massive sliding inlay bone graft for correction of ununited fractures of long bones. Amer. J. Surg. **91**, 486 (1956).

WAGNER, W.: Die Versorgung der pertrochanteren Oberschenkelbrüche mit dem Rundnagel nach LEZIUS. Zbl. Chir. **85**, 171 (1960).

WALTER, A. M., u. L. HEILMEYER: Antibiotika-Fibel. Stuttgart: Georg Thieme 1954.

WALTER, S.: Beitrag zur Behandlung der Ulnapseudarthrose. Chirurg **27**, 210 (1956).

WANKE, R., R. MAATZ, H. JUNGE u. W. LENTZ: Knochenbrüche und Verrenkungen. München u. Berlin: Urban & Schwarzenberg 1962.

WASL, H.: Eine Methode zur Einrichtung von Abduktions- und Luxationsfrakturen am proximalen Humerusende. Zbl. Chir. **84**, 1605 (1959).

WASSNER, U. J.: Zur operativen Versorgung der medialen Schenkelhalsfraktur. Chirurg **26**, 83 (1955).

— Wann ist die Behandlung der Tibiakopffraktur mit der komprimierenden Schraube indiziert? Chirurg **26**, 536 (1955).

WATSON-JONES, R.: Fractures and joint injuries, vol. I. Edinburgh: E. & S. Livingstone Ltd. 1955.

— J. G. BONNIN, T. KING, J. PALMER, H. SMITH, O. J. VAUGHAN-JACKSON, J. C. ADAMS, H. J. BURROW, and E. A. NICOLL: Medullary nailing of the fractures after fifty years, with a review of the difficulties and complications of the operation. J. Bone Jt Surg. **32**B, 694 (1950).

WEBER, B. G.: Grundlagen und Möglichkeiten der Zuggurtungsosteosynthese. Chirurg **35**, 81 (1964).

— u. H. VASEY: Osteosynthese bei Olecranonfraktur. Z. Unfallmed. Berufskrankh. **56**, 90 (1963).

WEIL, M. H., and B. S. MILLER: Studies on the effects of a vasopressor agent. Circulation **21**, 830 (1960).

WEIS, J.: Über die Technik der Schenkelhalsnagelung bei pertrochanteren Frakturen. Chirurg **21**, 44 (1950).

WELLER, S.: Über die Behandlung von Knöchelfrakturen mit Gabelsprengung und Subluxation des Talus. Medizinische **9**, 359 (1958).

— Über eine neue Art zur Festigung der Malleolengabel nach Ruptur des tibio-fibularen Bandapparates. Mschr. Unfallheilk. **61**, 339 (1958).

— Über ein neues Hilfsmittel zur exakten Einführung von Kirschnerdrähten. Münch. med. Wschr. **101**, 868 (1959).

— Betrachtungen zur operativen Osteosynthese. Dtsch. med. Wschr. **86**, 1966 (1961).

— Knöchelfrakturen mit Gabelsprengung und Subluxation des Talus. Sportarzt **2**, 37 (1963).

— Die Behandlung von Olecranonfrakturen. Med. Welt **25**, 1545 (1963).

—, E. KÖHNLEIN: Tierexperimentelle Erfahrungen mit Ostamer. Mschr. Unfallheilk. **64**, 450 (1961).

—, u. G. LEITZ: Das Schicksal des oberen Sprunggelenkes nach Knöchelfrakturen und die therapeutische Konsequenz hinsichtlich der Erstversorgung. Med. Welt **25**, 1338 (1963).

WERR, H.: Die operativ versorgte petrochantere Femurfraktur. Mschr. Unfallheilk. **62**, 138 (1959).

WEYAND, E.: Beitrag zur Behandlung der Schenkelhalsfraktur. Zbl. Chir. **77**, 1369 (1952).

— Vorteile und Nachteile der Küntschernagelung am allgemeinen Krankenhaus. Zbl. Chir. **78**, 689 (1953).

WHISTON, G.: Internal fixation for fractures and dislocations of the pelvis. J. Bone Jt Surg. **35**A, 701 (1953).

WHITE, E. H.: Employment of beaded wires in fractures of the forearm. Surg. Gynec. Obstet. **94**, 200 (1952).

— T. J. RADLEY, and N. N. EARLEY: Screw stabilization in fractures of the tibial shaft. J. Bone Jt Surg. **35**A, 749 (1953).

WIESER, C., and M. ALLGÖWER: La significance du cal dans la stabilité des ostéosynthèses. Méd. et Hyg. (Genève) **20**, 745 (1962).

— — Die Beurteilung der Knochenheilung nach stabiler Osteosynthese im Rö-bild. Radiol. clin. (Basel) **31**, 297 (1962).

WILLENEGGER, H.: Über die lokale Penicillinbehandlung der chronischen Osteomyelitis. Helv. chir. Acta 16, 270 (1949).

— Über Erfahrungen und Bedeutung der örtlichen Chemotherapie bei chirurgischen Infektionen. Helv. chir. Acta 18, 406 (1951).

— Fragen zur operativen Frakturenbehandlung. Arch. klin. Chir. 276, 173 (1953).

— Die Behandlung schwerer Hand- und Fingerinfektionen mit antibiotischer Spüldrainage. Chirurg 31, 8 (1960).

— Die Behandlung der Luxationsfrakturen des oberen Sprunggelenks nach biomechanischen Gesichtspunkten. Helv. chir. Acta 28, 225 (1961).

— Therapeutische Möglichkeiten und Grenzen der antibakteriellen Spüldrainage bei chirurgischen Infektionen. Arch. klin. Chir. 304, 670 (1963).

—, u. A. GUGGENBÜHL: Zur operativen Behandlung bestimmter Fälle von distaler Radiusfraktur, Helv. chir. Acta 26, 81 (1959).

— — Surgical treatment of certain cases of distal radial fracture (Colles' fracture). Yearb. Orthop. Traumat. Surg. 1959/60 Series. Chicago: The Yearb. Publ. 1961.

—, u. E. M. MÜLLER: Grundsätzliche Fragen zur operativen Frakturenbehandlung. Separatum nach einem Vortrag an der Unfallmed. Tagg. vom 4./5. 3. 1960 in Verh. Ber. Landesverb. Südwestdeutschland d. gewerbl. Berufsgenossenschaften in Heidelberg 1960, S. 73.

—, u. W. ROTH: Die antibakterielle Spüldrainage als Behandlungsprinzip bei chirurgischen Infektionen. Dtsch. med. Wschr. 30, 1485 (1962).

— R. SCHENK, F. STRAUMANN, M. MÜLLER, M. ALLGÖWER u. H. KRÜGER: Methodik und vorläufige Ergebnisse experimenteller Untersuchungen über die Heilvorgänge bei stabiler Osteosynthese. Arch. klin. Chir. 301, 846 (1962).

WILLIAMS, J. A., and J. FINE: A semiautomatic instrument for measuring blood volume. J. Amer. med. Ass. 178, 1097 (1961).

    Measurement of blood volume with a new apparatus. N. Engl. J. Med. 264, 842 (1961).

WILSON, M. J., H. G. COHEN, and J. H. MOWER: The double pin method in the treatment of fractures of the tibia and fibula. J. int. Coll. Surg. 29, 196 (1958).

WINKLER, L.: Ursachen der Gewebereaktion bei der Osteosynthese mit Metallen. Zbl. Chir. 77, 665 (1952).

WITT, A. N.: Zur operativen Behandlung der suprakondylären Humerusfraktur im Kindesalter. Chirurg 26, 488 (1955).

— Spätzustände nach Verletzungen des Fußgelenks und der Fußwurzel. Verh. Dtsch. Ges. Orthop. 44. Kongr. Beilageheft Z. Orthop 88, 288 (1957).

— Supramalleoläre Frakturen kombiniert mit Luxationsfrakturen des oberen Sprunggelenks, ihre Gefahren für die Zirkulation und ihre Behandlung. Wiederherstellungschir. u. Traum. 5, 15 (1960).

WONDRAK, E., u. J. VESELY: Die Monteggia-Fraktur. Zbl. Chir. 83, 1460 (1958).

WULF, A. DE: Le traitement des dislocations acromio-coracoclaviculaires. Acta orthop. belg. 21, 538 (1955).

WUSTMANN, O.: Die Chirurgie des Ellbogengelenkes. Berlin: W. de Gruyter & Co. 1954.

— Die Kompressionsosteosynthese. Ärztl. Prax. 6, 7 (1954).

YOUNG, J. S., and H. D. GRIFFITH: Dynamics of parenchymatous embolism in relationship to the dissemination of malignant tumours. J. Path. Bact. 62, 293 (1950).

ZELLWEGER, J.: Penicillinallergie und chirurgische Lokalbehandlung. Thesis Basel 1954.

ZENKER, R., u. F. GROLL: Erfahrungen mit der örtlichen Anwendung von Penicillin und Marbadal zur Verhütung und Behandlung von Infektionen. Arch. klin. Chir. 264, 190 (1950).

ZIEGLER, A.: Funktionelle Frakturbehandlung. Schweiz. Z. Unfallmed. Unfallrechtsprechung 10 (1916).

ZIEROLD, A. A.: Reaction of bone to various metals. Arch. Surg. 9, 365 (1924).

ZOLLINGER, F.: Richtlinien zur Vereinheitlichung der Meßmethodik. Beilage zu Nr. 7 der Mitt. der Med. Abt. der SUVA (Schweiz. Unfallversicherungs-Anstalt), Luzern 1940.

ZOPFF, G.: Die gelenkte Nagelung des Schenkelhalses. Z. Orthop. 80, 17 (1950/51).

ZORN, G.: Die Behandlung der Fersenbein-Stauchungsbrüche mit dem Schraubennagel nach BÜRKLE DE LA CAMP. Zbl. Chir. 85, 1245 (1960).

ZRUBECKY, G.: Bedeutung der Seitenverschiebung für die Wund- und Knochenbruchheilung beim offenen Unterschenkelbruch. Arch. orthop. Unfall-Chir. 47, 307 (1955).

ZUELZER, W. A.: Fixation of small but important bone fragments with a hook plate J. Bone Jt Surg. 33 A, 430 (1951).

ZUR VERTH, J.: Beidseitige subtrochantere Spontanfrakturen der Oberschenkel bei Tabes dorsalis. Arch. orthop. Unfall-Chir. 49, 516 (1958).

Subject Index